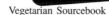

Learning Disabilities Sourcebook, 3rd Edition

Leukemia Sourcebook

Liver Disorders Sourcebook

Lung Disorders Sourcebook

Medical Tests Sourcebook, 3rd Edition

Men's Health Concerns Sourcebook, 2nd Edition

Mental Health Disorders Sourcebook, 4th Edition

Mental Retardation Sourcebook

Movement Disorders Sourcebook, 2nd Edition

Multiple Sclerosis Sourcebook

Muscular Dystrophy Sourcebook

Obesity Sourcebook

Osteoporosis Sourcebook

Pain Sourcebook, 3rd Edition

Pediatric Cancer Sourcebook

Physical & Mental Issues in Aging Sourcebook

Podiatry Sourcebook, 2nd Edition

Pregnancy & Birth Sourcebook, 2nd Edition

Prostate Cancer Sourcebook

Prostate & Urological Disorders Sourcebook

Reconstructive & Cosmetic Surgery Sourcebook

Rehabilitation Sourcebook

Respiratory Disorders Sourcebook, 2nd Edition

Sexually Transmitted Diseases Sourcebook, 3rd Edition

Sleep Disorders Sourcebook, 2nd Edition

Smoking Concerns Sourcebook

Sports Injuries Sourcebook, 3rd Edition

Stress-Related Disorders Sourcebook, 2nd Edition

Stroke Sourcebook, 2nd Edition

Surgery Sourcebook, 2nd Edition

Thyroid Disorders Sourcebook

Transplantation Sourcebook

Traveler's Health Sourcebook

Urinary Tract & Kidney Diseases & Disorders Sourcebook, 2nd Edition

Vegetarian Sourcebook

Women's Health Concerns Sourcebook, 3rd Edition

Workplace Health & Safety Sourcebook

Worldwide Health Sourcebook

# Teen Health Series

Abuse & Violence Information for Teens

Accident & Safety Information for Teens

Alcohol Information for Teens, 2nd Edition

Allergy Information for Teens

Asthma Information for Teens

Body Information for Teens

Cancer Information for Teens

Complementary & Alternative Medicine Information for Teens

Diabetes Information for Teens

Diet Information for Teens, 2nd Edition

Drug Information for Teens, 2nd Edition

Eating Disorders Information for Teens, 2nd Edition

Fitness Information for Teens, 2nd Edition

Learning Disabilities Information for Teens

Mental Health Information for Teens, 2nd Edition

Pregnancy Information for Teens

Sexual Health Information for Teens, 2nd Edition

Skin Health Information for Teens, 2nd Edition

Sleep Information for Teens

Sports Injuries Information for Teens, 2nd Edition

Stress Information for Teens

Suicide Information for Teens

Tobacco Information for Teens

# Child Abuse
## SOURCEBOOK

*Second Edition*

## Health Reference Series

*Second Edition*

# Child Abuse
## SOURCEBOOK

*Basic Consumer Health Information about the Maltreatment of Children, Including Statistics, Risk Factors, Symptoms, Therapies, and the Long-Term Consequences of Physical, Emotional, and Sexual Abuse and Neglect, Featuring Facts about Munchausen Syndrome by Proxy (MSBP), Abusive Head Trauma, Corporal Punishment, Parental Substance Abuse, Incest, and Child Exploitation*

*Along with Information about Child Protective Services, Reporting Abuse and Neglect, Legal Protections, Juvenile Court, Foster Care and Adoption, and Parenting Strategies, a Glossary of Related Terms, and Directories of Resources for Additional Help and Information*

*Edited by*
*Joyce Brennfleck Shannon*

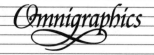

*Omnigraphics*

P.O. Box 31-1640, Detroit, MI 48231

Bibliographic Note

Because this page cannot legibly accommodate all the copyright notices, the Bibliographic Note portion of the Preface constitutes an extension of the copyright notice.

Edited by Joyce Brennfleck Shannon

*Health Reference Series*

Karen Bellenir, *Managing Editor*
David A. Cooke, MD, FACP, *Medical Consultant*
Elizabeth Collins, *Research and Permissions Coordinator*
Cherry Edwards, *Permissions Assistant*
EdIndex, Services for Publishers, *Indexers*

\* \* \*

Omnigraphics, Inc.

Matthew P. Barbour, *Senior Vice President*
Kevin M. Hayes, *Operations Manager*

\* \* \*

Peter E. Ruffner, *Publisher*
Copyright © 2009 Omnigraphics, Inc.
ISBN 978-0-7808-1037-2

Library of Congress Cataloging-in-Publication Data

Child abuse sourcebook : basic consumer health information about the maltreatment of children, including statistics, risk factors, symptoms, therapies, and the long-term consequences of physical, emotional, and sexual abuse and neglect, featuring facts about Munchausen syndrome by proxy (MSBP), abusive head trauma, corporal punishment, parental substance abuse, incest, and child exploitation; along with information about child protective services, reporting abuse and neglect, legal protections, juvenile court, foster care and adoption, and parenting strategies, a glossary of related terms, and directories of resources for additional help and information / edited by Joyce Brennfleck Shannon. -- 2nd ed.
    p. cm.
  Includes bibliographical references and index.
  Summary: "Provides basic consumer health information about abuse and neglect of children and adolescents, with information about prevention and intervention strategies. Includes index, glossary of related terms, and other resources"--Provided by publisher.
  ISBN 978-0-7808-1037-2 (hardcover : alk. paper) 1. Child abuse--United States. 2. Child abuse--United States--Prevention. 3. Abused children--United States. I. Shannon, Joyce Brennfleck.
  HV6626.52.C557 2009
  362.76--dc22
                                                                    2009027489

# Table of Contents

Visit www.healthreferenceseries.com to view *A Contents Guide to the Health Reference Series*, a listing of more than 15,000 topics and the volumes in which they are covered.

## Part II: Physical and Emotional Abuse of Children

## Part III: Sexual Abuse of Children

## Part IV: Intervention and Treatments for Child Maltreatment

## Part V: Preventing Child Maltreatment

## Part VI: Strategies for Positive Parenting

## Part VII: Additional Help and Information

# *Preface*

## *About This Book*

Maltreatment of children and adolescents occurs in all races, economic levels, religions, family structures, and communities. In the United States, more than one child in every hundred experiences neglect or abuse each year, with nearly 80% of the perpetrators being a parent of the victim. The national Administration on Children, Youth, and Families states that "abuse and neglect can have consequences for children, families, and society that last lifetimes, if not generations." To avoid the harm caused by child abuse and neglect, research has shown that parents and caregivers need support from family, friends, and community to help them provide safe and healthy homes for their children.

*Child Abuse Sourcebook, Second Edition* provides updated information about neglect and physical, emotional, and sexual abuse of children and adolescents. These include abusive head trauma, Munchausen syndrome by proxy, corporal punishment, bullying, aggression through technology, child exploitation, teen dating abuse, and parental substance abuse. Guidelines are provided on how to report abuse and who must report abuse. Information about the legal protections available through Child Protective Services, the court system, foster care, and adoption is described. Abuse prevention programs that provide education, respite and crisis care, and support groups for children, teens, adults, and communities are presented. A section on strategies for positive parenting discusses child discipline, anger management, leaving children home alone, and helping children who have been sexually abused. A glossary of related terms and directories of additional resources are also included.

## How to Use This Book

This book is divided into parts and chapters. Parts focus on broad areas of interest. Chapters are devoted to single topics within a part.

*Part I: Child Maltreatment* gives information about the number of children and youth affected by child abuse and neglect and the long-term effects they may experience. Warning signs and symptoms of child maltreatment are included along with information about how parental substance abuse, domestic violence, and foster care experiences increase the likelihood of child abuse and neglect.

*Part II: Physical and Emotional Abuse of Children* describes the actions that constitute these types of maltreatment. Topics presented include medical evaluation of physical abuse, abusive head trauma, Munchausen by proxy syndrome, corporal punishment, harassment, bullying, youth violence, aggression through technology, and teen dating abuse.

*Part III: Sexual Abuse of Children* identifies the risk indicators and warning signs of sexually victimized children and youth. It presents information about sexual abuse, including harmful contact and non-contact behaviors that may occur in families, at school, from other children, and online. A separate chapter explains female genital mutilation which is most common in regions of Africa, but is practiced among some immigrant communities in the United States.

*Part IV: Intervention and Treatments for Child Maltreatment* provides information about the help that is available for children and adolescents who are experiencing abuse or neglect. Legislation, how to report suspected abuse, the child welfare system, and investigations and assessments provided by Child Protective Services are explained. Information is presented about the court system, foster care, and adoption. Also, therapy and treatment guidelines for helping children and adults who may have experienced abuse as children are described.

*Part V: Preventing Child Maltreatment* describes strategies and programs which have been successful in reducing and preventing child abuse and neglect. It includes information for parents and community organizations about abuse prevention education, support groups, safe practices in youth-serving organizations, respite and crisis care, and home visiting programs. Tips about protecting family members from sex offenders living in the community are also provided.

*Part VI: Strategies for Positive Parenting* offers practical advice for parents and caregivers about age-appropriate child discipline, managing parental and child anger, and encouraging good sportsmanship. Guidance about leaving children home alone, handling bullying situations, and helping children who have experienced sexual abuse or violence is also included.

*Part VII: Additional Help and Information* provides a glossary of terms related to child abuse. State telephone numbers for reporting child abuse or neglect are included. Organizations that have information for victims and survivors of child sexual abuse, and adults and juveniles with sexual behavior problems are listed. Also, a directory of resources for additional information about child abuse prevention is offered.

## Bibliographic Note

This volume contains documents and excerpts from publications issued by the following U.S. government agencies: Administration for Children and Families; Centers for Disease Control and Prevention (CDC); Child Welfare Information Gateway; Federal Bureau of Investigation (FBI); FRIENDS National Resource Center for Community-Based Child Abuse Prevention (CBCAP); Health Resources and Services Administration (HRSA); Juvenile Justice Clearinghouse; National Center on Substance Abuse and Child Welfare (NCSACW); National Institute of Mental Health (NIMH); National Institute on Alcohol Abuse and Alcoholism (NIAAA); National Resource Center for Family-Centered Practice and Permanency Planning; Substance Abuse and Mental Health Services Administration (SAMHSA); and the U.S. Department of Justice.

In addition, this volume contains copyrighted documents from the following individuals and organizations: American Academy of Family Physicians; American Humane Association; Center for Law and Social Policy; Centres of Excellence for Children's Well-Being; Child Trends; Nora Ellen Groce; Lauren J. Litton and I.S.P. Consulting; National Alliance for Youth Sports; National Crime Victims Research and Treatment Center; Nemours Foundation; Parents and Teachers Against Violence in Education; Prevent Child Abuse America; Shaken Baby Task Force; South Eastern Centre Against Sexual Assault (SECASA); Stop It Now!; Texas Association Against Sexual Assault; Tolerance.org; University of North Carolina Medical Center News Office; and the World Health Organization.

## Acknowledgements

In addition to the listed organizations, agencies, and individuals who have contributed to this *Sourcebook*, special thanks go to managing editor Karen Bellenir, research and permissions coordinator Liz Collins, and document engineer Bruce Bellenir for their help and support.

## About the Health Reference Series

The *Health Reference Series* is designed to provide basic medical information for patients, families, caregivers, and the general public. Each volume takes a particular topic and provides comprehensive coverage. This is especially important for people who may be dealing with a newly diagnosed disease or a chronic disorder in themselves or in a family member. People looking for preventive guidance, information about disease warning signs, medical statistics, and risk factors for health problems will also find answers to their questions in the *Health Reference Series*. The *Series*, however, is not intended to serve as a tool for diagnosing illness, in prescribing treatments, or as a substitute for the physician/patient relationship. All people concerned about medical symptoms or the possibility of disease are encouraged to seek professional care from an appropriate health care provider.

## A Note about Spelling and Style

*Health Reference Series* editors use *Stedman's Medical Dictionary* as an authority for questions related to the spelling of medical terms and the *Chicago Manual of Style* for questions related to grammatical structures, punctuation, and other editorial concerns. Consistent adherence is not always possible, however, because the individual volumes within the *Series* include many documents from a wide variety of different producers and copyright holders, and the editor's primary goal is to present material from each source as accurately as is possible following the terms specified by each document's producer. This sometimes means that information in different chapters or sections may follow other guidelines and alternate spelling authorities. For example, occasionally a copyright holder may require that eponymous terms be shown in possessive forms (Crohn's disease *vs.* Crohn disease) or that British spelling norms be retained (leukaemia *vs.* leukemia).

## *Locating Information within the* Health Reference Series

The *Health Reference Series* contains a wealth of information about a wide variety of medical topics. Ensuring easy access to all the fact sheets, research reports, in-depth discussions, and other material contained within the individual books of the *Series* remains one of our highest priorities. As the *Series* continues to grow in size and scope, however, locating the precise information needed by a reader may become more challenging.

*A Contents Guide to the Health Reference Series* was developed to direct readers to the specific volumes that address their concerns. It presents an extensive list of diseases, treatments, and other topics of general interest compiled from the Tables of Contents and major index headings. To access *A Contents Guide to the Health Reference Series*, visit www.healthreferenceseries.com.

## *Medical Consultant*

Medical consultation services are provided to the *Health Reference Series* editors by David A. Cooke, MD, FACP. Dr. Cooke is a graduate of Brandeis University, and he received his MD degree from the University of Michigan. He completed residency training at the University of Wisconsin Hospital and Clinics. He is board-certified in Internal Medicine. Dr. Cooke currently works as part of the University of Michigan Health System and practices in Ann Arbor, MI. In his free time, he enjoys writing, science fiction, and spending time with his family.

## *Our Advisory Board*

We would like to thank the following board members for providing guidance to the development of this *Series*:

- Dr. Lynda Baker, Associate Professor of Library and Information Science, Wayne State University, Detroit, MI

- Nancy Bulgarelli, William Beaumont Hospital Library, Royal Oak, MI

- Karen Imarisio, Bloomfield Township Public Library, Bloomfield Township, MI

- Karen Morgan, Mardigian Library, University of Michigan-Dearborn, Dearborn, MI

- Rosemary Orlando, St. Clair Shores Public Library, St. Clair Shores, MI

## Health Reference Series *Update Policy*

The inaugural book in the *Health Reference Series* was the first edition of *Cancer Sourcebook* published in 1989. Since then, the *Series* has been enthusiastically received by librarians and in the medical community. In order to maintain the standard of providing high-quality health information for the layperson the editorial staff at Omnigraphics felt it was necessary to implement a policy of updating volumes when warranted.

Medical researchers have been making tremendous strides, and it is the purpose of the *Health Reference Series* to stay current with the most recent advances. Each decision to update a volume is made on an individual basis. Some of the considerations include how much new information is available and the feedback we receive from people who use the books. If there is a topic you would like to see added to the update list, or an area of medical concern you feel has not been adequately addressed, please write to:

Editor
*Health Reference Series*
Omnigraphics, Inc.
P.O. Box 31-1640
Detroit, MI 48231-1640
E-mail: editorial@omnigraphics.com

# Part One

# Child Maltreatment

# Chapter 1

# Child Abuse and Neglect Defined

## What Is Child Abuse and Neglect?

### *How is child abuse and neglect defined in federal law?*

Federal legislation lays the groundwork for states by identifying a minimum set of acts or behaviors that define child abuse and neglect. The Federal Child Abuse Prevention and Treatment Act (CAPTA), (42 U.S.C.A. §5106g), as amended by the Keeping Children and Families Safe Act of 2003, defines child abuse and neglect as, at minimum:

- any recent act or failure to act on the part of a parent or caretaker which results in death, serious physical or emotional harm, sexual abuse or exploitation; or
- an act or failure to act which presents an imminent risk of serious harm.

Most federal and state child protection laws primarily refer to cases of harm to a child caused by parents or other caregivers; they generally do not include harm caused by other people, such as acquaintances or strangers.

This chapter includes text excerpted from "What Is Child Abuse and Neglect," Child Welfare Information Gateway, U.S. Department of Health and Human Services (HHS), April 2008; and, excerpts from "Child Neglect: A Guide for Prevention, Assessment, and Intervention," Child Welfare Information Gateway, HHS, updated January 9, 2009.

## *What are the major types of child abuse and neglect?*

Within the minimum standards set by CAPTA, each state is responsible for providing its own definitions of child abuse and neglect. Most states recognize four major types of maltreatment: physical abuse, neglect, sexual abuse, and emotional abuse. Although any of the forms of child maltreatment may be found separately, they often occur in combination. In many states, abandonment and parental substance abuse are also defined as forms of child abuse or neglect.

The examples provided are for general informational purposes only. Not all states' definitions will include all of the examples listed, and individual states' definitions may cover additional situations not mentioned here.

**Physical abuse** is nonaccidental physical injury (ranging from minor bruises to severe fractures or death) as a result of punching, beating, kicking, biting, shaking, throwing, stabbing, choking, hitting (with a hand, stick, strap, or other object), burning, or otherwise harming a child, that is inflicted by a parent, caregiver, or other person who has responsibility for the child. Such injury is considered abuse regardless of whether the caregiver intended to hurt the child. Physical discipline, such as spanking or paddling, is not considered abuse as long as it is reasonable and causes no bodily injury to the child.

**Neglect** is the failure of a parent, guardian, or other caregiver to provide for a child's basic needs. Neglect may be:

- physical (failure to provide necessary food or shelter, or lack of appropriate supervision);

- medical (failure to provide necessary medical or mental health treatment);

- educational (failure to educate a child or attend to special education needs);

- emotional (inattention to a child's emotional needs, failure to provide psychological care, or permitting the child to use alcohol or other drugs).

These situations do not always mean a child is neglected. Sometimes cultural values, the standards of care in the community, and poverty may be contributing factors, indicating the family is in need of information or assistance. When a family fails to use information and resources, and the child's health or safety is at risk, then child welfare intervention may be required. In addition, many states provide an exception to the definition of neglect for parents who choose not to seek medical care for their children due to religious beliefs that may prohibit medical intervention.

**Sexual abuse** includes activities by a parent or caregiver such as fondling a child's genitals, penetration, incest, rape, sodomy, indecent exposure, and exploitation through prostitution or the production of pornographic materials.

**Emotional abuse** (or psychological abuse) is a pattern of behavior that impairs a child's emotional development or sense of self-worth. This may include constant criticism, threats, or rejection, as well as withholding love, support, or guidance. Emotional abuse is often difficult to prove and, therefore, child protective services may not be able to intervene without evidence of harm or mental injury to the child. Emotional abuse is almost always present when other forms are identified.

**Abandonment** is now defined in many states as a form of neglect. In general, a child is considered to be abandoned when the parent's identity or whereabouts are unknown, the child has been left alone in circumstances where the child suffers serious harm, or the parent has failed to maintain contact with the child or provide reasonable support for a specified period of time.

**Substance abuse** is an element of the definition of child abuse or neglect in many states. Circumstances that are considered abuse or neglect in some states include the following:

- Prenatal exposure of a child to harm due to the mother's use of an illegal drug or other substance

- Manufacture of methamphetamine in the presence of a child

- Selling, distributing, or giving illegal drugs or alcohol to a child

- Use of a controlled substance by a caregiver that impairs the caregiver's ability to adequately care for the child

## Definition and Scope of Neglect

Child neglect is the most common type of child maltreatment. Unfortunately, neglect frequently goes unreported and, historically, has not been acknowledged or publicized as greatly as child abuse. Even professionals often have given less attention to child neglect than to abuse. One study found that caseworkers indicated that they were least likely to substantiate referrals for neglect. In some respects, it is understandable why violence against children has commanded more attention than neglect. Abuse often leaves visible bruises and scars, whereas the signs of neglect tend to be less visible. However, the effects of neglect can be just as detrimental. In fact, some studies have shown that neglect may be more detrimental to children's early brain development than physical or sexual abuse.

Instances of neglect are classified as mild, moderate, or severe.

- **Mild neglect** usually does not warrant a report to child protective services (CPS), but might necessitate a community-based intervention (for example, a parent failing to put the child in a car safety seat).

- **Moderate neglect** occurs when less intrusive measures, such as community interventions, have failed or some moderate harm to the child has occurred (for example, a child consistently is inappropriately dressed for the weather, such as being in shorts and sandals in the middle of winter). For moderate neglect, CPS may be involved in partnership with community support.

- **Severe neglect** occurs when severe or long-term harm has been done to the child (for example, a child with asthma who has not received appropriate medications over a long period of time and is frequently admitted to the hospital). In these cases, CPS should be and is usually involved, as is the legal system.

The seriousness of the neglect is determined not only by how much harm or risk of harm there is to the child, but also by how chronic the neglect is. Chronicity can be defined as "patterns of the same acts or omissions that extend over time or recur over time." An example of chronic neglect would be parents with substance abuse problems who do not provide for the basic needs of their children on an ongoing basis.

## *Types of Neglect*

While neglect may be harder to define or to detect than other forms of child maltreatment, child welfare experts have created common categories of neglect, including physical neglect; medical neglect;

inadequate supervision; environmental, emotional, and educational neglect; and newborns addicted or exposed to drugs, as well as some newly recognized forms of neglect.

**Physical neglect** is one of the most widely recognized forms. It includes the following:

- **Abandonment:** The desertion of a child without arranging for his reasonable care or supervision. Usually, a child is considered abandoned when not picked up within two days.

- **Expulsion:** The blatant refusal of custody, such as the permanent or indefinite expulsion of a child from the home, without adequately arranging for his care by others or the refusal to accept custody of a returned runaway.

- **Shuttling:** When a child is repeatedly left in the custody of others for days or weeks at a time, possibly due to the unwillingness of the parent or the caregiver to maintain custody.

- **Nutritional neglect:** When a child is undernourished or is repeatedly hungry for long periods of time, which can sometimes be evidenced by poor growth. Nutritional neglect often is included in the category of "other physical neglect."

- **Clothing neglect:** When a child lacks appropriate clothing, such as not having appropriately warm clothes or shoes in the winter.

- **Other physical neglect:** Includes inadequate hygiene and forms of reckless disregard for the child's safety and welfare (for example, driving while intoxicated with the child, leaving a young child in a car unattended).

**Medical neglect** encompasses a parent or guardian's denial of or delay in seeking needed health care for a child as described:

- **Denial of health care:** The failure to provide or to allow needed care as recommended by a competent health care professional for a physical injury, illness, medical condition, or impairment.

- **Delay in health care:** The failure to seek timely and appropriate medical care for a serious health problem that any reasonable person would have recognized as needing professional medical attention.

**Inadequate supervision** encompasses a number of behaviors, including the following:

- **Lack of appropriate supervision:** Some states specify the amount of time children at different ages can be left unsupervised, and the guidelines for these ages and times vary. In addition, all children are different, so the amount of supervision needed may vary by the child's age, development, or situation.

- **Exposure to hazards:** Examples of exposure to in- and out-of-home hazards include:

  - safety hazards such as poisons, small objects, electrical wires, stairs, drug paraphernalia;

  - smoking and second-hand smoke, especially for children with asthma or other lung problems;

  - guns and other weapons that are kept in the house that are loaded and not locked up or are in reach of children;

  - unsanitary household conditions such as rotting food, human or animal feces, insect infestation, or lack of running or clean water; and,

  - lack of car safety restraints.

- **Inappropriate caregivers:** Another behavior that can fall under "failure to protect" is leaving a child in the care of someone who either is unable or should not be trusted to provide care for a child.

- **Other forms of inadequate supervision:** Additional examples of inadequate supervision include: not returning at agreed upon times or giving caregiver's necessary items for the child; leaving a child with a caregiver who is not adequately supervising the child; or allowing a child to engage in risky or harmful behaviors.

**Environmental neglect:** Some of the characteristics mentioned can be seen as stemming from environmental neglect, which is characterized by a lack of environmental or neighborhood safety, opportunities, or resources.

**Emotional neglect:** Typically, emotional neglect is more difficult to assess than other types of neglect, but is thought to have more severe and long-lasting consequences than physical neglect. It often occurs with other forms of neglect or abuse, which may be easier to identify, and includes the following:

- **Inadequate nurturing or affection:** The persistent, marked inattention to the child's needs for affection, emotional support, or attention.

- **Chronic or extreme spouse abuse:** The exposure to chronic or extreme spouse abuse or other domestic violence.

- **Permitted drug or alcohol abuse**: The encouragement or permission by the caregiver of drug or alcohol use by the child.

- **Other permitted maladaptive behavior:** The encouragement or permission of other maladaptive behavior (chronic delinquency, assault) under circumstances where the parent or caregiver has reason to be aware of the existence and the seriousness of the problem, but does not intervene.

- **Isolation**: Denying a child the ability to interact or to communicate with peers or adults outside or inside the home.

**Educational neglect:** Although state statutes and policies vary, both parents and schools are responsible for meeting certain requirements regarding the education of children. Types of educational neglect include the following:

- **Permitted, chronic truancy:** Permitting habitual absenteeism from school averaging at least five days a month if the parent or guardian is informed of the problem and does not attempt to intervene.

- **Failure to enroll or other truancy:** Failing to homeschool, to register, or to enroll a child of mandatory school age, causing the child to miss at least one month of school without valid reasons.

- **Inattention to special education needs:** Refusing to allow or failing to obtain recommended remedial education services or neglecting to obtain or follow through with treatment for a child's diagnosed learning disorder or other special education need without reasonable cause.

# Chapter 2

# *Recognizing Child Abuse and Neglect: Signs and Symptoms*

### *Recognizing Child Abuse: What Parents Should Know*

The first step in helping abused children is learning to recognize the symptoms of child abuse. Although child abuse is divided into four types—physical abuse, neglect, sexual abuse, and emotional maltreatment—the types are more typically found in combination than alone. A physically abused child for example is often emotionally maltreated as well, and a sexually abused child may be also neglected. Any child at any age may experience any of the types of child abuse. Children over age five are more likely to be physically abused and to suffer moderate injury than are children under age five.

### *Recognizing Child Abuse*

Experienced educators likely have seen all forms of child abuse at one time or another. They are alert to signs like these that may signal the presence of child abuse.

### *The Child*

- Shows sudden changes in behavior or school performance
- Has not received help for physical or medical problems brought to the parents' attention

"Recognizing Child Abuse: What Parents Should Know," © 2009 Prevent Child Abuse America (www.preventchildabuse.org). Reprinted with permission.

- Has learning problems that cannot be attributed to specific physical or psychological causes
- Is always watchful, as though preparing for something bad to happen
- Lacks adult supervision
- Is overly compliant, an overachiever, or too responsible
- Comes to school early, stays late, and does not want to go home

### The Parent

- Shows little concern for the child, rarely responding to the school's requests for information, for conferences, or for home visits
- Denies the existence of—or blames the child for—the child's problems in school or at home
- Asks the classroom teacher to use harsh physical discipline if the child misbehaves
- Sees the child entirely bad, worthless, or burdensome
- Demands perfection or a level of physical or academic performance the child cannot achieve
- Looks primarily to the child for care, attention, and satisfaction of emotional needs

### The Parent and Child

- Rarely touch or look at each other
- Consider their relationship entirely negative
- State that they do not like each other

None of these signs proves that child abuse is present in a family. Any of them may be found in any parent or child at one time or another. But when these signs appear repeatedly or in combination, they should cause the educator to take closer look at the situation and to consider the possibility of child abuse. That second look may reveal further signs of abuse or signs of a particular kind of child abuse.

## Signs of Physical Abuse

Consider the possibility of physical abuse when the child:

- has unexplained burns, bites, bruises, broken bones, or black eyes;
- has fading bruises or other marks noticeable after an absence from school;
- seems frightened of the parents and protests or cries when it is time to go home from school;
- shrinks at the approach of adults; or
- reports injury by a parent or another adult caregiver.

Consider the possibility of physical abuse when the parent or other adult caregiver:

- offers conflicting, unconvincing, or no explanation for the child's injury;
- describes the child as evil, or in some other very negative way;
- uses harsh physical discipline with the child; or
- has a history of abuse as a child.

## Signs of Neglect

Consider the possibility of neglect when the child:

- is frequently absent from school;
- begs or steals food or money from classmates;
- lacks needed medical or dental care, immunizations, or glasses;
- is consistently dirty and has severe body odor;
- lacks sufficient clothing for the weather;
- abuses alcohol or other drugs; or
- states there is no one at home to provide care.

Consider the possibility of neglect when the parent or other adult caregiver:

- appears to be indifferent to the child;
- seems apathetic or depressed;
- behaves irrationally or in a bizarre manner; or
- is abusing alcohol or other drugs.

## Signs of Sexual Abuse

Consider the possibility of sexual abuse when the child:

- has difficulty walking or sitting;
- suddenly refuses to change for gym or to participate in physical activities;
- demonstrates bizarre, sophisticated, or unusual sexual knowledge or behavior;
- becomes pregnant or contracts a venereal disease, particularly if under age fourteen;
- runs away; or
- reports sexual abuse by a parent or another adult caregiver.

Consider the possibility of sexual abuse when the parent or other adult caregiver:

- is unduly protective of the child, severely limits the child's contact with other children, especially of the opposite sex;
- is secretive and isolated; or
- describes marital difficulties involving family power struggles or sexual relations.

## Signs of Emotional Maltreatment

Consider the possibility of emotional maltreatment when the child:

- shows extremes in behavior, such as overly compliant or demanding behavior, extreme passivity or aggression;
- is either inappropriately adult (parenting other children, for example) or inappropriately infantile (frequently rocking or head-banging, for example);
- is delayed in physical or emotional development;
- has attempted suicide; or
- reports a lack of attachment to the parent.

Consider the possibility of emotional maltreatment when the parent or other adult caregiver:

- constantly blames, belittles, or berates the child;

14

- is unconcerned about the child and refuses to consider offers of help for the child's school problems; or

- overtly rejects the child.

## For More Information

### Prevent Child Abuse America
200 S. Michigan Ave., 17ᵗʰ Floor
Chicago, Illinois 60604
Phone: 312-663-3520
Fax: 312-939-8962
Website: http://www.preventchildabuse.org

# Chapter 3

# *Risk and Protective Factors for Child Abuse and Neglect*

## *Risk and Protective Factors*

Neglect occurs to children of all races, social and economic classes, religions, family structures, and communities. However, there are some factors that appear to make children more or less likely to be neglected. Having one or more risk factors does not necessarily mean that a child will be neglected; families and children react to personal and societal factors differently. But they are warning signs, nevertheless.

One or two major risk factors for neglect may have little effect on a child's development, but having three or more risk factors exponentially increases the potential for developmental problems. Risk factors may be cumulative so that the more risk factors a child or family is exposed to over the course of the child's development, the greater the potential for problems to arise. The risk and protective factors in a child or family's life also may interact with each other.

An instance of possible neglect may be related to one or more contributing factors. For example, if a child is exposed to lead paint in the home, there may be many contributing factors to the neglect. The parent may be unwilling or unable to move to a home where lead paint is not present, the landlord may be unwilling to remove the lead paint from the walls, the city may not have an adequate lead abatement

This chapter includes text from "Child Neglect: A Guide for Prevention, Assessment, and Intervention: Chapter 4," Child Welfare Information Gateway, U.S. Department of Health and Human Services (HHS), updated September 18, 2008.

program, or the community may not have placed enough emphasis on making sure that low-income housing is safe. The caseworker would need to assess the situation to determine if this is a case of neglect by the parent.

## Environmental Factors

Neglectful families do not exist in a vacuum; numerous environmental factors can contribute to child neglect. Some of these include poverty, community and society characteristics, and access to social supports. These factors may be interrelated (for example, families who are poor often live in high-risk or unsafe communities or lack social supports).

### Poverty

The level of child well-being in a state is strongly associated with its rate of child poverty. Compared to other types of child maltreatment, neglect is more directly associated with poverty. Of course, most poor people do not neglect or otherwise maltreat their children, but poverty, when combined with other risk factors, such as substance abuse, social isolation, financial uncertainty, continual family chaos, or a lack of available transportation and affordable child care can put a child at greater risk for neglect.

It is important to note that many poor families are well adjusted and competent; they have healthy marriages and do not express their stress in violent or otherwise hurtful ways. Many children who live in poverty are able to perform well in school, are socially well-adjusted, do not engage in illegal activities, and are not poor as adults. These children may have protective factors, such as affectionate parents, high self-esteem, or a role model, that help them to achieve these positive outcomes.

### Community Characteristics

Children who live in dangerous neighborhoods have been found to be at higher risk for neglect than children in safer neighborhoods. One study suggests a relationship between unsafe or dangerous housing conditions and the adequacy of children's physical needs being met in the areas of nutrition, clothing, and personal hygiene. These communities also are associated with less social contact or support, which is another risk factor for neglect. Other characteristics of these distressed neighborhoods include high levels of truancy, low academic achievement, high juvenile arrest rates, and high teen birth rates. When stressful living conditions continue over time, families in these neighborhoods are more likely to be reported to child protective services (CPS) for child neglect.

## Social Support

Families with healthy support networks have more access to models of suitable parental behavior. In addition, they have more friends, family, or neighbors who may be willing to act as alternative caregivers or to provide additional support or nurture to both the parent and the child. Impoverished communities often lack positive informal and formal support systems for families. Social support can take many forms, including:

- emotional support,
- tangible support,
- decision-making or problem-solving assistance,
- support related to self-esteem, and
- social companionship.

Social support is provided by:

- relatives,
- neighbors,
- friends,
- schools,
- employers,
- health and mental health service agencies,
- religious institutions,
- recreational programs,
- after-school programs and sports, and
- other community groups and organizations.

Studies on social isolation and child neglect have compared parents who maltreat their children with parents who do not. These studies found that parents who maltreat their children:

- report more isolation and loneliness;

19

- report less social support;
- have smaller social networks;
- receive less social and emotional support from their social networks;
- have fewer contacts with others in their social networks;
- perceive the support they receive as less positive than non-neglecting parents;
- may be more likely to distrust available social support; and,
- may perceive, rightly or wrongly, that their neighborhoods are less friendly and their neighbors less helpful.

Social support is important not only for parents but also for children. Social supports offer children both emotional and physical resources that may either protect them from neglect or help them to achieve better outcomes if they have been neglected. Research shows that the presence of one or more positive and significant individuals in a child's life may act as a buffer against negative outcomes due to child abuse or neglect. Supportive adults may be able to look out for children and possibly protect them from neglect. For a child who is in an out-of-home placement, a positive relationship with a foster parent might serve as a protective factor.

## Family Factors

Several family characteristics are associated with higher rates of neglect. Some life situations, such as marital problems, domestic violence, single parenthood, unemployment, and financial stress, can increase the likelihood that neglect will occur. Although these characteristics may not cause maltreatment, they are possible risk factors for neglect. Some family characteristics that may lead to neglect can be categorized as communication and interaction patterns, family composition, domestic violence, and family stress.

### Communication and Interaction Patterns

Characteristics of families that are more likely to have positive outcomes include cohesion; emotional support for one another; and parents or caregivers who are warm, involved with their children, and firm and consistent in their discipline methods. Families that share similar beliefs, rituals, or values in such matters as financial management and the use of leisure time also appear to offer some protection. Having a strong familial sense of culture and spirituality also helps. In addition, a father's involvement, support, and connection with his children have also been associated with more positive child outcomes. Even if parents are not able to provide a positive family environment, other relatives (such as older siblings or grandparents) may be able to step in and provide this for the children.

Neglectful families, however, often have problems communicating and interacting in positive or appropriate ways. These families are more chaotic, express fewer positive emotions, and have less empathy and openness. Additionally, they are more likely to lack emotional closeness, negotiation skills, and a willingness to take responsibility for their actions.

In neglectful families, there may be less engagement between the parent and the child and more negative interactions than in non-neglectful families. Parents who maltreat their children often are less supportive, affectionate, playful, or responsive than parents who do not maltreat their children.

### Religiosity and Social Support

Involvement in faith communities has been shown to have many positive effects for families. Families with access to a helpful community of people receive significant social, financial, emotional, and physical support. Parents who are connected with a religious community may experience higher levels of social support themselves and may afford their children greater opportunities for such support than do parents who do not participate. A consistent empirical finding is that adults who are part of a religious community are less socially isolated than are other adults. Such support enhances coping mechanisms and provides parents with a different perspective which helps them deal with stress and difficulties. A growing body of research highlights the role of religion and spirituality in helping parents cope with sick or emotionally or behaviorally disturbed children.

Religiosity has been found in several studies to be positively correlated with family cohesiveness and less incidence of interparental conflict. Parental religiosity has been linked to greater involvement, warmth and positivity in parent-child relationships. Religiousness is positively correlated with an authoritative parenting style, which is characterized by greater respect, warmth and affection, as well as clearly-communicated and well-defined rules for children. Additionally, many religions have proscriptions against excessive drug and alcohol use. Each of these characteristics promotes a healthy family environment.

### Family Composition

Single parenthood is associated with higher incidences of neglect. One study found that being in a single-parent household increased the risk of child neglect by 87 percent. Many factors may account for this. There is less time to accomplish the tasks of the household, including monitoring and spending time with children and earning sufficient money when there is only one parent or caregiver. Single parents often have to work outside the home, which might mean they are not always available to supervise their children. Single-parent families are also more likely to live in poverty than two-parent households. According to one analysis of the child poverty rate by family type, the poverty rate in 2003 was:

- 7.6 percent for children living with married parents;
- 34.0 percent for children living with a single parent; and,
- 21.5 percent of children living with both parents.

Of course, neglect also occurs in married, two-parent households, especially if there is a high level of marital discord.

The presence of fathers in families often has been left out of the research on child neglect. This may be because fathers typically are not seen as the person primarily responsible for providing for the needs of the children, or because many mothers are single parents or primary caregivers or are typically more accessible to researchers. However, research on fathers shows that the presence of a positive father or father figure decreases the likelihood of neglect in the home. Having a father in the household not only may provide children and the mother with an additional source of emotional support, but it also may provide the family with more money and other resources. Compared to their peers living with both parents, children in single-parent homes had:

- 87 percent greater risk of being harmed by physical neglect;
- 165 percent greater risk of experiencing notable physical neglect;
- 74 percent greater risk of suffering from emotional neglect; and,
- 120 percent greater risk of experiencing some type of maltreatment overall.

### Domestic Violence

Children living in a home where domestic violence is present are at a greater risk of being neglected. One study found that in 35 percent of neglect cases, domestic violence had occurred in the home. Caregivers who are victims of domestic violence may be abused to the point of being unable or unwilling to keep their abusers from also abusing the children. This type of neglect is often referred to as "failure or inability to protect the child from harm." In some cases, abused caregivers are afraid to defend the children in their care because doing so might put the caregiver's or children's lives in danger or provoke more abuse. Whether or not caregivers are charged with "failure or inability to protect" often depends on whether the caregivers knew or should have known that their children were being abused. Studies show that in 30 to 60 percent of homes with identified cases of domestic violence or child maltreatment, it is likely that both types of abuse exist.

**Effects of witnessing domestic violence on children:** In many families affected by domestic violence, the parents believe that their children are not witnessing the incidents, but reports from children show that between 80 and 90 percent are aware of the abuse and can provide detailed accounts of it. Children who witness domestic violence often suffer harmful consequences. The extent of the harm possibly depends upon the child's age, developmental stage, gender, and role in the family. With increasing recognition of the effect exposure to domestic violence can have on children, many child protection services (CPS) agencies consider it a form of emotional abuse.

### Family Stress

Neglectful families often have experienced stressful life events due to financial difficulties, substance abuse problems, housing problems, illness, or other challenges. Families that are coping with such problems may not have the time or emotional capacity to provide for the basic needs of their children or to participate in interventions. Neglectful families often report more day-to-day stress than non-neglectful families. In addition, particularly stressful life events (such as the loss of a job or the death of a family member) may exacerbate characteristics in the family, such as hostility, anxiety, or depression, which may increase levels of family conflict and child maltreatment.

## Parent or Caregiver Factors

Some parental or caregiver characteristics associated with child neglect include problematic childhoods, developmental histories, or personality factors; physical and mental health problems; substance abuse issues; and poor parenting or problem-solving skills. As with all risk factors, the presence of one or more of these factors does not mean that a parent or caregiver will be neglectful, but these are characteristics that are present more often in neglectful parents.

### Parent's Childhood, Developmental History, and Personality Factors

The way parents were reared can greatly affect the way they rear their own children. People who did not have their needs met by a parent when they were children may not know how to meet the needs of their own children. Some studies have found that neglectful parents are more likely to have been maltreated as children. Neglectful mothers were three times more likely to have been sexually abused than mothers who do not neglect their children; however, the majority of individuals who are maltreated as children do not maltreat their own children. In addition, there are individuals who were not abused or neglected as children who maltreat their children. It remains unclear why some previously maltreated people abuse and neglect their children while others do not.

Two other childhood factors that have been found to be associated with future neglect are running away from home and having been placed in foster care, which usually indicate a troubled childhood that can negatively affect one's ability to take care of one's own children. Growing up in unstable, hostile, non-nurturing homes can lead to unstable personalities when the children become adults, and can lead to stressful marriages and abusive parenting practices with their own children.

Children also may be at greater risk of harm if their parents are not aware of the neglect, deny that neglect took place, downplay their role in the neglect, or are unwilling to do anything to make sure the neglect does not recur. One study found that the most common response given by mothers for supervisory neglect was that there was nothing wrong with their behavior.

Some parental developmental and personality characteristics that can be considered protective factors include having secure attachments, stable relationships with their own parents, good coping skills, social competence, and reconciliation with their own history (if any) of childhood maltreatment.

## *Parenting and Problem-Solving Skills*

Parents need to have the cognitive resources to care adequately for a child. They also need certain educational abilities, such as literacy, to be able to care properly for their child (for example, to read prescription labels on their child's medication). Studies have found links between child neglect and parents' poor problem-solving skills, poor parenting skills, and inadequate knowledge of childhood development. Parents who are unaware of the developmental and cognitive abilities of children at different ages may have unrealistic expectations and be more likely to neglect their children. For example, a parent might expect that a 4-year-old child can be left alone for the evening because of unrealistic expectations of the child's abilities. Studies also have found that parents who are inconsistent with discipline or use harsh or excessive punishment can be at risk for neglecting their children. As would be expected, having parents who are engaged with their children and involved in their activities and education acts as a protective factor.

## *Substance Abuse*

Reported rates of substance abuse by maltreating parents vary; neglect, however, has the strongest association with substance abuse among all forms of maltreatment. One study found that children whose parents abused alcohol and other drugs were more than four times more likely to be neglected than children whose parents did not. According to one study of CPS caseworkers, 65 percent of maltreated children who had parents with substance abuse problems were maltreated while the parent was intoxicated. Also, the substance most likely to be abused by maltreating parents is alcohol (alone or in combination with an illicit drug).

Substance abuse also may be related to the recurrence of neglect. Studies have found that caregivers with substance abuse problems are more likely to neglect their children continually and to be re-referred to CPS than caregivers who do not abuse substances. Substance abuse also has been linked with as many as two-thirds of child maltreatment fatalities.

Substance abuse often co-occurs with other problems, which makes it difficult to assess its impact on child maltreatment. Parental substance abuse is likely to co-occur with the following problems that also are associated with child maltreatment:

- Lack of knowledge about child development
- Poor problem-solving and social skills
- Low maternal affection
- Poor attachment relationships
- Poor attention to the needs of an infant
- Disinterest in spending time with one's children
- Inconsistent disciplinary practices
- Social isolation
- Mental health problems, especially depression
- Anger toward or a lack of attention to one's children
- Difficulty maintaining employment
- Engagement in criminal behavior
- Failure to provide appropriately for the needs of their children (clothing, food, medical care, hygiene, and emotional attention)

### Mental Health

Certain mental health problems in parents have been associated with child neglect, although research results vary on this connection. For example, some studies have found that, when controlling for social variables and substance abuse, neglect and depression are not associated. Other studies have shown a link between child neglect and serious or postpartum depression. For example, mothers suffering from postpartum depression are less responsive and sensitive toward their infants and may be disengaged or withdrawn. Of course, numerous mental illnesses can affect an individual's ability to care for a child properly. As with any condition, mental illness occurs along a continuum of severity.

### Other Parental Factors

Other parental factors that may be associated with child neglect include: age, education, gender, employment, criminal activity, and prior involvement with CPS. Research on young parents has focused mostly on teenage mothers. Low parental education may also be associated with neglect, and young mothers may be less likely to attain a high level of education, thus limiting their work prospects and leading to financial stress. Other risk factors for neglect associated with young mothers include substance abuse, inadequate knowledge of childhood development, and poor parenting skills.

Because a lack of employment is related to so many other risk factors for child neglect, it is not surprising that both maternal and paternal lack of employment are associated with higher rates of child neglect. Parents who have committed a crime also may be more likely to neglect their children. Again, this may be because criminal activity is linked to other risk factors, such as substance abuse and poverty.

Parents' prior involvement with CPS has been linked to subsequent reports of neglect. These parents may be discouraged, less likely to think that their situation will change, less willing to receive services, or less motivated to change. However, families who have been involved with CPS and had positive experiences may be more motivated and open to receiving services. It is important that young parents, both mothers and fathers, obtain the support they need so that they can adequately attend to the needs of their children.

## Child Factors

Any child can be the victim of neglect, but some characteristics appear to be more highly represented among maltreated children, including being under the age of three years, having certain behavioral problems, and having special needs.

### Age

In 2004, children from birth to age three years had the highest rate of reported maltreatment (16.1 per 1,000 children). Research also shows that children under three years of age are most at risk for neglect, with rates decreasing as the age of the child increases.

### Temperament and Behavior

A child's temperament and behavior may be associated with child neglect. Children with an irritable temperament and who have difficulty being soothed may be more at risk for being neglected than other children, since having a difficult temperament may strain the parent-child relationship. One study found that a difficult child temperament (as perceived by the mother) was specifically associated with emotional neglect.

Neglected children also often demonstrate a distinct set of behaviors including being passive, nonassertive, or withdrawn. It is unclear whether children develop these behavior problems because they are neglected or if they are neglected because they have behavior problems.

Behavior problems can be categorized as either internalizing or externalizing. Internalizing behavior is a behavior or a feeling that is directed inward, such as depression. Such children may be overlooked because they rarely act out. Externalizing behavior is characterized by outward expressions of behaviors and feelings that are easily observable, such as being aggressive. These children often receive more attention than those who internalize because their behavior is often disruptive to others.

Maltreatment may cause internalized behaviors, such as:

- agitation,
- nightmares,
- avoidance of certain activities or people,
- difficulty falling asleep or staying asleep,
- sleeping too much,
- difficulty concentrating,
- hypervigilance,
- irritability,
- becoming easily fatigued,
- poor appetite or overeating,
- low self-esteem, or
- feelings of hopelessness.

The listed symptoms, if experienced persistently or if many of them are experienced all at once, should be cause for concern. Maltreatment also may cause externalized behaviors, including:

- difficulty paying attention,
- not listening when spoken to,
- difficulty organizing tasks and activities,
- being easily distracted,

- being forgetful,
- bedwetting,
- excessive talking,
- difficulty awaiting their turn,
- bullying or threatening others,
- being physically cruel to people or animals,
- playing with or starting fires,
- stealing, or
- destroying property.

It is important to keep the child's age and developmental level in mind when assessing a child for these symptoms. For example, bedwetting by a 13-year-old would cause more concern than bedwetting by a 2-year-old. If a child's internalized or externalized behaviors interfere with his normal functioning or if his behavior changes dramatically, then the child should be referred for further assessment.

### Special Needs

While the link between children with special needs and neglect is unclear, some studies have found higher rates of child abuse and neglect among children with disabilities. One study found such children to be 1.7 times more likely to be maltreated than children without disabilities. Another study, however, failed to find increased levels of maltreatment among a sample of children with moderate to severe retardation.

Children with special needs, such as those with physical or developmental challenges, may be more at risk for maltreatment because:

- their parents become overwhelmed with trying to take care of them and may respond with irritability, inconsistent care, or punitive discipline;

- children may be unresponsive or have limited ability to respond, interact, or show as much affection as parents expect, thereby disrupting parent-child attachments; and,

- society tends to devalue individuals with disabilities.

An alternate explanation for higher rates of maltreatment among children with special needs is that parents of children with special needs have more frequent contact with an array of professionals and thus may be under greater scrutiny. In any case, these parents may need more support and encouragement to help them provide for the needs of their children. For children with special needs, having a strong and secure attachment to their primary caregivers, in turn, may moderate the negative effects of the disability and provide protection from neglect.

### Other Child Characteristics

Other child characteristics associated with neglect include the following:

- Being born prematurely, with a low birth weight, or with birth anomalies
- Being exposed to toxins in utero
- Experiencing childhood trauma
- Having an antisocial peer group, such as being a gang member

Children who are premature or have low birth weights may be at risk for neglect because their parents may be confused, anxious, or feel helpless, which may make it harder for them to relate to the baby. These parents also may have fewer or less positive interactions with the infant, restricting the formation of positive attachments.

Some child characteristics that appear to be protective factors against neglect include the following:

- Good health
- A history of adequate development
- Above-average intelligence
- Hobbies and interests
- Humor
- A positive self-concept
- Good peer relationships
- An easy temperament
- A positive disposition
- An active coping style
- Good social skills

- An internal locus of control (believing one's behavior and life experiences are the result of personal decisions and efforts)
- A lack of self-blame
- A balance between seeking help and autonomy

Recently there has been a shift toward a strengths-based focus with a greater emphasis on resilience and protective factors and a movement away from focusing solely on risk factors, particularly for preventing neglect and its recurrence. The belief is that prevention strategies are most effective when they involve building up a family's strengths. However, research suggests that solely focusing on building up protective factors, while not resolving some of the risk factors, may not be a particularly effective strategy. Intervention strategies should address both risk and protective factors to provide the most help to families.

## *Resilience*

Resilience can be defined as the ability to thrive, mature, and increase competence in the face of adverse circumstances. Some children who are neglected are able not only to survive the neglect, but also to achieve positive outcomes despite it. What sets these children apart may be a greater number of protective factors related to either themselves, or their parents, or their environment. One important finding from research is that resiliency can be developed at any point in life. For example, teenagers who exhibit learning or behavior problems may become well-functioning, productive adults by the time they are thirty. Resilience is thought to stem from ordinary human processes, such as parenting, thinking skills, motivation, rituals of family and culture, and other basic systems that foster human adaptation and development. These ordinary processes should be recognized, promoted, and supported so that they work well and can help children.

# Chapter 4

# *Child Maltreatment Statistics*

## *Chapter Contents*

# Section 4.1

# *Victims of Child Abuse*

Excerpted from "Child Maltreatment 2006: Chapter 3," Administration for Children and Families (ACF), 2008. The complete report is available online at http://www.acf.hhs.gov/programs/cb/pubs/cm06/cm06.pdf.

## *Children Who Were Subjects of an Investigation*

Based on a rate of 47.8 per 1,000 children, an estimated 3.6 million children received an investigation by child protective services (CPS) agencies during the federal fiscal year (FFY) 2006. The rate of all children who received an investigation or assessment increased from 43.8 per 1,000 children for 2002 to 47.8 per 1,000 children for FFY 2006. The national estimates are based upon counting a child each time he or she was the subject of a CPS investigation.

The rate of victimization decreased from 12.3 per 1,000 during 2002, to 12.1 per 1,000 children during FFY 2006, which is a 1.6 percent decrease. State-specific, 5-year trends illustrate that 28 states decreased their rate from 2002 to 2006, while 22 states increased their rate. Two states were not able to provide data for this analysis.

## *Types of Maltreatment*

During FFY 2006:

- nearly three-quarters of victims (74.7%) had no history of prior victimization;

- 64.1 percent of victims experienced neglect;

- 16.0 percent were physically abused;

- 8.8 percent were sexually abused;

- 6.6 percent were psychologically maltreated;

- 2.2 percent were medically neglected; and

- 15.1 percent of victims experienced such other types of maltreatment as abandonment, threats of harm to the child, or congenital drug addiction.

States may code any condition that does not fall into one of the main categories—physical abuse, neglect, medical neglect, sexual abuse, and psychological or emotional maltreatment—as other. These maltreatment type percentages total more than 100 percent because children who were victims of more than one type of maltreatment were counted for each maltreatment.

The data for victims of specific types of maltreatment were analyzed in terms of the report sources. Of victims of physical abuse, 24.2 percent were reported by teachers, 23.1 percent were reported by police officers or lawyers, and 12.1 percent were reported by medical staff. Overall, 74.9 percent were reported by professionals and 25.1 percent were reported by nonprofessionals. The patterns of reporting of neglect and sexual abuse victims were similar—police officers or lawyers accounted for the largest report source percentage of neglect victims (27.1%) and the largest percentage of sexual abuse victims (28.1%).

## Sex and Age of Victims

For FFY 2006, 48.2 percent of child victims were boys, and 51.5 percent of the victims were girls. The youngest children had the highest rate of victimization. The rate of child victimization for the age group of birth to one year was 24.4 per 1,000 children of the same age group. The victimization rate for children in the age group of 1–3 years was 14.2 per 1,000 children in the same age group. The victimization rate for children in the age group of 4–7 years was 13.5 per 1,000 children in the same age group. Overall, the rate of victimization was inversely related to the age group of the child.

Nearly three-quarters of child victims (72.2%) ages birth to one year and age group of 1–3 years (72.9%) were neglected compared with 55.0 percent of victims ages 16 years and older. For victims in the age group of 4–7 years 15.3 percent were physically abused and 8.2 percent were sexually abused, compared with 20.1 percent and 16.5 percent, respectively, for victims in the age group of 12–15 years old.

## Race and Ethnicity of Victims

African-American children, American Indian or Alaska Native children, and children of multiple races had the highest rates of victimization at 19.8, 15.9, and 15.4 per 1,000 children of the same race or ethnicity, respectively. White children and Hispanic children had rates of approximately 10.7 and 10.8 per 1,000 children of the same race or ethnicity, respectively. Asian children had the lowest rate of 2.5 per 1,000 children of the same race or ethnicity.

One-half of all victims were White (48.8); almost one-quarter (22.8) were African-American; and 18.4 percent were Hispanic. For all racial categories except Native Hawaiian and Pacific Islander, the largest percentage of victims suffered from neglect.

## Living Arrangement of Victims

Data are incomplete for the living arrangement of victims. Slightly more than one-half of the states (28) reported on the living arrangement of victims during the alleged abuse or neglect. Among these 28 states, nearly 40.0 percent (37.3%) of the victims had unknown or missing data on living arrangement and were excluded from the analysis. Approximately 27 percent (26.7%) of victims were living with a single mother. Nearly 20 percent (19.7%) of victims were living with married parents, while approximately 22 percent of victims (21.6%) were living with both parents but the marital status was unknown.

## Reported Disability of Victims

Children who were reported with any of the following risk factors were considered as having a disability: mental retardation, emotional disturbance, visual or hearing impairment, learning disability, physical disability, behavioral problems, or another medical problem. In general, children with such risk factors are undercounted, as not every child receives a clinical diagnostic assessment from CPS agency staff. Nearly eight percent (7.7%) of victims had a reported disability. Three percent of victims had behavior problems and 1.9 percent of victims were emotionally disturbed. A victim could have been reported with more than one type of disability.

## Factors Influencing the Determination That a Child Is a Victim of Maltreatment

The determination as to whether or not a child is considered a victim of maltreatment is made during a CPS investigation. A multivariate analysis was conducted to examine whether some child characteristics or circumstances place children at a greater risk for being identified as victims during the investigation process. The odds ratio analyses indicate the likelihood that an allegation of maltreatment is confirmed by the CPS agency. Highlights of the findings follow:

- Children with allegations of multiple types of maltreatment were nearly four times more likely to be considered a victim of maltreatment than were children with allegations of physical abuse. Children with allegations of sexual abuse were nearly twice as likely to be considered victims, and children with allegations of neglect and other abuse types were also significantly more likely to be considered victims than children with allegations of physical abuse.

- Children who were reported as disabled were 54 percent more likely to be considered a victim of maltreatment than children who were not reported as disabled.

- The likelihood of being considered a victim declined, compared with infants, as the age of the children increased.

- Children who were reported by educational personnel were more than twice as likely to be considered a victim of maltreatment as children reported by social and mental health personnel.

## Recurrence

For many victims who have experienced repeat maltreatment, the efforts of the CPS system have not been successful in preventing subsequent victimization.

- Children who had been prior victims of maltreatment were 96 percent more likely to experience a recurrence than those who were not prior victims.

- Child victims who were reported with a disability were 52 percent more likely to experience recurrence than children without a disability.

- The oldest victims (16–21 years of age) were the least likely to experience a recurrence, and were 51 percent less likely than were infants (younger than age one year).

## Victims by Relationship to Perpetrators

Nearly 83 percent (82.4%) of victims were abused by a parent acting alone or with another person. Approximately, 40 percent (39.9%)

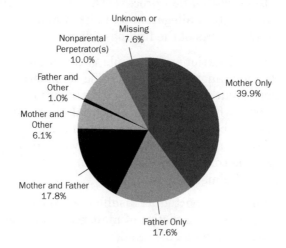

**Figure 4.1.** *Victims by Perpetrator Relationship, 2006*

## Table 4.1. Victims by Age Group and Maltreatment Type, 2006

| AGE GROUP | VICTIMS | NEGLECT | | PHYSICAL ABUSE | | MEDICAL NEGLECT | | SEXUAL ABUSE | |
|---|---|---|---|---|---|---|---|---|---|
| | | NUMBER | % | NUMBER | % | NUMBER | % | NUMBER | % |
| Age <1 | 100,139 | 72,314 | 72.2 | 14,328 | 14.3 | 3,629 | 3.6 | 445 | 0.4 |
| Age 1–3 | 172,940 | 125,997 | 72.9 | 18,731 | 10.8 | 3,948 | 2.3 | 4,558 | 2.6 |
| Age 4–7 | 213,194 | 138,886 | 65.1 | 32,697 | 15.3 | 3,843 | 1.8 | 17,539 | 8.2 |
| Age 8–11 | 170,944 | 103,964 | 60.8 | 29,312 | 17.1 | 3,233 | 1.9 | 18,314 | 10.7 |
| Age 12–15 | 170,635 | 94,910 | 55.6 | 34,348 | 20.1 | 3,447 | 2.0 | 28,138 | 16.5 |
| Age 16 and Older | 54,564 | 29,989 | 55.0 | 11,998 | 22.0 | 1,030 | 1.9 | 8,798 | 16.1 |
| Unknown or Missing | 2,829 | 1,727 | 61.0 | 627 | 22.2 | 50 | 1.8 | 328 | 11.6 |
| | | | | | | | | | |
| **Total** | **885,245** | **567,787** | | **142,041** | | **19,180** | | **78,120** | |
| **Percent** | | | **64.1** | | **16.0** | | **2.2** | | **8.8** |

| AGE GROUP | PSYCHOLOGICAL ABUSE | | OTHER ABUSE | | UNKNOWN | | TOTAL MALTREATMENTS | |
|---|---|---|---|---|---|---|---|---|
| | NUMBER | % | NUMBER | % | NUMBER | % | NUMBER | % |
| Age <1 | 3,967 | 4.0 | 16,300 | 16.3 | 1,097 | 1.1 | 112,080 | 111.9 |
| Age 1–3 | 10,262 | 5.9 | 29,016 | 16.8 | 2,114 | 1.2 | 194,626 | 112.5 |
| Age 4–7 | 14,555 | 6.8 | 31,833 | 14.9 | 2,570 | 1.2 | 241,923 | 113.5 |
| Age 8–11 | 13,647 | 8.0 | 25,406 | 14.9 | 1,947 | 1.1 | 195,823 | 114.6 |
| Age 12–15 | 12,372 | 7.3 | 23,465 | 13.8 | 1,950 | 1.1 | 198,630 | 116.4 |
| Age 16 and Older | 3,524 | 6.5 | 7,832 | 14.4 | 541 | 1.0 | 63,712 | 116.8 |
| Unknown or Missing | 250 | 8.8 | 126 | 4.5 | 2 | 0.1 | 3,110 | 109.9 |
| | | | | | | | | |
| **Total** | **58,577** | | **133,978** | | **10,221** | | **1,009,904** | |
| **Percent** | | **6.6** | | **15.1** | | **1.2** | | **114.1** |

*Based on data from 51 States*

of child victims were maltreated by their mothers acting alone; another 17.6 percent were maltreated by their fathers acting alone; and 17.8 percent were abused by both parents. Victims abused by non-parental perpetrators accounted for 10.0 percent. A nonparental perpetrator is defined as a caregiver who is not a parent and can include foster parent, child daycare staff, unmarried partner of parent, legal guardian, and residential facility staff.

The data for victims of specific maltreatment types were analyzed in terms of perpetrator relationship to the victim. Of the victims who experienced neglect, 86.7 percent were neglected by a parent. Of the victims who were sexually abused, 26.2 percent were abused by a parent and 29.1 percent were abused by a relative other than a parent.

**Table 4.2.** Victims by Perpetrator Relationship, 2006

| | VICTIMS | |
|---|---|---|
| PERPETRATOR | NUMBER | % |
| Mother Only | 284,326 | 39.9 |
| Father Only | 125,353 | 17.6 |
| Mother and Father | 126,992 | 17.8 |
| Mother and Other | 43,175 | 6.1 |
| Father and Other | 7,015 | 1.0 |
| Female Partner of Parent | 1,247 | 0.2 |
| Male Partner of Parent | 13,146 | 1.8 |
| Female Legal Guardian | 1,116 | 0.2 |
| Male Legal Guardian | 278 | 0.0 |
| | | |
| Relative | 34,675 | 4.9 |
| Foster Parent (Relative) | 320 | 0.0 |
| Foster Parent (Nonrelative) | 1,133 | 0.2 |
| Foster Parent (Unknown Relationship) | 768 | 0.1 |
| Residential Facility Staff | 1,185 | 0.2 |
| Daycare Staff | 3,615 | 0.5 |
| Other Professional | 903 | 0.1 |
| Friend or Neighbor | 2,940 | 0.4 |
| More than One Nonparental Perpetrator | 10,133 | 1.4 |
| Unknown or Missing | 53,876 | 7.6 |
| | | |
| **Total** | **712,196** | |
| **Percent** | | **100.0** |

*Based on data from 47 States.*

# Section 4.2

# *Child Abuse and Neglect Fatalities*

Excerpted from "Child Maltreatment 2006: Chapter 4," Administration for Children and Families (ACF), 2008. The complete report is available online at http://www.acf.hhs.gov/programs/cb/pubs/cm06/cm06.pdf.

Child fatalities are the most tragic consequence of maltreatment. The collection of accurate data regarding fatalities attributed to child abuse and neglect is challenging and requires coordination among many agencies. The National Child Abuse and Neglect Data System (NCANDS) case-level data are from public child protective services (CPS) agencies and, therefore, do not include information for deaths that are not investigated by a CPS agency. In this section, national estimates of the number and rate of child maltreatment deaths per 100,000 children are provided. The characteristics of these fatality victims also are discussed.

During federal fiscal year (FFY) 2006:

- there were an estimated 1,530 child fatality victims;

- approximately one-fifth (17.6%) of child fatality data were reported from agencies other than child welfare; and

- more than three-quarters (78.0%) of child fatality victims were younger than four years.

## *Number of Child Fatalities*

During FFY 2006, an estimated 1,530 children (compared to 1,460 children for FFY 2005) died from abuse or neglect—at a rate of 2.04 deaths per 100,000 children. The national estimate was based on data from state child welfare information systems, as well as other data sources available to the states. The rate of 2.04 is an increase from the rate for FFY 2005 of 1.96 per 100,000 children. This increase can be attributed to better reporting practices and is not necessarily an increase in the number of fatalities.

While most fatality data were obtained from state child welfare agencies, many agencies also received data from additional sources. For FFY 2006, nearly one-fifth (17.6%) of fatalities were reported through the agency file, which includes fatalities reported by health departments and fatality review boards. The coordination of data collection with other agencies contributes to a fuller understanding of the size of the phenomenon, as well as to better estimation.

## Age and Sex of Child Fatalities

More than three-quarters (78.0%) of children who were killed were younger than four years of age, 11.9 percent were 4–7 years of age, 4.8 percent were 8–11 years of age, and 5.4 percent were 12–17 years of age.

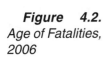
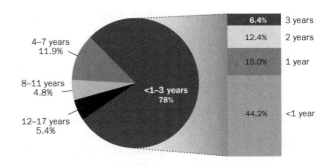

*Figure 4.2.*
*Age of Fatalities, 2006*

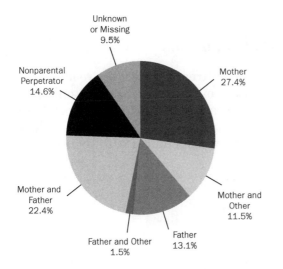

*Figure 4.3.* Perpetrator Relationships of Child Fatalities, 2006

The youngest children experienced the highest rates of fatalities. Infant boys (younger than one year) had a fatality rate of 18.5 deaths per 100,000 boys of the same age. Infant girls (younger than one year) had a fatality rate of 14.7 deaths per 100,000 girls of the same age. In general, fatality rates for both boys and girls decreased with age.

## Race and Ethnicity of Child Fatalities

Nearly one-half (43.0%) of all fatalities were White children. More than one-quarter (29.4%) were African-American children, and nearly one-fifth (17.0%) were Hispanic children. Children of American Indian or Alaska Native, Asian, Pacific Islander, other, and multiple race categories collectively accounted for 10.7 percent of fatalities.

## Perpetrator Relationships of Child Fatalities

Three-quarters (75.9%) of child fatalities were caused by one or more parents. More than one-quarter (27.4%) of fatalities were perpetrated by the mother acting alone. Nonparental perpetrators (for example, other relative, foster parent, residential facility staff, other, and legal guardian) were responsible for 14.7 percent of fatalities.

## Maltreatment Types of Child Fatalities

The three main categories of maltreatment related to fatalities were neglect (41.1%), combinations of maltreatments (31.4%), and physical abuse (22.4%). Medical neglect accounted for 1.9 percent of fatalities.

## Prior CPS Contact of Child Fatalities

Some children who died from maltreatment were already known to CPS agencies. Children whose families had received family preservation services in the past five years accounted for 13.7 percent of child fatalities. Slightly more than two percent (2.3%) of the child fatalities had been in foster care and were reunited with their families in the past five years.

## Section 4.3

# *Referrals, Reports, and Investigations of Child Abuse and Neglect*

Excerpted from "Child Maltreatment 2006: Chapter 2," Administration for Children and Families (ACF), 2008. The complete report is available online at http://www.acf.hhs.gov/programs/cb/pubs/cm06/cm06.pdf.

Child protective services (CPS) agencies have established two stages for responding to child abuse and neglect allegations. The first is the receipt of a referral from a professional or another person in the community. A referral is the initial notification to CPS alleging abuse or neglect of one or more children. Agency hotline or intake units screen out some referrals as not being appropriate for further investigation or assessment. The second stage is the investigation or assessment of the screened-in referral, which is called a report.

When an allegation reaches the second stage and is considered a report, the agency either initiates an investigation or pursues an alternative response. The purpose of an investigation is to determine if the child was maltreated—or is at risk of maltreatment—and to establish the appropriate intervention. Alternative responses emphasize an assessment of the family's needs and the prevention of future maltreatment, rather than making a formal determination of maltreatment. Regardless of which type of response the agency uses for a specific report, it must decide if further action is necessary to protect the child.

This section presents statistics regarding referrals, reports, and investigations or assessments. National estimates for federal fiscal year (FFY) 2006 are based on the child populations for the 50 states, the District of Columbia, and Puerto Rico. During FFY 2006:

- approximately 3.3 million allegations of child abuse and neglect including 6.0 million children were made to CPS agencies;

- about 62 percent (61.7%) of those allegations reached the report stage and either were investigated or received an alternative response; and

- nearly 30 percent (28.6%) of the investigations that reached the report stage determined that at least one child was a victim of child abuse or neglect.

## Screening of Referrals

The process of determining whether a referral meets a state's standard for an investigation or assessment is known as screening. Screening in a referral means that an allegation of child abuse or neglect met the state's standard for investigation or assessment and the referral reaches the second stage and is called a report. Screening out a referral means that the allegation did not meet the state's standard for an investigation or assessment. Reasons for screening out a referral may include the following: The referral did not concern child abuse or neglect; it did not contain enough information to enable an investigation or assessment to occur; the children in the referral were the responsibility of another agency or jurisdiction, for example, a military installation or a tribe; or the alleged victim was older than 18 years.

During FFY 2006, an estimated 3.3 million referrals, including approximately 6.0 million children, were made to CPS agencies. The national rate was 43.7 referrals per 1,000 children for FFY 2006 compared with 43.9 referrals per 1,000 children for FFY 2005.

During FFY 2006, CPS agencies screened in 61.7 percent of referrals and screened out 38.3 percent. These results were similar to FFY 2005 data, which indicated 62.1 percent were screened in and 37.9 percent were screened out.

## Report Sources

National Child Abuse and Neglect Data System (NCANDS) collects case-level information for all reports that received a disposition or finding within the year. The information includes the report source, the number of children in the investigation, and the disposition of the report.

Professionals submitted more than one-half (56.3%) of the reports. The term professional indicates that the person encountered the alleged victim as part of the report source's occupation. State laws require most professionals to notify CPS agencies of suspected maltreatment. The categories of professionals include teachers, legal staff or police officers, social services staff, medical staff, mental health workers, child daycare workers, and foster care providers. The three largest percentages of 2006 reports were from professionals—

teachers (16.5%), lawyers or police officers (15.8%), and social services staff (10.0%).

Nonprofessional sources submitted the remaining 43.7 percent of reports. These included parents, relatives, friends and neighbors, alleged victims, alleged perpetrators, anonymous callers, and other sources. NCANDS uses the term other sources for those categories that states are not able to cross-reference to any of the NCANDS terms. Other sources may include clergy members, sports coaches, camp counselors, bystanders, volunteers, and foster siblings. The three largest groups of nonprofessional reporters were anonymous (8.2%), other (8.0%), and other relatives (7.8%).

## Investigation or Assessment Results

CPS agencies assign a finding—also called a disposition—to a report after the circumstances are investigated and a determination is made as to whether the maltreatment occurred or the child is at risk of maltreatment. For FFY 2006, 1,907,264 investigations received a disposition. Each state establishes dispositions by policy and law. The major NCANDS disposition categories follow:

- **Alternative response non-victim:** A conclusion that the child was not identified as a victim when a response other than an investigation was provided.

- **Alternative response victim:** A conclusion that the child was identified as a victim when a response other than an investigation was provided.

- **Indicated:** An investigation disposition that concludes that maltreatment could not be substantiated under state law or policy, but there was reason to suspect that the child may have been maltreated or was at risk of maltreatment. This is applicable only to states that distinguish between substantiated and indicated dispositions.

- **Substantiated:** An investigation disposition that concludes that the allegation of maltreatment or risk of maltreatment was supported or founded by state law or state policy.

- **Unsubstantiated:** An investigation disposition that determines that there was not sufficient evidence under state law to conclude or suspect that the child was maltreated or at risk of being maltreated.

Two alternative response categories are provided in NCANDS. The category that is most commonly used by states is alternative response non-victim. Some states also use the alternative response victim category. During FFY 2006, 12 states used the alternative response non-victim category and two states used the alternative response victim category.

For nearly 30 percent of investigations, at least one child was found to be a victim of maltreatment with one of the following dispositions—substantiated (25.2%), indicated (3.0%), or alternative response victim (0.4%). The remaining investigations led to a finding that children were not victims of maltreatment and the report received one of the following dispositions—unsubstantiated (60.4%), alternative response non-victim (5.9%), other (3.2%), closed with no finding (1.7%), or intentionally false (0.1%). When the 2002 investigation rates were compared to the FFY 2006 rates for each state, it was noted that by FFY 2006, the majority of states had increased their investigation rates. Two states were unable to submit the data needed for this analysis.

## Report Dispositions by Report Source

Report dispositions are based on the facts of the report as found by the CPS worker. The type of report source may be related to the disposition of a report because of the reporter's knowledge and credibility. Case-level data submitted to NCANDS were used to examine this hypothesis. Based on more than 1.8 million reports, key findings follow:

- Approximately two-thirds of substantiated or indicated reports were made by professional sources. Approximately 30 percent of substantiated and indicated reports were made by legal staff and police officers.

- Nonprofessional report sources accounted for more than one-half of several categories of report disposition, indicating that children were not found to be victims of maltreatment. Those included alternative response non-victim (58.8%), intentionally false (76.1%), or closed with no finding (54.5%).

## Response Time from Report to Investigation

Most states set requirements for beginning an investigation into a report of child abuse or neglect. While some states have a single timeframe for responding to reports, many states establish priorities based on the information received from the report source. Of the states that establish priorities, many specify a high-priority response as within one hour or within 24 hours. Lower priority responses range from 24 hours to 14 days.

Because CPS agencies receive reports of varying degrees of urgency, average response times reflect the types of reports that are received, as well as the ability of workers to meet the time standards. The median response time from report to investigation was 66 hours or approximately 2–3 days. The average response time for these states was 86 hours or approximately four days. This is comparable to a median response time of 67 hours and an average response time of 89 hours for FFY 2005.

## *CPS Workforce and Workload*

Given the large number and complexity of investigations and assessments that are conducted each year, there is an ongoing interest in the nature of the workforce that performs CPS functions. In most agencies, the screening and investigation are conducted by different groups of workers. In many rural and smaller agencies, one worker may perform both those functions, and other functions not mentioned here.

States that reported significant numbers of specialized workers for intake, screening, investigation, and assessment were used to estimate the average number of cases that were handled by CPS workers. The average number of completed investigations per investigation worker was 62 per year. This compares with 67.5 in FFY 2005.

# Section 4.4

# *Perpetrators of Child Abuse*

Excerpted from "Child Maltreatment 2006: Chapter 5," Administration for Children and Families (ACF), 2008. The complete report is available online at http://www.acf.hhs.gov/programs/cb/pubs/cm06/cm06.pdf.

The National Child Abuse and Neglect Data System (NCANDS) defines a perpetrator as a person who is considered responsible for the maltreatment of a child. Thus, this section provides data about only those perpetrators of child abuse victims and does not include data about alleged perpetrators.

Given the definition of child abuse and neglect, which largely pertains to caregivers, not to persons unknown to a child, most perpetrators of child maltreatment are parents. Also included are relatives, foster parents, and residential facility staff. During federal fiscal year (FFY) 2006:

- nearly 80 percent (79.9%) of perpetrators were parents of the victim;

- approximately 60 percent (60.4%) of perpetrators were found to have neglected children; and

- approximately 58 percent (57.9%) of perpetrators were women, and 42 percent (42.1%) of perpetrators were men.

For the analyses in this section, a perpetrator may be counted multiple times if he or she has maltreated more than one child. A perpetrator is counted for each child in each report. This section presents data about the demographic characteristics of perpetrators, the relationship of perpetrators to their victims, and the types of maltreatment they committed.

## *Characteristics of Perpetrators*

For FFY 2006, 57.9 percent of the perpetrators were women and 42.1 percent were men. Women typically were younger than men. The

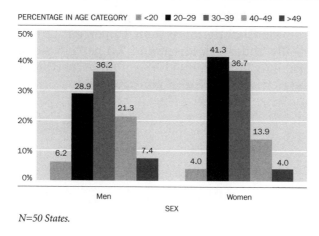

*N=50 States.*

**Figure 4.4.** *Age and Sex of Perpetrators, 2006*

median age of women was 31 years and 34 years for men. Of the women who were perpetrators, more than 40 percent (45.3%) were younger than 30 years of age, compared with one-third of the men (35.1%).

The racial distribution of perpetrators was similar to the race of their victims. During FFY 2006, more than one-half (53.7%) of perpetrators were White and one-fifth (20.7%) were African-American. Approximately 20 percent (19.5%) of perpetrators were Hispanic.

Nearly 80 percent (79.9%) of perpetrators were parents. Other relatives accounted for an additional 6.7 percent. Unmarried partners of parents accounted for 3.8 percent. Of the parents who were perpetrators, more than 90 percent (91.5%) were biological parents, 4.2 percent were stepparents, and 0.7 percent were adoptive parents.

**Table 4.3.** Perpetrators by Type of Maltreatment, 2006

| | PERPETRATORS | |
| MALTREATMENT TYPE | NUMBER | PERCENT |
| --- | --- | --- |
| Neglect | 569,348 | 60.4 |
| Physical Abuse | 97,533 | 10.3 |
| Multiple Maltreatments | 108,093 | 11.5 |
| Psychological Maltreatment, "Other," or Unknown | 101,518 | 10.8 |
| Sexual Abuse | 66,365 | 7.0 |
| **Total** | **942,857** | |
| **Percent** | | **100.0** |

*Based on data from 50 States.*

49

More than one-half (60.4%) of all perpetrators were found to have neglected children. Slightly more than 10 percent (10.3%) of perpetrators physically abused children, and 7.0 percent sexually abused children. More than 11 percent (11.5%) of all perpetrators were associated with more than one type of maltreatment.

# Chapter 5

# *Cost of Child Abuse and Neglect in the United States*

Child abuse and neglect are preventable, yet each year in the United States, close to one million children are confirmed victims of child maltreatment. An extensive body of research provides promising and best practices on what works to improve child safety and well-being outcomes and reduce the occurrence of child abuse and neglect. These efforts are essential as child abuse and neglect have pervasive and long-lasting effects on children, their families, and the society. Adverse consequences for children's development often are evident immediately, encompassing multiple domains including physical, emotional, social, and cognitive. For many children, these effects extend far beyond childhood into adolescence and adulthood, potentially compromising the lifetime productivity of maltreatment victims (Daro, 1988).

It is well documented that children who have been abused or neglected are more likely to experience adverse outcomes throughout their lifespan in a number of areas:

- Poor physical health (for example, chronic fatigue, altered immune function, hypertension, sexually transmitted diseases, obesity)

- Poor emotional and mental health (depression, anxiety, eating disorders, suicidal thoughts and attempts, post-traumatic stress disorder)

- Social difficulties (insecure attachments with caregivers, which may lead to difficulties in developing trusting relationships with peers and adults later in life)

- Cognitive dysfunction (deficits in attention, abstract reasoning, language development, and problem-solving skills, which ultimately affect academic achievement and school performance)

- High-risk health behaviors (a higher number of lifetime sexual partners, younger age at first voluntary intercourse, teen pregnancy, alcohol and substance abuse)

- Behavioral problems (aggression, juvenile delinquency, adult criminality, abusive or violent behavior) (Source: Child Welfare Information Gateway, 2006; Goldman, Salus, Wolcott, and Kennedy, 2003; Hagele, 2005)

The costs of responding to the impact of child abuse and neglect are borne by the victims and their families but also by society. This chapter updates an earlier publication documenting the nationwide costs as a result of child abuse and neglect (Fromm, 2001). Similar to the earlier document, this chapter places costs in two categories: direct costs, that is, those costs associated with the immediate needs of children who are abused or neglected; and indirect costs, that is, those costs associated with the long-term and/or secondary effects of child abuse and neglect. All estimated costs are presented in 2007 dollars. Adjustments for inflation have been conducted using the price indexes for gross domestic product published by the Bureau of Economic Analysis (http://www.bea.gov).

Based on data drawn from a variety of sources, the estimated annual cost of child abuse and neglect is $103.8 billion in 2007 value. This figure represents a conservative estimate as a result of the methods used for the calculation. First, only children who could be classified as being abused or neglected according to the Harm Standard in the *Third National Incidence Study of Child Abuse and Neglect (NIS-3)* are included in the analysis. The Harm Standard requirements, compared to the Endangerment Standard requirements used in NIS-3, are more stringent (Sedlak and Broadhurst, 1996). Second, only those costs related to victims are included. We have not attempted to quantify other costs associated with abuse and neglect, such as the costs of intervention or treatment services for the perpetrators or other members of the victim's family. Third, the categories of costs included in this analysis are by no means exhaustive. As examples, a large number of child victims require medical examinations

**Table 5.1.** Total Annual Cost of Child Abuse and Neglect in the United States

| Direct Costs | Estimated Annual Cost (in 2007 dollars) |
|---|---|
| Hospitalization | $6,625,959,263 |

Rationale: 565,000 maltreated children suffered serious injuries in 1993.[1] Assume that 50% of seriously injured victims require hospitalization.[2] The average cost of treating one hospitalized victim of abuse and neglect was $19,266 in 1999.[3] Calculation: 565,000 x 0.50 x $19,266 = $5,442,645,000.

| | |
|---|---|
| Mental Health Care System | $1,080,706,049 |

Rationale: 25% to 50% of child maltreatment victims need some form of mental health treatment.[4] For a conservative estimate, 25% is used. Mental health care cost per victim by type of maltreatment is: physical abuse ($2,700); sexual abuse ($5,800); emotional abuse ($2,700) and educational neglect ($910).[4] Cross referenced against NIS-3 statistics on number of each incident occurring in 1993.[1] Calculations: Physical Abuse—381,700 x 0.25 x $2,700 = $257,647,500; Sexual Abuse—217,700 x 0.25 x $5,800 = $315,665,000; Emotional Abuse—204,500 x 0.25 x $2,700 = $138,037,500; and Educational Neglect— 397,300 x 0.25 x $910 = $90,385,750; Total = $801,735,750.

| | |
|---|---|
| Child Welfare Services System | $25,361,329,051 |

Rationale: The Urban Institute conducted a study estimating the child welfare expenditures associated with child abuse and neglect by state and local public child welfare agencies to be $23.3 billion in 2004.[5]

| | |
|---|---|
| Law Enforcement | $33,307,770 |

Rationale: The National Institute of Justice estimated the following costs of police services for each of the following interventions: physical abuse ($20); sexual abuse ($56); emotional abuse ($20) and educational neglect ($2).[4] Cross referenced against NIS-3 statistics on number of each incident occurring in 1993.[1] Calculations: Physical Abuse—381,700 x $20 = $7,634,000; Sexual Abuse—217,700 x $56 = $12,191,200; Emotional Abuse—204,500 x $20 = $4,090,000; and Educational Neglect—397,300 x $2 = $794,600; Total = $24,709,800.

| | |
|---|---|
| **Total Direct Costs** | $33,101,302,133 |

**Table 5.2.** Total Annual Cost of Child Abuse and Neglect in the United States (*continued on next page*)

| Indirect Costs | Estimated Annual Cost (in 2007 dollars) |
|---|---|

**Special Education**        $2,410,306,242

Rationale: 1,553,800 children experienced some form of maltreatment in 1993.[1] 22% of maltreated children have learning disorders requiring special education.[6] The additional expenditure attributable to special education services for students with disabilities was $5,918 per pupil in 2000.[7] Calculation: 1,553,800 x 0.22 x $5,918 = $2,022,985,448.

**Juvenile Delinquency**        $7,174,814,134

Rationale: 1,553,800 children experienced some form of maltreatment in 1993.[1] 27% of children who are abused or neglected become delinquents, compared to 17% of children in the general population,[8] for a difference of 10%. The annual cost of caring for a juvenile offender in a residential facility was $30,450 in 1989.[9] Calculation: 1,553,800 x 0.10 x $30,450 = $4,731,321,000.

**Mental Health and Health Care**        $67,863,457

Rationale: 1,553,800 children experienced some form of maltreatment in 1993.[1] 30% of maltreated children suffer chronic health problems.[6] Increased mental health and health care costs for women with a history of childhood abuse and neglect, compared to women without childhood maltreatment histories, were estimated to be $8,175,816 for a population of 163,844 women, of whom 42.8% experienced childhood abuse and neglect.[10] This is equivalent to $117 [$8,175,816 divided by (163,844 x 0.428)] additional health care costs associated with child maltreatment per woman per year. Assume that the additional health care costs attributable to childhood maltreatment are similar for men who experienced maltreatment as a child. Calculation: 1,553,800 x 0.30 x $117 = $54,346,699.

**Adult Criminal Justice System**        $27,979,811,982

Rationale: The direct expenditure for operating the nation's criminal justice system (including police protection, judicial and legal services, and corrections) was $204,136,015,000 in 2005.[11] According to the National Institute of Justice, 13% of all violence can be linked to earlier child maltreatment.[4] Calculations: $204,136,015,000. x 0.13 = $26,537,681,950.

**Table 5.2.** Total Annual Cost of Child Abuse and Neglect in the United States (*continued on next page*)

| Indirect Costs | Estimated Annual Cost (in 2007 dollars) |
|---|---|
| Lost Productivity to Society | $33,019,919,544 |

Rationale: The median annual earning for a full-time worker was $33,634 in 2006.[12] Assume that only children who suffer serious injuries due to maltreatment (565,000[1]) experience losses in potential lifetime earnings and that such impairments are limited to 5% of the child's total potential earnings.[2] The average length of participation in the labor force is 39.1 years for men and 29.3 years for women;[13] the overall average 34 years is used. Calculation: $33,634 x 565,000 x 0.05 x 34 = $32,305,457,000.

| | |
|---|---|
| **Total Indirect Costs** | $70,652,715,359 |
| **Total Cost (Direct and Indirect Costs)** | $ 103,754,017,492 |

[1] Sedlak, A.J, and Broadhurst, D.D. (1996). *The third national incidence study of child abuse and neglect (NIS-3)*. U.S. Department of Health and Human Services. Washington, DC.

[2] Daro, D. (1988). *Confronting child abuse: Research for effective program design.* New York: Free Press.

[3] Rovi, S., Chen, P.H., and Johnson, M.S. (2004). The economic burden of hospitalizations associated with child abuse and neglect. *American Journal of Public Health*, 94, 586-590. Retrieved September 7, 2007 from http://www.ajph.org/cgi/reprint/94/4/586?ck=nck.

[4] Miller, T.R., Cohen, M.A., and Wiersema, B. (1996) *Victim costs and consequences: A new look.* The National Institute of Justice. Retrieved August 27, 2007 from http://www.ncjrs.gov/pdffiles/victcost.pdf.

[5] Scarcella, C.A., Bess, R., Zielewski, E.H., and Geen, R. (2006). *The cost of protecting vulnerable children V: Understanding state variation in child welfare financing.* The Urban Institute. Retrieved August 27, 2007 from http://www.urban.org/UploadedPDF/311314_vulnerable_children.pdf.

[6] Hammerle, N. (1992). *Private choices, social costs, and public policy: An economic analysis of public health issues.* Westport, CT: Greenwood, Praeger.

[7] Chambers, J.G., Parrish, T.B., and Harr, J.J. (2004). *What are we spending on special education services in the United States, 1999–2000*, Palo Alto, CA: American Institutes for Research. Retrieved August 28, 2007 from http://www.csefair.org/publications/seep/national/AdvRpt1.PDF.

**Table 5.2.** Total Annual Cost of Child Abuse and Neglect in the United States (*continued from previous pages*)

[8] Widom, C.S., and Maxfield, M.G. (2001). *An update on the "cycle of violence."* U.S. Department of Justice, the National Institute of Justice. Retrieved August 27, 2007 from http://www.ncjrs.gov/pdffiles1/nij/184894.pdf.

[9] U.S. Bureau of the Census (1993). *Statistical abstract of the United States, 1993 (113th edition.)* Washington, DC: Government Printing Office. Retrieved September 6, 2007 from http://www2.census.gov/prod2/statcomp/documents/1993-03.pdf.

[10] Walker, E.A., Unutzer, J., Rutter, C. Gelfand, A., Saunders, K., VonKorff, M., Koss, M., and Katon, W. (1999). Costs of health care use by women HMO members with a history of childhood abuse and neglect. *Archives of General Psychiatry*, 56, 609-613. Retrieved August 22, 2007 from http://archpsyc.ama-assn.org/cgi/reprint/56/7/609?ck=nck.

[11] U.S. Department of Justice (2007). *Key facts at a glance: Direct expenditures by criminal justice function, 1982–2005*. Bureau of Justice Statistics. Retrieved September 5, 2007 from http://www.ojp.usdoj.gov/bjs/glance/tables/exptyptab.htm.

[12] U.S. Department of Labor (2007). *National compensation survey: Occupational wages in the United States, June 2006*. U.S. Bureau of Labor Statistics. Retrieved September 4, 2007 from http://www.bls.gov/ncs/ocs/sp/ncbl0910.pdf.

[13] Smith, S.J. (1985). Revised worklife tables reflect 1979–80 experience. *Monthly Labor Review*, August 1985, 23-30. Retrieved September 4, 2007 from http://www.bls.gov/opub/mlr/1985/08/art3full.pdf.

or outpatient treatment for injuries not serious enough to require hospitalization; maltreated children are at greater risk of engaging in substance abuse and require alcohol and drug treatment services; and youth with histories of child abuse and neglect may be at greater risk of engaging in risky behaviors such as unprotected sexual activities as well as greater risk of teen pregnancy. We were not able to estimate these types of costs as data are not readily available.

Although the economic costs associated with child abuse and neglect are substantial, it is essential to recognize that it is impossible to calculate the impact of the pain, suffering, and reduced quality of life that victims of child abuse and neglect experience. These intangible losses, though difficult to quantify in monetary terms, are real and should not be overlooked. Intangible losses, in fact, may represent the largest cost component of violence against children and should be taken into account when allocating resources (Miller, 1993).

# Cost of Child Abuse and Neglect in the United States

## References

Bureau of Economic Analysis, U.S. Department of Commerce. National Income and Products Accounts (NIPS) Tables–Table 1.1.4. Price Indexes for Gross Domestic Product. Retrieved September 4, 2007 from http://www.bea.gov/national/nipaweb/TableView.asp?SelectedTable =4&FirstYear=2005&LastYear=2007&Freq=Qtr.

Child Welfare Information Gateway (2006). *Long-term consequences of child abuse and neglect*. Retrieved January 30, 2007, from http://www.childwelfare.gov/pubs/factsheets/long_term_consequences.cfm.

Daro, D. (1988). *Confronting child abuse: Research for effective program design*. New York: Free Press.

Fromm, S. (2001). *Total estimated cost of child abuse and neglect in the United States: Statistical evidence*. Chicago, IL: Prevent Child Abuse America. Retrieved September 4, 2007 from http://member .preventchildabuse.org/site/DocServer/cost_analysis .pdf?docID=144.

Goldman, J., Salus, M.K., Wolcott, D., and Kennedy, K.Y. (2003). *A coordinated response to child abuse and neglect: The foundation for practice*. Child Abuse and Neglect User Manual Series. Washington, DC: Government Printing Office. Retrieved January 29, 2007, from http://www.childwelfare.gov/pubs/usermanuals/foundation/foundation.pdf.

Hagele, D.M. (2005). The impact of maltreatment on the developing child. *North Carolina Medical Journal, 66*, 356-359. Retrieved September 11, 2007 from http://www.ncmedicaljournal.com/sept-oct-05/Hagele.pdf.

Miller, R.M., Cohen, M.A., and Wiersema, B. (1996). *Victim costs and consequences: A new look*. The National Institute of Justice. Retrieved August 27, 2007 from http://www.ncjrs.gov/pdffiles/victcost.pdf.

Sedlak, A.J., and Broadhurst, D.D. (1996). *The third national incidence study of child abuse and neglect (NIS-3)*. U.S. Department of Health and Human Services. Washington, DC.

# Chapter 6

# *Impact of Child Neglect*

The impact of neglect on a child may not be apparent at an early stage except in the most extreme cases. However, the effects of neglect are harmful and possibly long-lasting for the victims. Its impact can become more severe as a child grows older and can encompass multiple areas, including:

- health and physical development;
- intellectual and cognitive development;
- emotional and psychological development; and
- social and behavioral development.

Although there are four categories of neglect's effects on an individual, they often are related. For example, if a child experiences neglect that leads to a delayed development of the brain, this may lead to cognitive delays or psychological problems, which may manifest as social and behavioral problems. Because neglected children often experience multiple consequences that may be the result of neglect and related circumstances in their lives, it may be difficult to determine if the impact is related specifically to the neglect, is caused by another

This chapter includes text from "Child Neglect: A Guide for Prevention, Assessment, and Intervention: Chapter 3," Child Welfare Information Gateway, U.S. Department of Health and Human Services (HHS), updated September 18, 2008.

factor, or arises from a combination of factors. The impact of neglect can vary based on:

- the child's age,
- the presence and strength of protective factors,
- the frequency, duration, and severity of the neglect, and
- the relationship between the child and caregiver.

The negative impacts of neglect are often associated with the various outcomes children experience in the child welfare system. For example, some of the developmental and health problems linked to neglect are related to higher rates of placement in out-of-home care, a greater number of out-of-home placements, longer out-of-home placements, and a decreased likelihood of children residing with their parents when discharged from foster care.

Research shows that the first few years of children's lives are crucial and sensitive periods for development. During these years, neural synapses are formed at a very high rate. After the age of three, synapses start to be "pruned," and certain pathways that are not used may be discarded. Studies supporting the idea of a sensitive developmental period show that maltreated infants suffer from greater developmental disabilities than those children who were maltreated later in childhood. One example of this is the ability to form attachments with one's primary caregiver. If this process is disrupted early in children's lives, they may have difficulty forming healthy relationships throughout their lives. Although learning can happen throughout life, it often is more difficult for children who were deprived of certain types of early stimulation.

Programs, such as Early Head Start and other infancy and early childhood programs, acknowledge that the first few years of life are extremely significant for development. Child welfare laws and interventions, however, often do not provide or authorize the resources necessary to protect children from neglect during these critical years. Unless children show clear physical signs of neglect, intervention often is unlikely to be mandated. Thus, for many cases of emotional neglect, and especially for young children who cannot tell others about the neglect, interventions may occur too late or not at all. If interventions finally occur, the children may be past critical developmental points and could suffer from deficiencies throughout their lives. Therefore, it is important that professionals working with young children be able to recognize the possible signs of neglect in order to intervene and to keep children from suffering further harm.

## Health and Physical Development

Studies show that neglected children can be at risk for many physical problems, including failure to thrive, severe diaper rash and other skin infections, recurrent and persistent minor infections, malnourishment, and impaired brain development. Because neglect includes medical neglect, other health problems can arise from the failure of the parents to obtain necessary medical care for their children. If children do not receive the proper immunizations, prescribed medications, necessary surgeries, or other interventions, there can be serious consequences, such as impaired brain development or poor physical health. The impact of a delay in or lack of treatment might be noticeable immediately or may not be apparent for several weeks, months, or even years. For example, a child who does not receive proper dental care might be all right in the short term, but suffer from tooth decay and gum disease later in life. Children with diabetes may be fine without treatment for a short while, but an extended delay in treatment could have serious consequences and possibly result in death.

### *Impaired Brain Development*

In some cases, child neglect has been associated with a failure of the brain to form properly, which can lead to impaired physical, mental, and emotional development. The brain of a child who has been maltreated may develop in such a way that it is adaptive for the child's negative environment, but is maladaptive for functional or positive environments. A maltreated child's brain may adapt for day-to-day survival, but may not allow the child to develop fully healthy cognitive and social skills. In one study, neglected children had the highest proportion of later diagnoses of mental retardation, which may be due to not getting the necessary care and stimulation for proper brain development. Children who are neglected early in life may remain in a state of "hyper-arousal" in which they are constantly anticipating threats, or they may experience dissociation with a decreased ability to benefit from social, emotional, and cognitive experiences. To be able to learn, a child's brain needs to be in a state of "attentive calm," which is rare for maltreated children. If a child is unable to learn new information, this may cause some areas of the brain to remain inactive, possibly resulting in delayed or stunted brain growth. It also can impair functioning later in life and may lead to the child being anxious, acting overly aggressive, or being withdrawn.

61

Children who have experienced global neglect, defined as neglect in more than one category, may have significantly smaller brains than the norm. This could be indicative of fewer neuronal pathways available for learning and may lead the children to be at an intellectual disadvantage for their entire lives.

## *Poor Physical Health*

The physical problems associated with neglect may start even before an infant is born, such as when the mother has had little or no prenatal care or smoked during pregnancy. These children may be born prematurely and have complications at birth. Neglected children also can have severe physical injuries, possibly due to the inattention of their parents, such as central nervous system and craniofacial injuries, fractures, and severe burns. They also may be dirty and unhygienic, leading to even more health problems, such as lice or infections. Children also may be exposed to toxins that could cause anemia, cancer, heart disease, poor immune functioning, and asthma. For example, exposure to indoor and outdoor air pollutants, such as ozone, particulate matter, and sulfur dioxide, can cause the development of asthma or increase the frequency or severity of asthma attacks. Additionally, children may have health problems due to a lack of medical attention for injury or illness, including chronic health problems. Neglected children may suffer from dehydration or diarrhea that can lead to more severe problems if unattended.

A medical condition associated with child neglect is "failure to thrive," which can be defined as "children whose growth deviates significantly from the norms for their age and gender." This condition typically occurs in infants and toddlers under the age of two years. Failure to thrive can be manifested as significant growth delays, as well as these:

- Poor muscle tone
- Unhappy or minimal facial expressions
- Decreased vocalizations
- General unresponsiveness

Failure to thrive can be caused by organic or nonorganic factors, but some doctors may not make such a sharp distinction because physical and behavioral causes often appear together. With organic failure to thrive, the child's delayed growth can be attributed to a physical cause, usually a condition that inhibits the child's ability to

62

take in, digest, or process food. When failure to thrive is a result of the parent's neglectful behavior, it is considered nonorganic.

Treatment for failure to thrive depends on the cause of the delayed growth and development, as well as the child's age, overall health, and medical history. For example, delayed growth due to nutritional factors can be addressed by educating the parents on an appropriate and well-balanced diet for the child. Additionally, parental attitudes and behavior may contribute to a child's problems and need to be examined. In many cases, the child may need to be hospitalized initially to focus on implementation of a comprehensive medical, behavioral, and psychosocial treatment plan. Even with treatment, failure to thrive may have significant long-term consequences for children, such as growth retardation, diminished cognitive ability, mental retardation, social and emotional deficits, and poor impulse control.

### Impact on the Brain of Prenatal Exposure to Alcohol and Drugs

Exposure to alcohol and drugs in utero may cause impaired brain development for the fetus. Studies have shown that prenatal exposure to drugs may alter the development of the cortex, reduce the number of neurons that are created, and alter the way chemical messengers function. This may lead to difficulties with attention, memory, problem solving, and abstract thinking. However, findings are mixed and may depend on what drug is abused. Alcohol abuse has been found to have some of the most detrimental effects on infants, including mental retardation and neurological deficits. One problem with determining the impact of substance abuse on a fetus is isolating whether the negative outcomes are directly associated with the alcohol or drug exposure or with other factors, such as poor prenatal care or nutrition, premature birth, or adverse environmental conditions after birth.

### Impact of Malnutrition on Children

Malnutrition, especially early in a child's life, has been shown to lead to stunted brain growth and to slower passage of electrical signals in the brain. Malnutrition also can result in cognitive, social, and behavioral deficits. Iron deficiency, the most common form of malnutrition in the United States, can lead to the following problems:

- Cognitive and motor delays
- Anxiety

- Depression

- Social problems

- Problems with attention

## Intellectual and Cognitive Development

Research shows that neglected children are more likely to have cognitive deficits and severe academic and developmental delays when compared with non-neglected children. When neglected children enter school, they may suffer from both intellectual and social disadvantages that cause them to become frustrated and fall behind. One study found that individuals at 28 years of age who suffered from childhood neglect scored lower on intelligence quotient (IQ) and reading ability tests, when controlling for age, sex, race, and social class, than people who were not neglected as children. Other studies have found that, although both abused and neglected children exhibited language delays or disorders, the problems were more severe for neglected children. Furthermore, neglected children have the greatest delays in expressive and receptive language when compared with abused and non-maltreated children. When compared to physically abused children, neglected children have academic difficulties that are more serious and show signs of greater cognitive and social and emotional delays at a younger age. These academic difficulties may lead to more referrals for special education services.

There are also language problems associated with neglect. In order for babies to learn language, they need to hear numerous repetitions of sounds before they can begin making sounds and eventually saying words and sentences. Language development may be delayed if the parent or other caregiver does not provide the necessary verbal interaction with the child.

### Impact of Neglect on Academic Performance

Neglect can negatively affect a child's academic performance. Studies have found the following results:

- Children placed in out-of-home care because of abuse or neglect have below-average levels of cognitive capacity, language development, and academic achievement.

- Neglected children demonstrated a notable decline in academic performance upon entering junior high school.

- Children who were physically neglected were found to have significantly lower IQ scores at 24 and 36 months and the lowest scores on standardized tests of intellectual functioning and academic achievement in kindergarten when compared with children who had experienced either no maltreatment or other forms of maltreatment.

- Neglected children, when compared with non-maltreated children, scored lower on measures of overall school performance and tests of language, reading, and math skills.

- Neglected boys, but not girls, were found to have lower full-scale IQ scores than physically abused and non-maltreated children.

## Emotional, Psychosocial, and Behavioral Development

Neglect can have a strong impact on, and lead to problems in, a child's emotional, psychosocial, and behavioral development. As with other effects already mentioned, these may be evident immediately after the maltreatment or not manifest themselves until many months or years later.

### Emotional and Psychosocial Consequences

All types of neglect, and emotional neglect in particular, can have serious psychosocial and emotional consequences for children. Some of the short-term emotional impacts of neglect, such as fear, isolation, and an inability to trust, can lead to lifelong emotional and psychological problems, such as low self-esteem.

A major component of emotional and psychosocial development is attachment. Children who have experienced neglect have been found to demonstrate higher frequencies of insecure, anxious, and avoidant attachments with their primary caregivers than non-maltreated children. In fact, studies have demonstrated that 70 to 100 percent of maltreated infants form insecure attachments with their caregivers. Often, emotionally neglected children have learned from their relationships with their primary caregivers that they will not be able to have their needs met by others. This may cause a child not to try to solicit warmth or help from others. This behavior may in turn cause teachers or peers not to offer help or support, thus reinforcing the negative expectations of the neglected child. One mitigating factor, however, may be having an emotionally supportive adult, either within or outside of the family, such as a grandparent or a teacher, available during childhood. Another mitigating factor may be having a loving, accepting spouse or close friend later in life.

Neglected children who are unable to form secure attachments with their primary caregivers may:

- become more mistrustful of others and may be less willing to learn from adults;

- have difficulty understanding the emotions of others, regulating their own emotions, or forming and maintaining relationships with others;

- have a limited ability to feel remorse or empathy, which may mean that they could hurt others without feeling their actions were wrong;

- demonstrate a lack of confidence or social skills that could hinder them from being successful in school, work, and relationships; and

- demonstrate impaired social cognition, which is one's awareness of oneself in relation to others and an awareness of other's emotions. Impaired social cognition can lead a person to view many social interactions as stressful.

### *Neglect May Result in Emotional, Psychosocial, and Behavioral Problems*

Neglected children, even when older, may display a variety of emotional, psychosocial, and behavioral problems which may vary depending on the age of the child. Some of these include the following:

- Displaying an inability to control emotions or impulses, usually characterized by frequent outbursts

- Being quiet and submissive

- Having difficulty learning in school and getting along with siblings or classmates

- Experiencing unusual eating or sleeping behaviors

- Attempting to provoke fights or solicit sexual interactions

- Acting socially or emotionally inappropriate for their age

- Being unresponsive to affection

- Displaying apathy

- Being less flexible, persistent, and enthusiastic than non-neglected children
- Demonstrating helplessness under stress
- Having fewer interactions with peers than non-neglected children
- Displaying poor coping skills
- Acting highly dependent
- Acting lethargic and lackluster
- Displaying self-abusive behavior (for example, suicide attempts or cutting themselves)
- Exhibiting panic or dissociative disorders, attention-deficit/hyperactivity disorder, or post-traumatic stress disorder
- Suffering from depression, anxiety, or low self-esteem
- Exhibiting juvenile delinquent behavior or engaging in adult criminal activities
- Engaging in sexual activities leading to teen pregnancy or fatherhood
- Having low academic achievement
- Abusing alcohol or drugs

### Societal Consequences

Society pays for many of the consequences of neglect. There are large monetary costs for maintaining child welfare systems, judicial systems, law enforcement, special education programs, and physical and mental health systems that are needed to respond to and to treat victims of child neglect and their families. Many indirect societal consequences also exist, such as increased juvenile delinquency, adult criminal activity, mental illness, substance abuse, and domestic violence. There may be a loss of productivity due to unemployment and underemployment associated with neglect. Additionally, supporting children who have developmental delays because of malnutrition often is much more costly than providing adequate nutrition and care to poor women and children.

### Behavioral Consequences

Neglected children may suffer from particular behavioral problems throughout life. Research shows that children who are exposed to poor family management practices are at a greater risk of developing conduct disorders and of participating in delinquent behavior. Neglected children also may be at risk for repeating the neglectful behavior with their own children. Research also shows that neglected children do not necessarily perceive their upbringing to be abnormal or dysfunctional and may model their own parenting behavior on the behavior of their parents. One study estimates that approximately one-third of neglected children will maltreat their own children.

# Chapter 7

# *Maltreatment of Infants*

During October 2005–September 2006 (federal fiscal year [FFY] 2006), approximately 905,000 U.S. children were victims of maltreatment that was substantiated by state and local child protective services (CPS) agencies. Substantiated maltreatment is defined as maltreatment by a parent or other caregiver deemed to have occurred after thorough investigation by a qualified staff member from a CPS agency with jurisdiction over the geographic area in which the maltreatment took place. Approximately 19% of child maltreatment fatalities occurred among infants (persons aged less than one year), and homicide statistics suggest that fatality risk might be greatest in the first week of life. However, the risk for nonfatal maltreatment among infants has not been examined previously at the national level. To determine the extent of nonfatal infant maltreatment in the United States, CDC and the federal Administration for Children and Families (ACF) analyzed data collected in fiscal year 2006 (the most recent data available) from the National Child Abuse and Neglect Data System (NCANDS). This chapter summarizes the results of that analysis, which indicated that, in fiscal year 2006, a total of 91,278 infants aged less than one year (rate: 23.2 per 1,000 population) experienced nonfatal maltreatment, including 29,881 (32.7%) who were aged less than one week. Neglect was the maltreatment category cited

Text in this chapter is from "Nonfatal Maltreatment of Infants—United States, October 2005–September 2006," *MMWR Weekly,* *57*(13);336–339, Centers for Disease Control and Prevention (CDC), April 4, 2008.

for 68.5% of infants aged less than one week, but NCANDS data did not permit further characterization of the nature of this neglect. Developing effective measures to prevent maltreatment of infants aged less than one week will require more detailed characterization of neglect in this age group.

NCANDS is a national data collection and analysis system created in response to the federal Child Abuse Prevention and Treatment Act—Public Law 93–247 as amended. Data have been collected annually from states and reported since 1993. States submit case-level data as child-specific records for each report of alleged child maltreatment for which a completed investigation or assessment by a CPS agency has been made during the reporting period. Individual CPS agencies are responsible for determining the type of maltreatment and outcome of the maltreatment investigation based on state and federal laws. However, no standardized definitions of maltreatment are used consistently by all states; therefore, each state maps its own classification of maltreatment onto NCANDS definitions before sending the final data file to NCANDS. Categories of maltreatment in NCANDS are as follows: physical abuse, neglect or deprivation of necessities, medical neglect, sexual abuse, psychological or emotional maltreatment, other, and unknown. For this report, neglect or deprivation of necessities and medical neglect were combined into one category; other and unknown maltreatments also were combined into one category. Once a state submits its data to NCANDS, a technical validation review is conducted by a staff supervised by the ACF Children's Bureau to assess the internal consistency of the data and to identify probable causes for missing data. States are requested to make corrections as needed.

In fiscal year 2006, 49 states, the District of Columbia, and Puerto Rico provided case-level data to NCANDS. For this report, data from five states (Alaska, Maryland, North Dakota, Pennsylvania, and Vermont) were not available for analysis. Only data regarding victims with a CPS agency disposition of substantiated maltreatment issued during fiscal year 2006 were analyzed. Among the approximately 3.6 million children aged less than 18 years who were subjects of maltreatment investigations in fiscal year 2006, maltreatment was substantiated by CPS agencies in approximately 905,000 (25.1%) children. Substantiated maltreatment data were analyzed for victims aged less than one year by the age of the infant victim at the time of first report, sex, race/ethnicity, type of maltreatment, and source of the report.

A total of 91,278 unique victims of substantiated maltreatment were identified in CPS agency dispositions in fiscal year 2006 among infants aged less than one year, an annual rate of 23.2 per 1,000 population.

A total of 47,117 (51.6%) victims were male. By race/ethnicity, 39,768 (43.6%) infant victims were White; 23,008 (25.2%) were Black or African American; 17,582 (19.3%) were Hispanic; 1,141 (1.3%) were American Indian or Alaska Native; and 583 (0.6%) were Asian. Multiple race/ethnicity was identified for 2,874 (3.1%) of the infant victims, and 6,322 (6.9%) were of unknown race/ethnicity.

Among the 91,278 infant victims of substantiated maltreatment, 35,455 (38.8%) were aged less than one month. Of these, 29,881 (84.3%) were aged less than one week. Among maltreated infants aged less than one week, 20,472 (68.5%) were categorized as victims of neglect (including deprivation of necessities or medical neglect), and 3,957 (13.2%) as victims of physical abuse.

Among the 29,881 infant victims aged less than one week, 25,964 (86.9%) victims were reported to CPS agencies by professionals, including 19,486 (65.2%) by medical personnel and 5,542 (18.5%) by social services personnel. Medical personnel also reported the greatest percentage 21,545 (60.8%) of victims aged less than one month. Of infant victims aged less than one year, 29,462 (32.3%) were reported by medical personnel, followed by law enforcement personnel 19,574 (21.4%), social services personnel 13,740 (15.1%), parents/other relatives 8,058 (8.8%), and friends/neighbors 2,927 (3.2%).

The findings in this report indicate that, in fiscal year 2006, 23.2 children per 1,000 population aged less than one year experienced substantiated nonfatal maltreatment in the United States. Among these infants, neglect was the maltreatment category most commonly cited, experienced by 68.5% of victims. Among infant victims aged less than one year who experienced substantiated maltreatment, 32.7% were aged less than one week, and 30.6% were aged less than four days. Neglect also was the maltreatment category most often cited among children aged less than one week.

The concentration of reports of neglect in the first few days of life and the preponderance of reports from medical professionals during the same period suggest that neglect often was identified at birth. One hypothesis for the concentration of maltreatment and neglect reports in the first few days of life is that the majority of reports resulted from maternal or newborn drug tests. Although tracking of prenatal substance exposure and hospital postnatal toxicology-screening practices vary among states and within states, positive maternal or neonatal drug test results routinely are reported to CPS agencies as child neglect. Additional research is needed to clearly define the causes of substantiated neglect and maltreatment among newborns and to determine the best strategies for intervention.

**Table 7.1.** Number and percentage of infants aged less than or equal to one week who were victims of substantiated maltreatment,* by type of maltreatment and source of report—National Child Abuse and Neglect Data system, United States, October 2005–September 2006**

| Source of report | Neglect*** | Physical abuse | Sexual abuse | Psychological or emotional maltreatment | Other maltreatment[a] | Total (%) |
|---|---|---|---|---|---|---|
| **Professionals** | | | | | | |
| Medical personnel | 13,456 | 2,845 | 12 | 39 | 3,134 | 19,486 (65.2) |
| Social services personnel | 2,796 | 854 | 8 | 18 | 1,866 | 5,542 (18.5) |
| Mental health personnel | 436 | 46 | 1 | 6 | 22 | 511 (1.7) |
| Legal, law enforcement, criminal justice personnel | 208 | 23 | 3 | 3 | 60 | 297 (0.9) |
| Education personnel/ Day care providers/ Foster care providers | 83 | 10 | | | 35 | 128 (0.4) |
| Total (%) | 16,979 (56.8) | 3,778 (12.6) | 24 (0.1) | 66 (0.2) | 5,117 (17.1) | 25,964 (86.9) |

| Community members/nonprofessionals | | | | | |
|---|---|---|---|---|---|
| Parents/other relatives | 220 | 27 | 2 | 3 | 72 | 324 (1.1) |
| Friends/neighbors | 185 | 11 | 1 | | 18 | 215 (0.7) |
| Alleged perpetrators | 2 | | | | 1 | 3 (0.0) |
| Other/unknown/anonymous reporters | 3,086 | 141 | 2 | 8 | 138 | 3,375 (11.3) |
| Total (%) | 3,493 (11.6) | 179 (0.6) | 5 (0.0) | 11 (0.0) | 229 (0.8) | 3,917 (13.1) |
| Overall total (%) | 20,472 (68.5) | 3,957 (13.2) | 29 (0.1) | 77 (0.3) | 5,346 (17.9) | 29,881 (100) |

*Defined as maltreatment by a parent or other caregiver deemed to have occurred after thorough investigation by a qualified staff member from a child protective services agency with jurisdiction over the geographic area in which the maltreatment took place. Additional information available at http://www.acf.hhs.gov/programs/cb/pubs/cm05/index.htm

**Data from five states (Alaska, Maryland, North Dakota, Pennsylvania, and Vermont) were not available for analysis.

***Includes deprivation of necessities and medical neglect.

a Includes infants who were victims of more than one type of maltreatment.

The percentage of substantiated reports categorized as physical abuse among infants aged less than one week (13.2%) is similar to the percentage among maltreated children of all ages (16%). Physical abuse is defined by CDC and NCANDS as the intentional use of physical force by a parent or caregiver against a child that results in, or has the potential to result in, physical injury. Physical abuse includes beating, kicking, biting, burning, shaking, or otherwise harming a child. Although the act is intentional, the consequence might be intentional or unintentional (for example, resulting from excessive discipline or physical punishment). One type of physical abuse, shaken baby syndrome/abusive head trauma (SBS/AHT), is a cause of severe physical injury and death in infants, occurring in 21.0–32.2 infants aged less than one year per 100,000 population. More detailed study of contextual information is needed to determine the causes of physical abuse in infants reported to NCANDS and to develop additional prevention strategies.

The findings in this report are subject to at least two other limitations, in addition to the lack of specific information about maltreatment circumstances. First, underreporting or delayed reporting might influence the findings. Both mandated reporters and the public might lack sufficient knowledge or training that supports reporting possible child maltreatment. To assist healthcare professionals in better reporting child maltreatment, CDC developed uniform definitions and recommended data elements to promote and improve consistency of child maltreatment reporting and serve as a technical reference for the collection of data. Second, data collection and reporting practices vary among states, and data from certain states were not available for analysis.

Serious injury resulting from physical abuse of infants can be decreased by efforts focusing on reduction of SBS/AHT through in-hospital programs aimed at parents of newborns. These programs have produced a substantial reduction in reported SBS/AHT in localized areas, and CDC is supporting research to evaluate the replicability of these results in diverse settings. In addition, home-visitation and parent-training programs, particularly those that 1) begin during pregnancy, 2) provide social support to parents, and 3) teach parents about developmentally appropriate infant behavior and age-appropriate disciplinary communication skills, have been determined to reduce risk for child maltreatment.

# Chapter 8

# *Maltreatment of Children with Disabilities*

According to researchers, children with a physical, sensory, intellectual, or mental health impairment are at increased risk of becoming victims of violence. While the amount of research available on this population is extremely limited, particularly for disabled children in the developing world, current research indicates that violence against disabled children occurs at annual rates at least 1.7 times greater than their non-disabled peers.[1] More targeted studies also indicate reasons for serious concern. For example, one group of researchers report that 90% of individuals with intellectual impairments will experience sexual abuse at some point in their life, and a national survey of deaf adults in Norway found 80% of all deaf individuals surveyed report sexual abuse at some point in their childhood.[2, 3]

The specific type and amount of violence against disabled children will vary depending upon whether it occurs within the family, in the community, in institutional settings, or in the work place.[4] There are however, several key issues that appear time and again when such violence occurs. Most striking is the issue of reoccurring stigma and prejudice.

Throughout history many—although not all—societies have dealt poorly with disability. Cultural, religious, and popular social beliefs

Excerpted from *Summary Report: Violence against Disabled Children*. UN Secretary Generals Report on Violence against Children, Thematic Group on Violence against Disabled Children–Findings and Recommendations, July 28, 2005. © 2005 Nora Ellen Groce, PhD. Reprinted with permission.

often assume that a child is born with a disability or becomes disabled after birth as the result of a curse, bad blood, an incestuous relationship, a sin committed in a previous incarnation, or a sin committed by that child's parents or other family members.

A child born in a community where such beliefs exist is at risk in a number of ways. A child born with a disability or a child who becomes disabled may be directly subject to physical violence, or sexual, emotional, or verbal abuse in the home, the community, institutional settings, or in the workplace. A disabled child is more likely to face violence and abuse at birth and this increased risk for violence reappears throughout the lifespan. This violence compounds already existing social, educational, and economic marginalization that limits the lives and opportunities of these children. For example, disabled children are far less likely than their non-disabled peers to be included in the social, economic, and cultural life of their communities; only a small percentage of these children will ever attend school; a third of all street children are disabled children. Disabled children living in remote and rural areas may be at increased risk.

## Settings

### *Violence in the Home and Family: Causes of Violence and Resulting Behaviors*

In societies where there is stigma against those with disability, research indicates that some parents respond with violence because of the shame the child had brought on the family, or respond with violence because a lack of social support leads to intense stress within the family. Among the violent manifestations of this are the following:

**Infanticide and mercy killings:** Disabled children may be killed either immediately at birth or at some point after birth; and sometimes years after birth. The rational for such killings is either: 1) the belief that the child is evil, or will bring misfortunate to the family or the community; or 2) the belief that the child is suffering or will suffer and is better off dead. Often called mercy killings, such murders are usually a response to societal beliefs about disability and lack of social support systems for individuals with disability and their family, not the actual physical condition of the child him or herself. In mercy killings, a parent or caretaker justifies withholding basic life sustaining supports (usually food, water, and/or medication) or actively takes the child's life through suffocation, strangulation, or some other means, with the intention of ending suffering.

76

What links such behaviors together is that the cause of death is not the child's disability, but actions taken on the part of the child's parent or caretaker. Importantly, the actions of the parent or caretaker are often not taken in isolation. The decision to end the life of a disabled child may be prompted either directly with advice and counsel of medical, social, and religious leaders, or family members. It may be prompted indirectly through lack of social, economic, and medical support networks that leave parents feeling isolated, depressed, and desperate. Cases where parents decide to end the life of a disabled child because they themselves are ill or aging and fear their child will be subjected to abuse or neglect after their own deaths are particularly heartrending. That communities often do not prosecute such forms of homicide, or let the perpetrator go with a reduced punishment, is recognition from the surrounding society of the lack of support and encouragement given to caring for and raising a disabled child. Importantly, in some societies, there are also often gender differences with disabled girl infants and girl children more likely to die through mercy killings than are boy children of the same age with comparable disabling conditions.

**Physical violence, sexual, emotional, and/or verbal abuse of the disabled child in a violent household:** While many parents are violent towards children where no disability exists, when a disabled child lives in a violent setting his or her disability often serves to compound and intensify the nature and extent of the abuse. For example, a mobility impaired child may be less able to flee when physically or sexually assaulted. A child who is deaf may be unable to communicate about the abuse he or she faces to anyone outside his or her household, unless these outsiders speak sign language or understand the home signs the child uses. (And when the abuser is the one interpreting the child's statement to someone outside the household, this further limits the child's ability to report abuse or ask for help). A child who is intellectually impaired may not be savvy enough to anticipate a parent's growing anger or know when to leave the room to avoid being struck.

**Theory of child-induced stress leading to violence:** Several theories of child abuse state that a disabled child faces increased risk as the result of child-produced stress. It is hypothesized that this cycle of increasing tensions can begin long before the child is diagnosed as having a disability. For example, a child with a hearing impairment may be regarded as disobedient; a child with vision problems may not make eye contact and appear to be unresponsive, a child with a neurological disorder may be difficult to comfort or feed. Other researchers suggest that parents who become violent towards their disabled child are reacting not to the child's condition alone, but to the social isolation and stigma they encounter from surrounding family, friends, and neighbors. Parents of disabled children often lack social supports as family and friends distance themselves; they can find no school willing to take their child, or they live in communities where there are few or no social services to help them with their child's needs. It is possible that both child-produced stressors and social isolation are compounded to produce a stressful and potentially violent situation in a household coping with a disabled child. It is also true that not all households with disabled children are violent and even within the same communities there are coping mechanisms in some families that prevent violence, while children with identical disabilities in other households are subjected to violence. As with many aspects of violence towards disabled children, at this point, much more research is needed to allow us to adequately understand the factors that inhibit or foster violence towards these children.

**Neglect as a precursor to violence:** Parents may respond to the stress of caring for a disabled child with neglect rather than active violence; however, when this neglect involves denial of food, medicine, and other life-sustaining services, it must be considered a form of violence. For example:

- **Neglect in providing basic/life-sustaining care:** The disabled child in a household may receive less food, medical care, or other services. This can be subtle, for example, parents or caretakers may wait a few additional days before spending scarce money for medicine or the child may receive less food or less nutritious food than his or her sibling. The response can also be direct: refusal to continue to feed, house, or cloth a child after he or she has been disabled.[5] Such neglect can lead to further impairments in a vicious feedback cycle in which the disabled child continually loses ground developmentally.

- **Neglect to provide disability-specific care**: Disability-specific health concerns are exacerbated through neglect. For example, bed sores go unattended resulting in a potentially deadly systemic infection, or a disabled child who needs assistance eating will become malnourished because no one takes enough time to adequately feed him or her.

- **Refusal to intervene:** Family, neighbors, health care professionals, or social service experts may be aware that a disabled child is being abused by parents or caretakers in the home, but are unwilling to intervene, rationalizing such violence by citing stress on parents or lack of alternative care arrangements. While deciding when to intervene to stop violence against children in the home is an issue in many societies, the neglect highlighted here is when a community does not stop violence against a disabled child that would be considered intolerable if perpetrated against a non-disabled child.

- **Gender specific neglect:** Such neglect may be further exacerbated by gender—for example, in a study from Nepal, the survival rate for boy children several years after they have had polio is twice that for girl children, despite the fact that polio itself affects equal numbers of males and females. Neglect, in the form of the lack of adequate medical care, less nutritious food, or lack of access to related resources is the apparent cause of these deaths.[6]

**Violence and abuse linked to social isolation:**

- **Child is shunned within the household:** Few family members talking to him or her or overseeing his or her safety.

- **The child is not allowed to leave the house or household compound:** In some cases, the child is kept home to ensure his or her own safety, as parents fear that the child may be struck by a cart or abused by someone in the neighborhood. But, in many other instances, a child is kept isolated because the family fears the reaction from other members of the community. Children in some communities are kept shackled in windowless storerooms, hot household courtyards, or dark attics for weeks, months, or years, often with little or no interaction, even by those within the household. Next door neighbors may not know of the child's existence and family members across town may be told that the child has long since died.

**Abuse by support staff within the home:** Parents and caretakers of disabled children must often call upon informal networks of family, friends, and neighbors, or formal networks of in-home nursing and attendant care to help with child care, rehabilitative, or medical support. In such instances:

- physical, sexual, verbal, and emotional abuse may take place by caregivers without the parent's knowledge or while the parent is away; or

- parents may be aware of or suspect abuse, but feel there are no alternatives to help with the care of the disabled child and thus be unwilling to admit, confront, or cancel the services they receive.

**Barriers to intervention:** Social service and child advocacy agencies may be aware that a disabled child is the victim of violence or neglect, but choose to keep that child in the household because there are few or no alternative foster care or safe, temporary residential care facilities that are disability accessible or willing to take in a disabled child The response of disabled children themselves to on-going violence within the home is dictated by a number of factors.

- They may be unaware that the abuse and neglect is unacceptable, in part because unlike the non-disabled child, they have little contact with others outside the household.

- They may be aware that this type of behavior is unacceptable, but be unable to physically contact or communicate with individuals outside the household who could help them.

- They may be aware that this type of behavior is unacceptable, but fear loss of relationship with caregiver or family member. While this is an issue for many children in violent households, for disabled children dependent on their abusers for physical care, communication with the outside world, or other disability-specific concerns, these issues are more complex.

- They may be aware that this type of behavior is unacceptable, seek to alert authorities, but are not listened to or believed.

### *Violence in Educational and Custodial Settings*

Millions of disabled children around the world spend part or all of their lives in institutional settings, be it in schools within their communities, disability-related residential schools, institutions or hospitals, or in the criminal justice system. In all cases, being disabled increases and compounds their risk for becoming victims of violence.

**Non-residential schools:** Sadly, victimization of disabled children in school can begin even before the child enters the schoolhouse door:

- **Traveling to and from school:** Because educational facilities for disabled children are rare, many children travel long distances to school. Reports of physical and sexual abuse by those responsible for transportation to and from school are common. For example, a recent study in the United States reported that 5% of all disabled students reporting sexual abuse were abused by bus drivers on their way to or from their schools.[7]

- **Physical threat of violence:** Disabled children are often bullied, teased, or subjected to physical violence (being beaten, stoned, spit upon, and so forth) by members of the community on their way to and from school.

- **Victims of crime:** Disabled children are often targeted by predators on their way to and from school. For example, perpetrators of violent crimes, including robbery and rape, often target students on their way to schools for the disabled, believing them to be more vulnerable and less likely or able to report crime or abuse. Students with sensory impairments (deafness or blindness) and students with intellectual disabilities seem to be at particular risk.

**Violence inside the classroom:**

- **Teachers:** Disabled children are often beaten, abused, or bullied by teachers, particularly untrained teachers who do not understand the limitations of some disabled children. Children with intellectual disabilities and children with hearing impairments are particularly at risk, but reports worldwide find that all disabled children are potential victims. Sexual abuse by teachers is also widely reported for both male and female students.

- **Fellow students:** Teachers that humiliate, bully, or beat children not only directly cause harm to the child, but model such behavior for other children in their classroom, who may follow the teacher's lead in physically harming, bullying, and socially isolating the targeted disabled child. Sexual abuse by fellow students is also a concern and is often linked to physical violence and bullying behaviors by such classmates.

- **School staff:** Individuals who work as teacher's aides or attendants for disabled children, or help transport, feed, or care for such children are often underpaid, overworked, and largely unsupervised. While many who undertake such career choices do so out of the best of motives, others choose these jobs because it allows easy access to the most vulnerable of children. A study from the United States, found that 11% of all those working as teachers' aides, transportation staff, or school janitorial staff in programs that served disabled children had previous criminal records, many related to child abuse or sexual abuse.[8]

- **Lack of reporting mechanism:** Few schools have mechanisms in place that allow students, parents, or caregivers to complain about violence or victimization. This is all the more serious because in many communities there are only a handful of schools or educational programs that are available for disabled children. Parents, caregivers, or children may hesitate to complain about violent or abusive behavior in the school, fearing that they will be dismissed from a program when no alternative exists. Of equal concern, few schools have systems in place to allow school staff to report abuse they have observed on the job.

**Violence in residential schools:** In a number of countries, children with specific types of disabilities, (particularly children who are deaf, blind, or intellectual impaired) are educated in residential schools, where they may live away from their families for months or years. In addition to the potential for victimization noted for disabled children in the classroom, additional concerns for violence against disabled children must be noted for residential schools:

- **Housing at residential schools:** Children who live in dormitories or are boarded out with local families are often subject to both physical violence and sexual abuse.

- **Lack of reporting mechanisms:** Reporting mechanisms for such violence is limited or non-existent for most children. Children in residential schools often have little or no regular contact with the parents—(and in some cases, such as with deaf children, may have parents who are unable to speak sign language or otherwise effectively communicate with them). Often there is also no adult caretaker or teacher in the school to whom the child can report abuse.

## References

1. American Academy of Pediatrics. 2001. Assessment of Maltreatment of Children with Disabilities. *Pediatrics*, 108:2:508–52.

2.  Valenti-Hein D., Schwartz L. 1995. *The Sexual Abuse of Those with Developmental Disabilities*. Santa Barbara, CA: James Stanfeld Co.

3.  Kvam M. 2000. Is Sexual Abuse of Children with Disabilities Disclosed?: A retrospective analysis of child disability and the likelihood of sexual abuse among those attending Norwegian hospitals. *Child Abuse and Neglect*, 24:8:1073–1084.

4.  One in Ten. 2003. *Violence and Children with Disabilities*. Vol. 24, 1: 2–19. New York: Rehabilitation International/UNICEF. http://www.rehab-international.org/publications/10_24.htm.

5.  UNICEF. 1999. *Global Survey of Adolescents with Disability: An overview of young people living with disabilities: their needs and their rights*. New York: UNICEF Inter-Divisional Working Group on Young People, Programme Division.

6.  Helander E. 1999. *Prejudice and Dignity: An introduction to community-based rehabilitation*. New York: UNDP. Second edition.

7.  Helander E. 2004. *The World of the Defenseless: A Global Overview of the health of maltreated children, effects of interventions, human rights issues and development strategies.*

8.  Sobsey D., Doe T. 1991. Patterns of Sexual Abuse and Assault. *Journal of Sexuality and Disability*. 9:3:243–259.

Chapter 9

# Long-Term Consequences of Child Abuse and Neglect

An estimated 905,000 children were victims of child abuse or neglect in 2006 (U.S. Department of Health and Human Services, 2008). While physical injuries may or may not be immediately visible, abuse and neglect can have consequences for children, families, and society that last lifetimes, if not generations.

The impact of child abuse and neglect is often discussed in terms of physical, psychological, behavioral, and societal consequences. In reality, however, it is impossible to separate them completely. Physical consequences, such as damage to a child's growing brain, can have psychological implications such as cognitive delays or emotional difficulties. Psychological problems often manifest as high-risk behaviors. Depression and anxiety, for example, may make a person more likely to smoke, abuse alcohol or illicit drugs, or overeat. High-risk behaviors, in turn, can lead to long-term physical health problems such as sexually transmitted diseases, cancer, and obesity.

This chapter provides an overview of some of the most common physical, psychological, behavioral, and societal consequences of child abuse and neglect, while acknowledging that much crossover among categories exists.

---

Text in this chapter is excerpted from "Long-Term Consequences of Child Abuse and Neglect," Child Welfare Information Gateway, updated December 31, 2008. The complete document is available online at http://www.childwelfare.gov/pubs/factsheets/long_term_consequences.cfm.

## *Factors Affecting the Consequences of Child Abuse and Neglect*

Not all abused and neglected children will experience long-term consequences. Outcomes of individual cases vary widely and are affected by a combination of factors, including the following:

- The child's age and developmental status when the abuse or neglect occurred

- The type of abuse (physical abuse, neglect, sexual abuse, and so forth)

- The frequency, duration, and severity of abuse

- The relationship between the victim and his or her abuser

Researchers also have begun to explore why, given similar conditions, some children experience long-term consequences of abuse and neglect while others emerge relatively unscathed. The ability to cope, and even thrive, following a negative experience is sometimes referred to as "resilience." A number of protective and promotive factors may contribute to an abused or neglected child's resilience. These include individual characteristics, such as optimism, self-esteem, intelligence, creativity, humor, and independence, as well as the acceptance of peers and positive individual influences such as teachers, mentors, and role models. Other factors can include the child's social environment and the family's access to social supports. Community well-being, including neighborhood stability and access to safe schools and adequate health care, are other protective and promotive factors.

## *Physical Health Consequences*

The immediate physical effects of abuse or neglect can be relatively minor (bruises or cuts) or severe (broken bones, hemorrhage, or even death). In some cases the physical effects are temporary; however, the pain and suffering they cause a child should not be discounted. Meanwhile, the long-term impact of child abuse and neglect on physical health is just beginning to be explored. According to the National Survey of Child and Adolescent Well-Being (NSCAW), more than one-quarter of children who had been in foster care for longer than 12 months had some lasting or recurring health problem. Following are some outcomes researchers have identified:

**Shaken baby syndrome:** Shaking a baby is a common form of child abuse. The injuries caused by shaking a baby may not be immediately noticeable and may include bleeding in the eye or brain, damage to the spinal cord and neck, and rib or bone fractures.

**Impaired brain development:** Child abuse and neglect have been shown, in some cases, to cause important regions of the brain to fail to form or grow properly, resulting in impaired development. These alterations in brain maturation have long-term consequences for cognitive, language, and academic abilities. NSCAW found more than three-quarters of foster children between one and two years of age to be at medium to high risk for problems with brain development, as opposed to less than half of children in a control sample.

**Poor physical health:** Several studies have shown a relationship between various forms of household dysfunction (including childhood abuse) and poor health. Adults who experienced abuse or neglect during childhood are more likely to suffer from physical ailments such as allergies, arthritis, asthma, bronchitis, high blood pressure, and ulcers.

## Psychological Consequences

The immediate emotional effects of abuse and neglect—isolation, fear, and an inability to trust—can translate into lifelong consequences, including low self-esteem, depression, and relationship difficulties. Researchers have identified links between child abuse and neglect and the following:

**Difficulties during infancy:** Depression and withdrawal symptoms were common among children as young as three years who experienced emotional, physical, or environmental neglect.

**Poor mental and emotional health:** In one long-term study, as many as 80 percent of young adults who had been abused met the diagnostic criteria for at least one psychiatric disorder at age 21. These young adults exhibited many problems, including depression, anxiety, eating disorders, and suicide attempts. Other psychological and emotional conditions associated with abuse and neglect include panic disorder, dissociative disorders, attention-deficit/hyperactivity disorder, depression, anger, posttraumatic stress disorder, and reactive attachment disorder.

**Cognitive difficulties:** NSCAW found that children placed in out-of-home care due to abuse or neglect tended to score lower than the general population on measures of cognitive capacity, language development, and academic achievement. A 1999 LONGSCAN study also found a relationship between substantiated child maltreatment and poor academic performance and classroom functioning for school-age children.

**Social difficulties:** Children who experience rejection or neglect are more likely to develop antisocial traits as they grow up. Parental neglect is also associated with borderline personality disorders and violent behavior.

## Behavioral Consequences

Not all victims of child abuse and neglect will experience behavioral consequences. However, behavioral problems appear to be more likely among this group, even at a young age. An NSCAW survey of children ages 3–5 years in foster care found these children displayed clinical or borderline levels of behavioral problems at a rate of more than twice that of the general population. Later in life, child abuse and neglect appear to make the following more likely:

**Difficulties during adolescence:** Studies have found abused and neglected children to be at least 25 percent more likely to experience problems such as delinquency, teen pregnancy, low academic achievement, drug use, and mental health problems. Other studies suggest that abused or neglected children are more likely to engage in sexual risk-taking as they reach adolescence, thereby increasing their chances of contracting a sexually transmitted disease.

**Juvenile delinquency and adult criminality:** According to a National Institute of Justice study, abused and neglected children were 11 times more likely to be arrested for criminal behavior as a juvenile, 2.7 times more likely to be arrested for violent and criminal behavior as an adult, and 3.1 times more likely to be arrested for one of many forms of violent crime (juvenile or adult).

**Alcohol and other drug abuse:** Research consistently reflects an increased likelihood that abused and neglected children will smoke cigarettes, abuse alcohol, or take illicit drugs during their lifetime. According to a report from the National Institute on Drug Abuse, as many as two-thirds of people in drug treatment programs reported being abused as children.

**Abusive behavior:** Abusive parents often have experienced abuse during their own childhoods. It is estimated approximately one-third of abused and neglected children will eventually victimize their own children.

## Societal Consequences

While child abuse and neglect almost always occur within the family, the impact does not end there. Society as a whole pays a price for child abuse and neglect, in terms of both direct and indirect costs.

**Direct costs:** Direct costs include those associated with maintaining a child welfare system to investigate and respond to allegations of child abuse and neglect, as well as expenditures by the judicial, law enforcement, health, and mental health systems. A 2001 report by Prevent Child Abuse America estimates these costs at $24 billion per year.

**Indirect costs:** Indirect costs represent the long-term economic consequences of child abuse and neglect. These include costs associated with juvenile and adult criminal activity, mental illness, substance abuse, and domestic violence. They can also include loss of productivity due to unemployment and underemployment, the cost of special education services, and increased use of the health care system. Prevent Child Abuse America estimated these costs at more than $69 billion per year.

## Summary

Much research has been done about the possible consequences of child abuse and neglect. The effects vary depending on the circumstances of the abuse or neglect, personal characteristics of the child, and the child's environment. Consequences may be mild or severe; disappear after a short period or last a lifetime; and affect the child physically, psychologically, behaviorally, or in some combination of all three ways. Ultimately, due to related costs to public entities such as the health care, human services, and educational systems, abuse and neglect impact not just the child and family, but society as a whole.

Chapter 10

# Effects of Childhood Stress on Health across the Lifespan

Stress is an inevitable part of life. Human beings experience stress early, even before they are born. A certain amount of stress is normal and necessary for survival. Stress helps children develop the skills they need to cope with and adapt to new and potentially threatening situations throughout life. Support from parents and/or other concerned caregivers is necessary for children to learn how to respond to stress in a physically and emotionally healthy manner.

The beneficial aspects of stress diminish when it is severe enough to overwhelm a child's ability to cope effectively. Intensive and prolonged stress can lead to a variety of short- and long-term negative health effects. It can disrupt early brain development and compromise functioning of the nervous and immune systems. In addition, childhood stress can lead to health problems later in life including alcoholism, depression, eating disorders, heart disease, cancer, and other chronic diseases.

The purpose of this chapter is to summarize the research on childhood stress and its implications for adult health and well-being. Of particular interest is the stress caused by child abuse, neglect, and repeated exposure to intimate partner violence (IPV).

---

Text in this chapter is excerpted from "The Effects of Childhood Stress on Health Across the Lifespan," by Jennifer S. Middlebrooks and Natalie C. Audage, Centers for Disease Control and Prevention (CDC), 2008. The complete report is available online at http://www.cdc.gov/ncipc/pub-res/pdf/Childhood _Stress.pdf.

## Types of Stress

Following are descriptions of the three types of stress that the National Scientific Council on the Developing Child has identified based on available research:

**Positive stress** results from adverse experiences that are short-lived. Children may encounter positive stress when they attend a new daycare, get a shot, meet new people, or have a toy taken away from them. This type of stress causes minor physiological changes including an increase in heart rate and changes in hormone levels. With the support of caring adults, children can learn how to manage and overcome positive stress. This type of stress is considered normal and coping with it is an important part of the development process.

**Tolerable stress** refers to adverse experiences that are more intense but still relatively short-lived. Examples include the death of a loved one, a natural disaster, a frightening accident, and family disruptions such as separation or divorce. If a child has the support of a caring adult, tolerable stress can usually be overcome. In many cases, tolerable stress can become positive stress and benefit the child developmentally. However, if the child lacks adequate support, tolerable stress can become toxic and lead to long-term negative health effects.

**Toxic stress** results from intense adverse experiences that may be sustained over a long period of time—weeks, months, or even years. An example of toxic stress is child maltreatment, which includes abuse and neglect. Children are unable to effectively manage this type of stress by themselves. As a result, the stress response system gets activated for a prolonged amount of time. This can lead to permanent changes in the development of the brain. The negative effects of toxic stress can be lessened with the support of caring adults. Appropriate support and intervention can help in returning the stress response system back to its normal baseline.

## The Effects of Toxic Stress on Brain Development in Early Childhood

The ability to manage stress is controlled by brain circuits and hormone systems that are activated early in life. When a child feels threatened, hormones are released and they circulate throughout the body. Prolonged exposure to stress hormones can impact the brain and impair functioning in a variety of ways.

- Toxic stress can impair the connection of brain circuits and, in the extreme, result in the development of a smaller brain.

- Brain circuits are especially vulnerable as they are developing during early childhood. Toxic stress can disrupt the development of these circuits. This can cause an individual to develop a low threshold for stress, thereby becoming overly reactive to adverse experiences throughout life.

- High levels of stress hormones, including cortisol, can suppress the body's immune response. This can leave an individual vulnerable to a variety of infections and chronic health problems.

- Sustained high levels of cortisol can damage the hippocampus, an area of the brain responsible for learning and memory. These cognitive deficits can continue into adulthood.

## The Effects of Toxic Stress on Adult Health and Well-Being

Research findings demonstrate that childhood stress can impact adult health. The Adverse Childhood Experiences (ACE) Study is particularly noteworthy because it demonstrates a link between specific violence-related stressors, including child abuse, neglect, and repeated exposure to intimate partner violence and risky behaviors and health problems in adulthood.

### The ACE Study

The ACE Study, a collaboration between the Centers for Disease Control and Prevention (CDC) and Kaiser Permanente's Health Appraisal Clinic in San Diego, uses a retrospective approach to examine the link between childhood stressors and adult health. Over 17,000 adults participated in the research, making it one of the largest studies of its kind. Each participant completed a questionnaire that asked for detailed information on their past history of abuse, neglect, and family dysfunction as well as their current behaviors and health status. Researchers were particularly interested in participants' exposure to the following ten adverse childhood experiences:

- Abuse
  - Emotional
  - Physical
  - Sexual
- Neglect
  - Emotional
  - Physical
- Household Dysfunction
  - Mother treated violently
  - Household substance abuse
  - Household mental illness
  - Parental separation or divorce
  - Incarcerated household member

### General ACE Study Findings

The ACE Study findings have been published in more than 30 scientific articles. The following are some of the general findings of the study: Childhood abuse, neglect, and exposure to other adverse experiences are common (Table 10.1). Almost two-thirds of study participants reported at least one ACE, and more than one in five reported three or more (Table 10.2).

The ACE score is the total number of adverse childhood experiences that each study participant reported. It is used to assess negative experiences during childhood. For example, experiencing physical neglect would be an ACE score of one. Experiencing physical neglect and witnessing a parent being treated violently would be an ACE score of two.

The short- and long-term outcomes of ACE include a multitude of health and behavioral problems. As the number of ACE a person experiences increases, the risk for the following health outcomes also increases:

- Alcoholism and alcohol abuse
- Chronic obstructive pulmonary disease
- Depression
- Fetal death
- Illicit drug use

- Ischemic heart disease
- Liver disease
- Risk for intimate partner violence
- Multiple sexual partners
- Sexually transmitted diseases
- Smoking
- Suicide attempts
- Unintended pregnancies

ACE are also related to risky health behaviors in childhood and adolescence, including pregnancies, suicide attempts, early initiation of smoking, sexual activity, and illicit drug use.

As the number of ACE increases, the number of co-occurring health conditions increases.

**Table 10.1.** Prevalence of Individual Adverse Childhood Experiences

| ACE Category | Women (N=9,367) | Men (N=7,970) | Total (N=17,337) |
|---|---|---|---|
| Abuse | | | |
| Emotional abuse | 13.1% | 7.6% | 10.6% |
| Physical abuse | 27.0% | 29.9% | 28.3% |
| Sexual abuse | 24.7% | 16.0% | 20.7% |
| Neglect | | | |
| Emotional neglect* | 16.7% | 12.4% | 14.8% |
| Physical neglect* | 9.2% | 10.7% | 9.9% |
| Household Dysfunction | | | |
| Mother treated violently | 13.7% | 11.5% | 12.7% |
| Household substance abuse | 29.5% | 23.8% | 26.9% |
| Household mental illness | 23.3% | 14.8% | 19.4% |
| Parental separation or divorce | 24.5% | 21.8% | 23.3% |
| Incarcerated household member | 5.2% | 4.1% | 4.7% |

*Collected during the second survey wave only (N=8,667).

**Table 10.2.** ACE Score

| Number of Adverse Childhood Experiences (ACE Score) | Women | Men | Total |
|---|---|---|---|
| 0 | 34.5% | 38.0% | 36.1% |
| 1 | 24.5% | 27.9% | 26.0% |
| 2 | 15.5% | 16.4% | 15.9% |
| 3 | 10.3% | 8.6% | 9.5% |
| 4 or more | 15.2% | 9.2% | 12.5% |

## *Violence-Related ACE Study Findings*

Findings from the ACE Study confirm what we already know—that too many people in the United States are exposed early on to violence and other childhood stressors. The study also provides strong evidence that being exposed to certain childhood experiences, including being subjected to abuse or neglect or witnessing intimate partner violence (IPV), can lead to a wide array of negative behaviors and poor health outcomes. In addition, the ACE Study has found associations between experiencing ACE and two violent outcomes: suicide attempts and the risk of perpetrating or experiencing IPV.

## *Child Maltreatment and Its Impact on Health and Behavior*

- Twenty-five percent of women and 16% of men reported experiencing child sexual abuse.

- Participants who were sexually abused as children were more likely to experience multiple other ACE.

- The ACE score increased as the child sexual abuse severity, duration, and frequency increased and the age at first occurrence decreased.

- Women and men who experienced child sexual abuse were more than twice as likely to report suicide attempts.

- A strong relationship was found between frequent physical abuse, sexual abuse, and witnessing of IPV as a child and a male's risk of involvement with a teenage pregnancy.

- Women who reported experiencing four or more types of abuse during their childhood were 1.5 times more likely to have an unintended pregnancy at or before the age of twenty.

- Men and women who reported being sexually abused were more at risk of marrying an alcoholic and having current marital problems.

### Witnessing Intimate Partner Violence (IPV) as a Child and Its Impact on Health and Behavior

- Study participants who witnessed IPV were two to six times more likely to experience another ACE.

- As the frequency of witnessing IPV increased, the chance of reported alcoholism, illicit drug use, injected drug use, and depression also increased.

- Exposure to physical abuse, sexual abuse, and IPV in childhood resulted in women being 3.5 times more likely to report IPV victimization.

- Exposure to physical abuse, sexual abuse, and IPV in childhood resulted in men being 3.8 times more likely to report IPV perpetration.

### The Link between ACE and Suicide Attempts

- Of study participants, 3.8% reported having attempted suicide at least once.

- Experiencing one ACE increased the risk of attempted suicide two to five times.

- As the ACE score increased so did the likelihood of attempting suicide.

- The relationship between ACE and the risk of attempted suicide appears to be influenced by alcoholism, depression, and illicit drug use.

### ACE and Associated Health Behaviors

Associations were found between ACE and many negative health behaviors. A partial list of behaviors follows:

- Participants with higher ACE scores were at greater risk of alcoholism.

- Those with higher ACE scores were more likely to marry an alcoholic.

- Study participants with higher ACE scores were more likely to initiate drug use and experience addiction.

- Those with higher ACE scores were more likely to have 30 or more sexual partners, engage in sexual intercourse earlier, and feel more at risk of contracting acquired immune deficiency syndrome (AIDS).

- Higher ACE scores in participants were linked to a higher probability of both lifetime and recent depressive disorders.

Chapter 11

# Parental Substance Abuse as Child Maltreatment

## Chapter Contents

## Section 11.1

# *The Relationship between Substance Abuse and Child Maltreatment*

Text in this section is excerpted from "Child Welfare and Substance Abuse: Current Issues and In-Depth TA," National Center on Substance Abuse and Child Welfare (NCSACW), www.ncsacw.samhsa.gov, June 16, 2005; and from, "Methamphetamine Addiction, Treatment, and Outcomes: Implications for Child Welfare Workers (Draft)," NCSACW, April 2006.

## *Children with Prenatal Substance Exposure*

### *Number of Children Prenatally Exposed to Substances*

- Approximately 410,000 infants have prenatal substance exposure.

- There are approximately 86,000 total child victims under one year old.

- Approximately 41,000 children under one year old enter out-of-home care.

Where did they all go? Most go home from the hospital. More than 80% are undetected and go home without assessment and needed services.

- Many doctors and hospitals do not test, or may have inconsistent implementation of state policies.

- Tests detect only very recent substance use.

- Inconsistent follow-up for woman identified as substance using or at-risk, but with no positive test at birth.

## *Children of Substance Abusers Who Are Also Victims of Child Abuse and/or Neglect*

### *Documenting Substance Use Disorders in Child Welfare*

Parental substance use disorders were a factor in 16% to 48% of children and family service reviews. Child welfare workers (CWW) misclassify caregivers who are substance dependent most of the time, for example:

- 71% of caregivers who are alcohol dependent are classified by the CWW as not having an alcohol problem; and,

- 73% of caregivers who are drug dependent are classified by the CWW as not having a drug problem.

**Table 11.1.** Children Living with One or More Substance Abusing Parent

| Substance use by parent | Number of affected children (in millions) |
|---|---|
| Used illicit drug in past year | 10.6 |
| Used illicit drug in past month | 8.4 |
| Depending on alcohol and/or needs treatment for illicit drugs | 8.3 |
| Abused or dependent on alcohol or illicit drug in past month | 6.0 |
| Dependent on alcohol and other drugs (AOD) | 7.5 |
| Dependent on alcohol | 6.2 |
| Dependent on illicit drugs | 2.8 |
| Need treatment for illicit drug abuse | 4.5 |

## Parents Who Use or Abuse Methamphetamine

In 2004, an estimated 418,000 (0.2 percent aged 18 or older) had used methamphetamine in the past month. Given the number of adults who currently use methamphetamine, episodic parental use or abuse of methamphetamine is the most common means by which children are affected by parental methamphetamine use. This method of exposure accounts for the highest number of children exposed to methamphetamine, compared to the numbers found in the other categories.

Parents under the influence of stimulants, including methamphetamine, pose a danger their children. When high, the parent may exhibit poor judgment, confusion, irritability, paranoia, and increased violence; they may fail to provide adequate supervision. The family and social environment may be poor, and the children may be at risk of abuse and neglect due to the family dynamics associated with substance use.

In households where a family member smokes the substance, children may be exposed to secondhand methamphetamine smoke. They may accidentally ingest the substance if it is kept in the home. Because methamphetamine users typically use other substances at the same time, including alcohol, tobacco, and other drugs, the risks to their children accumulate, and it becomes difficult to attribute a particular effect to a particular substance.

## Parents with Methamphetamine Dependence

When the parent is dependent on methamphetamine, chronic neglect of the children becomes more likely, and the family and social environment is more likely to be inadequate. The children are exposed to the drug-affected parent more frequently and for longer periods of time. They may be found living in poor conditions, lacking food, water, gas, and electricity. They may lack medical care, dental care, and immunizations. These children are also at greater risk of abuse.

## Prenatal Exposure

Pregnant methamphetamine users appear to know less about the potential harm to themselves or the fetus, compared to users of crack cocaine or heroin. Crack cocaine users were more likely than the other two groups to fear the negative effects of their drug use on their fetus. Heroin-using women were concerned about the effects of their drug use, but primarily concerned with avoiding potential parental custody problems. Women in all three groups tended to avoid prenatal care clinics.

Since the crack epidemic of the late 1980s, researchers have been aware that prenatal stimulant exposure has both direct and indirect effects. The fetus is directly affected by the cocaine that enters its system, and it is indirectly affected by the decrease in the mother's blood flow that results from cocaine use. Many of the effects of prenatal exposure to methamphetamine have also been documented among infants exposed to other substances, particularly cocaine/crack. Many studies of the effects of prenatal exposure however compare methamphetamine-exposed infants to non-exposed infants without also comparing them to cocaine-exposed or other stimulant-exposed infants, so it is not known whether the effects are associated with methamphetamine in particular or with all stimulants.

Stimulant-exposed children may also be affected by other substances used by the mother, and by environmental risk factors such as the mother's nutritional and health status. Recent surveys indicate that 12–14% of all pregnant women consume alcohol and two-thirds of female smokers continue to smoke during pregnancy. Among meth using pregnant women, nicotine use is nearly universal while marijuana and alcohol were secondary drugs used by 60% of the women. The cumulative effects of the use of multiple substances and other environmental risk factors have significant adverse effects on the newborn. These effects may be greater than the effects of stimulant use alone. Prenatal substance exposure can cause birth defects, fetal death, growth retardation, premature birth, low birthweight, developmental disorders, difficulty sucking and swallowing, and hypersensitivity to touch after birth.

Methamphetamine exposure during pregnancy can jeopardize the development of the fetal brain and other organs. An echoencephalographic study of neonates who were exposed prenatally to methamphetamine or cocaine indicated higher rates of bleeding, decay, and lesions in the brain. A high dose of methamphetamine taken during pregnancy can cause a rapid rise in temperature and blood pressure in the brain of the fetus, which can lead to stroke or brain hemorrhage. Infants prenatally exposed to methamphetamine are significantly smaller for their gestational age compared with unexposed infants, and methamphetamine-exposed infants whose mothers also smoked tobacco had significantly decreased growth, compared with infants exposed to methamphetamine alone.

Earlier studies of infants prenatally exposed to cocaine, methamphetamine, or both revealed no significant differences in perinatal variables among the three drug-exposed groups. All three groups had altered neonatal behavioral patterns, characterized by abnormal sleep patterns, poor feeding, tremors, and hypertonia (excessive muscle tension). All three groups also had significantly higher rates of prematurity and intrauterine growth retardation, and had smaller head circumferences, compared to the drug-free comparison group. Infants exposed prenatally to methamphetamine are more likely than other prenatally exposed infants to experience feeding problems due to difficulty in sucking and swallowing. Shah found that 34.4% of methamphetamine exposed infants had feeding problems compared to 9.4% of infants prenatally exposed to cocaine. These difficulties suggest that infants prenatally exposed to methamphetamine may be at risk for failure to thrive issues.

Longer-term effects of prenatal methamphetamine exposure may be similar to other substances: long-term cognitive deficits, learning disabilities, and poor social adjustment in older children. Over-stimulation and self-regulation difficulties have been observed with cocaine-exposed children, and these effects may be seen in children exposed to other stimulants. A study showed alterations of brain chemistry in children that may be related to findings that some cocaine-exposed children are more impulsive and easily distracted than their non-exposed peers. Additional research is needed to determine if the same effects are found in methamphetamine-exposed children. Shah describes the symptoms of prenatal exposure to methamphetamine in children 18 months–5 years include less focused attention, easily distracted, poor anger management, and aggressive outbursts.

### Home Labs

Some parents produce relatively small quantities of methamphetamine in their homes for their own use or small-scale distribution. Children in these homes are subject to the same risks noted in the sections on parents who use, abuse and are dependent on the drug, but they have additional risks associated with the substances used in the production of methamphetamine and the method of production. The children may be exposed to toxic chemicals, contaminated food, fumes released during the cooking process, and the danger of fire or explosion from the manufacturing process.

The risk of toxic exposure for children in homes where methamphetamine is manufactured is high. Children are more likely than adults to suffer health effects from exposure to chemicals. They have higher metabolic rates; their skeletal systems and nervous systems are developing; their skin is not as thick as an adult's skin which means they absorb chemicals faster; and children tend to put things in their mouths and use touch to explore the world. Some fumes or gases are heavier than air, and will sink down to the child's level, increasing their exposure. Children also tend to imitate adult behavior and are vulnerable in chaotic and unsafe environments. A review by Kolecki revealed that pediatric patients with methamphetamine poisoning often exhibited rapid heartbeat, agitation, inconsolable crying, irritability, and vomiting.

### Trafficking

Parents who traffic in methamphetamine by selling, transporting, or distributing it, expose their children to an increased risk of violence and abuse associated with drug trafficking. There may be weapons in the home. The parent's associates or customers may carry weapons, putting the children at risk for violence. These children are also at increased risk of physical and sexual abuse by those who visit the home.

### Superlabs

Superlabs are methamphetamine laboratories where methamphetamine is produced on a large scale. Children are sometimes found in these superlabs, but they are less likely to be present in superlabs than in the homes where smaller quantities are produced. From 2000 to 2003, there were 7,513 known cases of children present at seized methamphetamine laboratory sites nationwide, with only 2,881 taken into protective custody.

Children in methamphetamine labs are exposed to great risk. They are exposed to the chemicals used in the production of methamphetamine. They may be at increased risk for severe neglect, and may be physically or sexually abused by family members or others who frequent the lab. They are exposed to the toxic effects of methamphetamine manufacturing such as fire explosions, toxic gas, and toxic waste. A child can also be harmed by consuming a chemical from a container or ingesting methamphetamine.

Child welfare workers should be aware of the symptoms of methamphetamine exposure so that they can identify children affected by methamphetamine labs or their own exposure to toxic chemicals. Because of the creation of toxic waste at methamphetamine labs, many first response personnel incur injury when dealing with the hazardous substances. Medical evaluation and treatment may be indicated if symptoms of illness develop following contact with methamphetamine lab chemicals or residual toxins. Symptoms include the following:

- Chronic cough
- Chest pain or tightness
- Shortness of breath
- Dizziness
- Headache
- Skin and eye irritation
- Chemical burns
- Nausea
- Lethargy

In addition to the toxic effects, there are other signs that could signal the presence of a methamphetamine lab. These include the following:

- Unusual, strong odors (like cat urine, ether, ammonia, acetone, or other chemicals) coming from sheds, outbuildings or other structures, orchards, campsites, or vehicles

- Possession of unusual materials, such as large amounts of over-the-counter allergy/cold/diet medications (including ephedrine or pseudoephedrine), or large quantities of solvents (such as acetone, Coleman fuel, or toluene)

- Discarded items such as ephedrine bottles, coffee filters with oddly-colored stains, lithium batteries, antifreeze containers, lantern fuel cans, and propane tanks

- The mixing of unusual chemicals in house, garage, or barn, or the possession of chemical glassware by persons not involved in the chemical industry

- Heavy traffic during late hours

- Residences with operating fans in windows in cold weather or blacked out windows

- Renters who pay their landlords in cash

The considerations are complicated for child welfare workers dealing with a case where a methamphetamine lab is involved. Family reunification considerations must address the issues of child safety and well-being based on the child's potential exposure to toxic substances. Reunifying families where the home environment is literally toxic is problematic. Child welfare workers must also consider the possibility of methamphetamine use among potential relative caregivers.

Methamphetamine-using parents may have needs beyond treatment for addiction, such as needs for mental health services, medical services, housing, and employment. Their children may have needs beyond safety from immediate harm. The most effective approach to the problem of methamphetamine-using parents and their at-risk children is a comprehensive, integrated services strategy, where treatment includes a range of services that support the parent in leaving addiction behind and stepping into the role of a positive, successful parent.

# Section 11.2

# *Alcohol and Pregnancy: Legal Significance for Child Abuse and Neglect*

Text in this section is from "Alcohol and Pregnancy:
Legal Significance for Child Abuse/Child Neglect," National Institute
on Alcohol Abuse and Alcoholism (NIAAA), September 18, 2008.

## *Legal Ramifications of Alcohol Use during Pregnancy*

Scientific research has established that alcohol consumption during pregnancy is associated with adverse health consequences. Fetal alcohol spectrum disorder (FASD) is the term used to describe the range of birth defects caused by maternal alcohol consumption during pregnancy. FASD is considered the most common nonhereditary cause of mental retardation. Included in FASD is the diagnosis often referred to as fetal alcohol syndrome (FAS), which is the most severe form of FASD. It is characterized by facial defects, growth deficiencies, and central nervous system dysfunction. Also included in FASD are other types of alcohol-induced mental impairments that are just as serious, if not more so, than in children with FAS. The term alcohol-related neurodevelopmental disorder (ARND) has been developed to describe such impairments. Prenatally exposed children can also have other alcohol-related physical abnormalities of the skeleton and certain organ systems; these are known as alcohol-related birth defects (ARBD).

The legal significance of a woman's conduct prior to birth of a child and of damage caused *in utero* varies considerably across jurisdictions. Some states have adopted statutes and/or regulations that clarify the rules for evidence of prenatal alcohol exposure in child welfare proceedings (for example, those alleging child abuse, child neglect, child deprivation, or child dependence, or concerning termination of parental rights).

## *States That Address Alcohol Use during Pregnancy as Potential Child Abuse or Neglect*

The following states have legal provision pertaining to the use of alcohol during pregnancy being considered as possible child abuse or neglect.

- Alabama
- Arizona
- Colorado
- Florida
- Illinois
- Indiana
- Louisiana
- Maine
- Maryland
- Massachusetts
- Nevada
- North Dakota
- Oklahoma
- South Carolina
- South Dakota
- Texas
- Utah
- Virginia
- Wisconsin

## Alcohol and Pregnancy: Civil Commitment

State and federal governments have established various policies in response to the risks associated with drinking during pregnancy. Civil commitment refers either to involuntary commitment of a pregnant woman to treatment or involuntary placement of a pregnant woman in protective custody of the state for the protection of a fetus from prenatal exposure to alcohol. As of January 1, 2008, five jurisdictions have statutory authorization for the civil commitment of women who abuse alcohol during pregnancy: Minnesota, North Dakota, Oklahoma, South Dakota, and Wisconsin.

There are two types of civil commitments—emergency and judicial. Emergency commitments are short in duration and may be imposed by the administrator of an appropriate mental health facility. Emergency commitment laws are not included in this research or in the coding of this policy topic except as described in this policy description. Judicial commitments are typically lengthier and must be ordered by a court.

The involuntary civil commitment arrangements in North Dakota, Oklahoma, and South Dakota provide for committing pregnant alcohol abusers to treatment facilities. The procedures in those three states are similar.

Minnesota provides two types of civil commitment procedures— early intervention and judicial commitment. Early intervention is of shorter duration and involves a less intrusive program than the standard judicial commitment procedure.

Wisconsin's child welfare laws provide for involuntary civil commitment to a variety of placements including a treatment facility, jail, and a relative's home. In Wisconsin, there are three stages leading to a judicial commitment. In the first stage, a woman is taken into protective custody, usually by law enforcement or child protective services. In the second stage, in cases in which there is a substantial health risk to the fetus, the woman may be held (detained) in protective custody for up to 48 hours. In the third stage, if custody is sought for a sustained period of time (i.e., a period longer than provided for in the second stage), the woman is entitled to legal representation and a hearing at which a court determines whether it will enter an order for her continued custody.

Despite their differences, all of these commitment and custody provisions are designed to protect the fetus via the involuntary restriction of the pregnant woman's action or conduct.

Chapter 12

# The Co-Occurrence of Domestic Violence and Child Abuse and Neglect

When families are in court because of allegations of child abuse and neglect, a commitment of time and understanding is required by all those involved. Some issues a family faces can be more complicated than others; that is the case with domestic violence. Domestic violence is pervasive in family court caseloads and can impact families in both apparent and subtle ways. The co-occurrence of domestic violence and child abuse and neglect creates a situation where there are several family members at risk, and decisions on how and if to intervene, can be extremely difficult and dangerous. It is essential that court professionals are aware of these issues and subtleties and wherever possible work in coordination in order to protect both the child and the parent who is the victim of the domestic violence.

Historically, communities treated the abuse of a parent and the abuse of a child in the same family as separate problems having little to do with each other. Intervening in intimate partner violence was widely viewed as secondary to the goal of protecting abused children. Philosophical and historical differences regarding the mission and mandates of child welfare institutions and domestic violence agencies created mistrust, tension, and lack of collaboration between fields. The

---

Text in this chapter is excerpted from: Litton, Lauren, J., Helping St. Louis County Families: A Guide for Court Professionals on the Co-Occurrence of Domestic Violence and Child Abuse/Neglect, St. Louis County Greenbook Initiative (2007). http://www.ispconsults.com/resourcesfiles/St_Louis_Family_Court_Guide .pdf. Reprinted with permission.

differing opinion about whose safety was paramount led to misconceptions and criticisms, producing disjointed and often contradictory interventions for families. In the end, it was the adult victim of abuse who was left to manage the many mandates of the various systems, even when the mandates conflicted or posed safety risks to the victim and his or her children.

## Co-Occurrence and Effects of Domestic Violence on Children

For the purposes of this chapter, co-occurrence exists when a child is independently abused or neglected in a family where domestic violence is also occurring. The abuse or neglect may or may not be related to the domestic violence. The fact that there is an intersection between domestic violence and child abuse is undeniable. For example:

- Missouri Department of Social Services reported that in 2005, 4.4% of the families investigated, and 6.7% of the substantiated cases, involved domestic violence;

- annually, between 3.3 and 10 million children witness domestic violence in the United States;

- approximately 50% of men who frequently assaulted their wives indicated they also abused their children;

- more than half of the victims of domestic violence reside with children under the age of 12;

- domestic violence may be the single major precursor to child abuse and neglect fatalities in this country;

- 80–90% of children living in homes with domestic violence are aware of the violence; and

- children who witness violence suffer greater rates of depression, anxiety, post traumatic stress disorder, alcohol and drug abuse, are at greater risk of entering the juvenile and criminal justice system, and have significantly lower academic achievement.

Domestic violence may appear in a child abuse case in several different ways. The most common ways are: domestic violence was the underlying factor that brought the family to the system's attention and led to the abuse of the child (for example, the child was physically injured when he or she got in the middle of a fight); the children were abused or neglected in an unrelated manner and during the course of interviews or pendency of the case the fact that domestic violence is occurring in the home has come to the attention of a professional involved in the case; or there is a history of domestic violence between the biological parents who are no longer together but the court notification of the dependency proceedings either reestablishes contact or provides further access for the battering parent to the child and abused parent.

Children are resilient, yet growing up in a violent home can affect a child's life and development. There are an abundance of studies available that provide documentation of various types of problems experienced by children who have been exposed to domestic violence. The level of risk in each family varies and domestic violence can have a multitude of complicated effects on children. Symptoms developed by children who have witnessed domestic violence are both internalized and externalized and may include the following:

- Sleep disorders
- Delinquency
- Anxiety
- Depression
- Bedwetting
- Learning problems
- Physical ailments
- Isolation
- Post traumatic stress
- Truancy
- Aggressive behavior

In spite of this, we know that when properly identified and addressed, the effects of domestic violence on children can be mitigated. Many children have developed sophisticated strategies to protect themselves from being physically and emotionally injured. There is not one typical way a child responds to intimate partner violence. Each child has a distinct reaction and even children within the same family can be affected differently. The way in which a child responds to the violence is based on a combination of their age, gender, temperament, level of involvement in the violence, interpretation of the experience, coping skills, and availability of support systems (friends, relatives, and other adults). While the impact of domestic violence on children is real and often palpable, a surprising number of children show significant resiliency in the face of this violence. Research demonstrates a critical connection between resiliency and a strong relationship between the child and the victimized parent. Other components of resiliency include extended support through community, family, and cultural connections and opportunities for success through recreation, school, or other activities. Accounting for resilience is imperative and should be incorporated into a risk assessment in order to determine the most effective and least harmful interventions.

Co-occurrence is unique and warrants special consideration because there is more than one person's safety at stake and interventions into a family can put the children and victimized parent in harm's way. Whenever possible, strategies should not be employed that compromise the vulnerability of one family member at the expense of another. The safety of the child can be promoted by enhancing the safety of the adult victim. Court professionals should focus on what is safe and appropriate for the child given the nature of the alleged child abuse or neglect the child has suffered, the age of the child, the child's relationship with each parent, and the history of intimate partner violence.

An often overlooked impact on children is the influence that the batterer exerts over the child's relationship with the victimized parent. Victims of domestic violence may be undermined in their parenting role. The battering can corrode the battered parent's relationship with his or her children. Perpetrators of domestic violence may thwart their former partner's parenting in ways both obvious and insidious. A batterer may: involve the children in further controlling or harming the victim (for example, have the children monitor the victimized parent); sabotage the other parent's authority through constant criticism or negative remarks; engage in activities with the children that the abused parent has forbidden; destroy the children's belongings when the abused parent counters his authority; or tell the children that the victimized parent does not love or want them.

Judges, attorneys, and other court professionals should not be surprised if they encounter children who have a closer bond with the battering parent than with the abused parent. Children may have adopted the philosophies that support intimate partner violence and may begin to model similar behaviors. For example, they blame the victimized parent for the abuse and problems in the family, use violence to resolve conflicts, or inflict abuse (emotional or physical) on the victimized parent or siblings. Ideally, each child should be referred to an expert in domestic violence and trauma who can determine what supportive services are needed to help the child cope with the violence that has occurred in the family. There are no existing tools that have been proven to adequately measure a child's exposure to adult domestic violence. Adaptations of other known tests vary greatly and leave the field with no standard method of measuring prevalence or individual incidents of exposure. When ordering or incorporating child assessments and counseling into a service plan, the following is recommended:

- Courts and social service providers only refer to mental health professionals who use a model of mental health assessment and treatment that combines a thorough knowledge of early childhood development, trauma, and the effects of domestic violence on all family members.

- Mental health providers work collaboratively with domestic violence advocates, community-based culturally specific services, and court professionals on behalf of children and families.

- Courts and social service providers ensure that children and non-offending parent are offered a range of services, like individual assessment and treatment, support groups, and educational materials, recognizing that children are affected differently by exposure to violence.

Domestic violence is a risk factor for children but not all families experiencing domestic violence should be referred to child protective services (CPS), nor should CPS respond to all reports of domestic violence. Court and social service professionals must examine factors that can lead to a child safely remaining with the family or the battered parent. Some of these factors may include whether the caregiver demonstrates protective capacities; the children show minimal behavioral or emotional effects; the children have formed a relationship with a supportive adult; an adequate safety plan is in place for the children; and the violence is not currently escalating.

## Post-Separation Violence and Battering Tactics

Post-separation violence is common in intimate partner violence situations and separation can serve as an impetus for increased or a renewal of abuse. Systems, service providers, and the community must be ready to address the ongoing possibility of harm that exists for victims of domestic violence when they are no longer residing or involved with their abusive partner. Victims have reported that after separation, their former partners have stalked, harassed, verbally and emotionally abused, beaten, and sexually assaulted them. Thus, the time during which a victim is pursuing a protection order or a divorce, or taking other steps to extricate from an abusive relationship is an extremely dangerous period. After separation, children remain the link between the battering and victimized parent. Custody and visitation arrangements are potentially dangerous for both the abused parent and children. Post-separation acts of violence are not solely directed toward the former partner. Other targets commonly include children, the victim's new partner, and individuals identified as aligning with the victim.

The legal system is effectively used by batterers as a way to exert and maintain control over a victim through continual litigation on child custody and visitation issues. Litigation is an opportunity to reassert the control batterers feel themselves losing as the relationship ends. Batterers can attempt to intimidate their partners by threatening to take the children away (for example, by making false reports to CPS, kidnapping, or maintaining ongoing litigation around custody or parent-child contact). Countering such actions can be financially devastating for victims. The battering parent may use the following tactics (many which involve the children) in order to try to retain power and control over the victimized parent:

### Related to Undermining Parenting

- Telling the children that they cannot be a family because of the victim

- Telling the children that the victimized parent is an alcoholic, addict, or mentally ill

- Sabotaging the victim parent's rules for the children

- Telling the children that the abused parent is to blame for the violence

- Getting the children to take his side

- Yelling at the victim when the children misbehave

### Related to Child Visitation

- Keeping the children longer than agreed

- Threatening to abduct the children

- Showing up unexpectedly to see the children
- Picking the children up at school without informing the abused parent beforehand
- Showering the children with gifts during visits
- Changing visitation plans without notice
- Not coming to see the children and blaming the victim
- Harassing the victim during exchanges

## Using the Children

- Calling the victim constantly under the guise of talking to or about the children
- Asking the children what the victimized parent is doing and who she is seeing
- Threatening to take custody away from the victim if she does not agree to reconcile
- Battering or threatening to hurt or kill the victimized parent in front of the children
- Telling the victimized parent that no one will believe him or her, everyone will think he or she is crazy, and he or she will lose custody of the children

## Related to Children Generally

- Keeping court cases active by frequent filings
- Physically abusing the children and ordering them not to tell their mother
- Abusing his new partner in front of the children
- Not permitting the abused parent access to proper health care for the children
- Driving recklessly with the children and/or the victim in the car
- Abusing drugs/alcohol in front of the children
- Withholding child support or quitting a job or remaining under-employed in order to avoid paying child support
- Recruiting relatives to speak negatively about the victim to the children

## Other

- Criticizing, assaulting, or threatening the victim's new partner
- Stalking the victim, children, and victim's friends or family
- Threatening to commit suicide
- Abusing or killing the family pets
- Threatening to call the police to have the victim arrested

Domestic violence is about power and control. Batterers are able to decide when, where, and how they are going to inflict abuse. This means that many professionals will never see the violent side of an individual. Professionals regularly report that men who batter are charming in their interactions and are able to manipulate situations in their favor. As systems and professionals become involved with a family, the abusive partner may look for ways to get these individuals to collude with him against the victim. In some cases, perpetrators actively employ the legal system as a means of maintaining ongoing control of their victims. Simultaneous misuse of the child protection system is not uncommon in these cases; excessive court filings or reports to CPS on minimal grounds may indicate the tendency to use official systems for harassment purposes. Hence, courts and professionals can inadvertently become tools for batterers to continue their abusive behavior. Judges, attorneys, volunteers, and social service providers may find batterers involved in the following actions:

- Presenting as the victim
- Using statements of remorse or guilt as a way to avoid consequences
- Alleging the partner is an alcoholic or chemically dependent
- Alleging the partner has mental illness
- Describing the protective actions by the victim (leaving or calling police) as ways to make the batterer look bad, get a leg up in court, or hurt the batterer (retribution for infidelity)
- Presenting as the more stable and calm partner (using the victim's anger about the situation as an example while on the other hand, the batterer is extremely cooperative)
- Denying or minimizing abuse
- Blaming the victim for the batterer's actions

- Avoiding responsibility by blaming alcohol, drugs, financial or marital problems, or other stress-related issues

- Presenting himself or herself as the provider for the family, both financially and emotionally

- Presenting the victim's behavior in a negative way in order to shift focus from the batterer

- Stating that the victim parent has been the barrier to resolving the family's problems (he or she won't go to counseling) and all the batterer wants to do is be a good parent and keep the family together.

- Presenting battering behaviors as being misunderstood (batterer is protecting the victim)

## Barriers to Leaving

Everyone deserves to live without violence. Many victims of domestic violence simply want the violence to stop. In the face of abuse and assaults, a battered parent often confronts difficult decisions. How will they protect themselves and their children from the physical dangers posed by the partner? How will he or she provide for her children? How will he or she manage the complex, and for many families, enduring relationship with the batterer over time? The barriers to escaping may be invisible to those outside of the victim's world, but they are extremely powerful. Victims of domestic violence stay in abusive relationships for many reasons, some include the following:

- Love

- Belief that the violence is the victim's fault

- Hope that the batterer will change

- Poverty and economic dependence (including lack of safe housing, loss of income and ability to provide for the children, loss of employment due to domestic violence, lack of job skills, and loss of health insurance benefits for children)

- Social and geographic isolation

- Fear of further violence (previous attempts to leave may have resulted in an escalation in the abuse)

- Ongoing intimidation, stalking, or coercion

- Use of weapons or following through on threats (knowing that the batterer is very dangerous and may be more so if the victim leaves)

- Language barriers

- Protection of the children

- Lack of knowledge about resources and how to access help

- Negative experiences with systems and friends (The victim may have tried to talk to others about what is happening in the home and received unhelpful or judgmental responses. Or, if there was prior system involvement, the police and court may have failed to hold the perpetrator accountable for violence, reinforcing the messages the abuser has sent the victim about his or her ability to remain above the law.)

- Emotional dependence (conflicting feelings of fear, shame, bewilderment, hope that things will improve, and a commitment to the relationship)

- Lack of confidence (After living with an abusive partner, the self-esteem of most individuals has been eroded to the point where they no longer have confidence in themselves, including their ability to survive alone, and may believe that there are no other options.)

- Belief systems and fear of bringing shame on family or cultural group

- Legal status (If a person is undocumented they may be afraid of identifying him- or herself to authorities for fear of deportation. The abuser may have withheld filing the proper paper work in order to keep the victim under control. If the victim is an immigrant/refugee, they may not be aware of legal options and believe they will have no way to support themselves and their children.)

Victims of domestic violence may face additional barriers in accessing services if they are members of a group typically underserved by traditional agencies. Legal and child protection systems have not been as responsive to victims whose primary language is not English or victims with disabilities. Identifying culturally appropriate and accessible services is a crucial part of creating safety mechanisms and effective interventions for families.

## Decision-Making and Protective Strategies of Victims of Domestic Violence

The most customary response by the community, law enforcement, the courts and social service agencies to domestic violence is requesting that the victim leave the abuser. The inference is that stopping the abuse is the victim's responsibility. It not only places the focus of interventions on the victim's behavior, but also assumes:

1. That leaving is a viable solution.

2. That ending the relationship is what the victim desires.

3. That ending the relationship is in the child's best interest.

4. That leaving will stop the violence.

Usually, one or more of these assumptions is not true.

Victims of domestic violence may attempt to protect themselves through a variety of mechanisms short of leaving the abusive relationship. Involvement with CPS or a formal case in juvenile court can lead battered parents to become vulnerable to: further manipulation from their batterers; depression and feelings of shame; termination of parental rights; economic hardship; pressure to compromise on access to children; and the feeling that they must choose whose safety to prioritize—their children's or their own—as they make decisions. Attorneys for battered parents must be ready to assist them in understanding how best to work with CPS so as to minimize the above issues and keep the safety of battered parents and their children implicitly linked. Thus, victims of domestic violence are often in survival mode. Without a sufficient understanding of domestic violence, volunteers and professionals may rely on their subjective interpretations of a battered parent's demeanor. Historically, adult victims' decisions or behaviors have been misinterpreted as instability, apathy, uncooperativeness, or even vindictiveness. A victim's choice not to leave a relationship or to use formal system assistance has been misinterpreted as failing to want to protect or care for her child. It is well documented that separation does not equal safety and willingness to separate from the abusive parent cannot function as a barometer of willingness to protect a child.

Victims of domestic violence are usually in the best position to determine what measures will increase or decrease their safety and the safety of their children. It is important that this determination and autonomy be valued and respected. Supportive, non-coercive, and empowering interventions, that promote the safety of both the adult victim and their children, should be incorporated into child abuse and neglect proceedings. It is in the child's best interest that court professionals support the victimized parent and help heal the child/parent bond. It is important to work with battered parents as part of the team to help children heal in addition to providing education about the effects of domestic violence on the children. When a battered parent is protected from abuse, he or she is then better able to protect the abused child. Even if the abusive relationship dissolves, frequently victims want their children to have a relationship with the abusive parent if it can be done in a way that does not compromise personal safety or the safety of the children.

Recognizing a battered parent's survival strategies and developing recommendations and service plans that build on those strategies will increase the likelihood of success for protecting children. It is imperative to acknowledge the protective behaviors of battered parents that may be overlooked or viewed in other circumstances as neglectful. The fear on the part of many battered parents of being blamed for the violence, or having disclosure of the violence lead to further state intervention may cause domestic violence to be identified late in the progression of a dependency case. Therefore, it is important to consider the history of abuse and the abused parent's efforts to manage existing safety threats and prevent additional safety threats to the children from arising. The following examples are ways an adult victim may try to protect themselves and their children:

- Fighting back and defying perpetrator (could have led to victim's arrest)
- Trying to improve the relationship with the partner
- Sending the children away from the home
- Pleasing and placating the perpetrator, complying with demands
- Remaining silent and not telling anyone about the violence for fear of making it worse
- Calling the police, seeking help from family members, obtaining a protection order, going to a shelter, or trying to find help for the perpetrator
- Dropping the protection order or withdrawing from help

- Learning to be devious as a way to survive

- Encouraging the perpetrator to drink so they'll pass out and not hurt anyone

- Leaving or returning to the relationship to try to make things better

- Enduring a beating or having unwanted sex to keep the batterer from attacking the children

- Establishing safety plans with her children)

- Avoiding the perpetrator (for example, working separate shifts)

- Reasoning with the perpetrator and expressing disapproval of his behavior

- Drinking and using drugs to numb the pain

- Lying about the perpetrator's criminal activity or child abuse so that they will not further hurt the victim or the children

Even with intervention, some families will want and choose to remain together. Court professionals will be challenged in these situations to consider options that keep children safe within that family dynamic, if at all possible. It is recommended that when both an adult victim and perpetrator have independently indicated that it is their intent to work together to rebuild their family, that this is discussed during case meetings and that strategies be used that do not punish a family for pursuing this option. Attorneys for battered parents and children should work closely with their clients to create safety plans that attend to potential risks when and if the batterer lives in the home.

Chapter 13

# The Legacy of Childhood Maltreatment and Foster Care Experience

## The Impact of Child Maltreatment and Foster Care

Child maltreatment is a devastating reality for millions of children in the United States. There are a number of trajectories that a child may follow after experiencing abuse or neglect. Some children may receive support and care from family members, foster parents, and other individuals, as well as specific services to address their particular needs. These children are likely to be on a trajectory that allows them to heal and thrive. The goal of the child welfare system is to have as many children on this trajectory as possible.

Unfortunately, a number of children are on a completely different trajectory because they receive little or no help or support. Their abuse or neglect may go undetected—research suggests that the true incidence of maltreatment is two or three times greater than what is officially substantiated. Alternatively, some children may receive no services despite detection of maltreatment. In fact, for a number of years now, nearly 40 percent of children who are determined by child protective services to have been abused or neglected receive no services at all. These children are not provided mental health services, follow-up visits, or foster care. While it is possible to imagine that some

Text in this chapter is from "Healthy Marriage and the Legacy of Child Maltreatment: A Child Welfare Perspective," by Tiffany Conway and Rutledge Q. Hutson. © 2008 Center for Law and Social Policy (www.clasp.org). Reprinted with permission.

children who experience maltreatment need no services to ameliorate harm or that they receive the needed help from family members, it is implausible to believe that 40 percent of maltreated children need no services and supports to recover from their trauma. For many children who get no help, the future offers a continuing set of challenges and difficulties.

A similar trajectory exists for children who are provided some services (such as foster care) but fail to receive other critical services, such as mental health treatment. These children may be removed from immediate harm, but denied the services and supports they need to heal and succeed in life. Similarly, the instability that often results from foster care may exacerbate the challenges a child faces and subject him to additional trauma. For children whose experience following abuse or neglect is fragmented, with inadequate services and instability, their trajectory is likely to be one of continuing challenges and difficulties into adulthood.

The *Adverse Childhood Experiences Study* (ACES) conducted by the Centers for Disease Control and Prevention indicates that adverse childhood experiences, including childhood maltreatment and other trauma, are associated with an increased risk for a host of problems— many of which are likely to interfere with achieving a healthy marriage later in life. For example, adverse childhood experiences increase the likelihood of alcohol abuse, illicit drug use, depression, suicide attempts, multiple sexual partners, unintended pregnancy, and risk for intimate partner violence. A study of foster care alumni who were in care for at least 12 continuous months between the ages of 14 and 18—the *Northwest Foster Care Alumni Study* (hereafter identified as *Northwest Alumni*)—illustrates the challenges faced by young people who have spent time in foster care. Another study of former foster youth, the *Midwest Evaluation of the Adult Functioning of Former Foster Youth* (hereafter identified as *Midwest Evaluation*) confirms these challenges are significant.

Compared to their counterparts in the general population, foster care alumni, including those who aged out of foster care may experience the following:

**Attain fewer years of education:** *Northwest Alumni:* Foster care alumni in this study were dramatically less likely to obtain a bachelor's or higher degree. Twenty-seven and a half percent of the general population between the ages of 25 and 34 hold a bachelor's degree or higher, while 1.8 percent of foster alumni do. *Midwest Evaluation:* Twenty-three percent of 21-year-old former foster youth have neither a general educational development (GED) nor a high school diploma, compared to 10.8 percent of the general population.

**Are more likely to be poor:** *Northwest Alumni:* Foster care alumni are less likely to be employed (80.1% versus 95%), more likely to live in poverty (33.2% versus 14.4%) and more likely to have experienced homelessness than the general population (11–22% versus 1%). *Midwest Evaluation:* Although the vast majority of the young adults in this study had held a job at some point, only half were currently employed (compared to 64% of their peers in the general population) suggesting a lack of financial security. Additionally, about half of these youth report experiencing economic hardship, compared to 27.5% of young people in the general population.

**Are more likely to experience mental health problems:** *Northwest Alumni*: Over half (54.4 percent) of foster care alumni had ongoing mental health disorders, compared to 22.1 percent of the general population. The rates of posttraumatic stress disorder (25.2%) were not only higher than the general population (4%) but were even higher than the rates for United States' war veterans (6–15%). Foster care alumni also may be less likely to recover (or take longer to recover) from certain mental health problems.

**Are more likely to use drugs:** *Northwest Alumni:* They are more likely to report symptoms of drug (21% versus 4.2%) and alcohol (11.3% versus 7%) dependence.

**Are more likely to be involved with the criminal justice system:** *Midwest Evaluation:* Young men who were formerly in foster care were more likely to have ever been arrested (79.4% versus 20.1%) and ever convicted (52.6% versus 12.1%). Similarly, young women who were formerly in foster care were significantly more likely than young women in the general population to have ever been arrested (56.7% versus 4.3%) and ever convicted (24.5% versus 1.3%).

**Are more likely to have children young, before marriage, or as teens:** *Midwest Evaluation:* Seventy-one percent of the young women who were former foster youth had been pregnant by the age of 21, the majority (61.9%) reporting two or more pregnancies. In comparison, at age 21, only a third of women in the general population report having ever been pregnant and most report only one pregnancy.

## The Impact of Instability and Disconnection

Placement in foster care may compound the difficulties that victims of child maltreatment face when that care is marked by instability and inadequate services. Unfortunately, children who are removed from their families and placed in foster care may not get the other services they need. For example, research indicates that about half of children in foster care have clinically significant emotional or behavioral problems, but only about one-quarter receive mental health services. In fact, only about half the children who enter care even receive a mental health assessment to determine their needs. Similarly, the families of children in care may not receive the services they need. National data suggest that more than three-quarters of those caring for children when they were placed in care needed substance abuse treatment services, but services were provided to only slightly more than one-quarter of these caregivers. When such treatment services are not available, children linger in foster care waiting for their parents to recover.

For too many children the experience of foster care is fraught with instability as they move from home to home. The *Northwest Alumni* study found that throughout the course of their foster care experience about one-third (31.9%) of foster care alumni had three or fewer placements, another third (35.8%) had four to seven placements, while the remaining third (32.3%) had eight or more placements. These placement changes mean not only a new family but, often also a new school with new teachers, new neighbors, a new doctor, and the need to make new friends. The *Northwest Alumni* study found that almost one-third of foster care alumni experienced ten or more school changes from elementary through high school. Children may also lose connections to people whom they feel very close to as a result of moves. Such instability can compromise a child's ability to form strong attachments, contribute to a number of behavioral problems, and, among other things, compromise a child's educational attainment. For children with mental health problems, such instability is associated with a greater likelihood that these problems will persist into adulthood.

Children in foster care may also have poor relationships with other key adults in their lives. Caseworkers may provide little continuity and stability because they typically carry more than double the recommend caseload and turnover is high—20 to 40 percent per year. These factors make it challenging for caseworkers to establish supportive relationships with children and help them heal. Similarly, there is concern that some foster parents lack the preparation, experience, time, or inclination to nurture the children in their care. The evidence on this point is mixed. For example, one third of foster care alumni in the *Northwest Alumni* study report maltreatment of some kind by a foster parent or other adult present in the foster home. On the other hand, official reports of maltreatment of children in foster care suggest that less than one percent of children experience substantiated maltreatment. Whatever the true incidence of repeat abuse or neglect, it is clear that some children in foster care experience additional adults who cannot be counted on to meet their needs—thus potentially exacerbating issues of trust and attachment.

Upon reaching the age of majority, youth in foster care, previously provided with at least some level of support, are frequently on their own. Youth who age-out of care report being told, on the morning of their 18th birthdays, that they must leave their foster homes. Around 20,000 to 25,000 young people age-out of the system each year. Many 18-year-olds in the general population are not prepared to support themselves and all that entails. Yet, a youth who experienced maltreatment, who may or may not have gotten adequate treatment to address that maltreatment, and who has no family to turn to for support, is expected to make it on his or her own. Not surprisingly, many of these youth experience significant difficulties.

While virtually all of the negative outcomes experienced by child victims, those who spent time in foster care and particularly those who age-out of care, are concerning in and of themselves, many of them also have the potential to further disrupt the child's life by interfering with the attainment and maintenance of a healthy marriage or other intimate adult relationships. The experience of low educational attainment, unemployment, poverty, mental health and substance abuse problems create barriers to achieving healthy marriage, as do non-marital births and involvement with the criminal justice system. These barriers must be addressed if a child who experienced abuse or neglect is to enjoy a satisfying, healthy marriage characterized by safety, communication, and commitment.

# Part Two

# Physical and Emotional Abuse of Children

# Chapter 14

# *Child Physical Abuse*

## What Is Child Physical Abuse?

Child physical abuse refers to a situation in which a child suffers, or is likely to suffer, significant harm from an injury inflicted by the child's parent or caregiver. The injury may be inflicted intentionally or may be the inadvertent result of physical punishment or physically aggressive treatment of a child.

Behavior by a parent or caregiver which may cause significant harm to a child, and is therefore physical abuse, includes:

- hitting,
- biting,
- shaking,
- punching,
- burning,
- administering poison,
- suffocating, and
- drowning.

Physical abuse may lead to bruises, cuts, welts, burns, fractures, internal injuries, or poisoning. In the most extreme cases, physical abuse results in the death of a child.

There are grounds for statutory intervention when a child has suffered, or is likely to suffer, significant harm as a result of physical

---

This chapter includes text from "What is child physical abuse?" © 2007 South Eastern Centre Against Sexual Assault SECASA (www.secasa.com.au). Reprinted with permission. Additional text from the American Humane Association is cited separately within the chapter.

abuse and the child's parents or caregivers have failed to protect the child, or are unlikely to protect the child, from harm of that type. Physical abuse of children is usually regarded as a criminal offense.

**Note:** While this chapter is concerned with physical injury which results from abuse, physical injury and significant harm may also result from neglect by a parent or caregiver. The failure of a parent or caregiver to ensure the safety of a child may expose the child to dangerous or even life-threatening situations which result in physical injury to the child.

### Physical Indicators

If you observe signs of physical injury on a child, you need to consider several factors before you decide whether or not they indicate possible physical abuse. The following physical indicators should raise concern:

- The location, nature, or extent of the injury do not fit with the explanation given.

- The child's age or developmental stage is not consistent with the type of injury. The severity or type of the injury itself is of concern.

Physical indicators include the following:

- Bruises and welts: These may appear on the face, back, bottom, genitals, and arms. Bruises or welts in unusual configurations may pattern the instrument used to inflict them, for example: hand or fingerprints or the linear marks of a cane. Cluster bruises and bruises of various colors may indicate repeated abuse, although it is difficult to date a bruise according to its color. Bruising on babies and young children is of significant concern.

- Fractures: Any fracture in a child under the age of two years is a serious concern. Fractures are not often detected without x-ray, although the child may have a swollen joint and appear to be in pain or irritable.

- Burns and scalds: These may show the shapes of the item used to inflict them. For example, iron, grill, or cigarette burns. Other types of burns include boiling water, oil, or flame burns.

- Abdominal injuries: Torn liver or spleen or ruptured intestines may be present without any outward signs of bruising on the abdominal wall. The signs are pain, vomiting, restlessness, and fever.

- Head or brain injuries: There may be no outward signs that these injuries are present. They are usually observed by health professionals and include subdural hematoma and other brain injuries which may lead to permanent brain damage; eye damage caused by shaking; and absence of hair which may indicate that hair has been pulled out.

- Lacerations and abrasions to the head, face, and mouth: The shape may indicate the implement used, for example, fingernail scratches leave parallel linear marks.

- Human bite marks.

- Multiple injuries: These may be both old and new.

- A history of repeated injuries.

- Any injury to a very young baby.

**Important:** When a protective worker from child protective services investigates a case of alleged physical abuse and any of the above physical indicators are present, they will arrange a medical examination by a forensic physician or specialist medical practitioner.

### Behavioral Indicators

Sometimes a child's behavior can be an indication that something is wrong. Behavioral indicators must be interpreted with regard to the individual child's level of functioning and developmental stage. The following are some of the behavioral indicators which may suggest possible physical abuse:

- The child is unusually wary of physical contact with adults.

- The child seems to be unduly frightened of a parent or another adult.

- The child does not show emotion when hurt.

- The child offers unlikely, implausible explanations of injuries.

- The child is habitually absent from school without an explanation—the parent/caregiver may be keeping the child at home until physical evidence of abuse has disappeared.

- The child wears inappropriate long-sleeved clothing on hot days (to hide bruising or other injuries).
- The child may be overly compliant, shy, withdrawn, passive, and uncommunicative.
- The child may be hyperactive, aggressive, disruptive, and destructive towards him/herself and others.
- The child displays regressed behavior, such as bedwetting or soiling.

Other behavioral indicators, which may be more common to adolescents than younger children, include:

- running away,
- criminal behavior,
- drug abuse, and
- acting out behavior.

The adolescent may appear as if they completely reject or lack trust in the world.

Parents may try to deny or conceal physical abuse. For example, they may:

- accuse the child or adolescent of lying about the abuse;
- provide an explanation for the injury which is unbelievable, inadequate, or illogical (for example, the parent may say, "He bruises easily," "Her brother hits her all the time and causes bruising," "He is so clumsy and prone to accidents");
- change their explanation for the injury over time;
- appear unconcerned about the child's condition;
- delay seeking medical assistance;
- attempt to conceal the child's injury;
- take the child to several different doctors and hospitals, or to out-of-region services for treatment; or,
- fail to attend school or health center appointments.

### When does physical punishment become physical abuse?

The level of punishment which can be inflicted on a child is subject to legal regulation. Physical punishment of children for the purpose of discipline, by parents or caregivers, is permitted by law provided it falls within the bounds of reasonable chastisement, is seen as moderate, and is administered for the purpose of correcting behavior. Reasonable chastisement is a term which is difficult to define precisely. Reasonableness is a flexible concept which involves taking all relevant factors into account. Whether chastisement is reasonable, according to the law will depend on:

- age of the child;
- stature of the child;
- health and intellectual capacity of the child;
- method of and reason for, inflicting the punishment; and,
- the harm caused to the child.

Child physical abuse is often the inadvertent result of physical punishment administered by an angry, frustrated parent. Sometimes, however, physical discipline is intended to harm the child.

Physical punishment which results, intentionally or unintentionally, in injury or tissue damage to the child or young person is physical abuse and may become the grounds for a charge of assault as well as the grounds for protective intervention by Child Protective Services.

The fact that our society is now concerned with the problem of child abuse does not mean that parents have suddenly taken to beating their children, but that our tolerance to child maltreatment has declined, and we are now appalled by acts to which our ancestors would have been indifferent. It is part of a growing human awareness that the human rights, dignity, and integrity of every man, woman, and child should be protected.

## Child Physical Abuse Information

Excerpted from "Child Discipline," © 2007 American Humane Association (www.americanhumane.org). Reprinted with permission.

According to the National Child Abuse and Neglect Data System (NCANDS), in 2005, an estimated 3.3 million reports of alleged abuse and/or neglect involving approximately six million children were made to local child protective services (CPS) agencies across the country. An estimated 899,000 of these children were determined to be victims of abuse and/or neglect (U.S. Department of Health and Human Services [HHS], 2007). Of these, 16.6 percent were determined to be victims of physical abuse. Further, an estimated 1,460 children died in

2005 as a result of child abuse and neglect (HHS, 2007). NCANDS data collection saw a large increase in child maltreatment numbers during its data collection in 2005 largely due to the inclusion of Alaska and Puerto Rico.

## What can you do?

**Discipline effectively:** Remember that kids will be kids. Children can be loud, unruly, and destructive. They will break things, interrupt telephone conversations, track mud through the house, not pick up their toys or clean their rooms, struggle over eating their vegetables, or pester routinely. Children will inevitably do things that may make their parents feel irritated, frustrated, disappointed, and angry. Changing a child's behavior is not easy. However, children should not be disciplined through violence.

It is better to deny children privileges when they do something unacceptable, as well as reward them when they do something good. This teaches children that there are consequences for their actions.

**Regain control:** Child abuse is a symptom of having difficulty coping with stressful situations. If you feel you are losing control, ask someone to relieve you for a few minutes. Then try these tips:

- Count to ten
- Take deep breaths
- Phone a friend
- Look through a magazine or newspaper
- Listen to music
- Exercise
- Take a walk (first make certain that children are not left without supervision)
- Take a bath
- Write a letter
- Sit down and relax
- Lie down

**Get help:** Support is available for families at risk of abuse through local child protection services agencies, community centers, churches, physicians, mental health facilities, and schools.

**Report, report, report:** If you suspect child abuse is occurring, first report it to the local child protective services agency (often called social services or human services) in your county or state. Professionals who work with children are required by law to report reasonable suspicion of abuse or neglect. Furthermore, in 20 states, citizens who suspect abuse or neglect are required to report it. "Reasonable suspicion" based on objective evidence, which could be firsthand observation or statements made by a parent or child, is all that is needed to report.

## What is NCANDS?

NCANDS, the National Child Abuse and Neglect Data System, is the primary source of national information on abused and neglected children known to public child protective services agencies. American Humane has provided technical assistance to this project since its beginning in 1990.

## References

U.S. Department of Health and Human Services, Administration on Children, Youth, and Families. (2007). *Child maltreatment 2005*. Washington, DC: U.S. Government Printing Office.

## Resources

Cohn, A. H., and Gordon, T. (1986). *Tips on parenting*. Chicago, IL: The National Center for the Prosecution of Child Abuse (NCPCA).

Dubowitz, H. (2000). What is physical abuse? In H. Dubowitz and D. DePanfilis (Eds.), *Handbook for child protection practice*. Thousand Oaks, CA: Sage.

Jaudes, P., and Mitchel, L. (1992). *Physical child abuse*. Chicago, IL: The National Center for the Prosecution of Child Abuse (NCPCA).

U.S. Advisory Board on Child Abuse and Neglect. (1995). *A nation's shame: Fatal child abuse and neglect in the United States*. Washington, DC: U.S. Advisory Board on Child Abuse and Neglect.

Winterfeld, A., and Hunt., D. E. (2003). The legal framework for child protective services. In C. Brittain and D. E. Hunt (Eds.), *Helping in child protective services: A competency-based casework handbook*. New York: Oxford University Press.

Chapter 15

# Medical Evaluation of Physical Abuse in Children

Physical abuse of children in our society is a serious problem that has only recently been recognized by the medical community. The first published report in contemporary medical literature was in 1946,[1] and the term "battered-child syndrome" was coined in 1962.[2] Reports of child abuse are increasing as the medical profession gains experience in recognizing the signs and symptoms of physical abuse. Anyone involved in the care of children is likely to see children who have been physically abused. In 1996, approximately one million children were confirmed to be victims of maltreatment, and 1,185 children died from their injuries.[3]

The physician evaluating children who may have been abused is faced with special challenges. In addition to providing the diagnosis and treatment, the physician plays a new role when providing care for victims of physical abuse. In these cases, the physician must also ensure the child's safety and assist in the collection of evidence for possible litigation. The physician is mandated to report any suspected abuse to the state child protective services agency.

In the face of these new and often unaccustomed roles, hostile families may challenge physicians when the possibility of physical abuse is broached. Preconceived ideas regarding racial, cultural, or economic

Reprinted with permission from "Evaluation of Physical Abuse in Children," by David M. Pressel, MD, PhD, May 15, 2000, American Family Physician. Copyright © 2000 American Academy of Family Physicians. All Rights Reserved. Reviewed in March, 2009 by David A. Cooke, MD, FACP.

norms as well as the strong feelings elicited when children may have been intentionally injured are confounding factors complicating the evaluation of suspected child abuse.

This chapter will review the physician's role in caring for children who are suspected victims of physical abuse. Typical features of the history, physical examination, and focused laboratory and radiologic studies help physicians in diagnosing physical abuse in children. In addition, physicians caring for children must remain cognizant of the many medical conditions whose presentation can mimic signs of physical abuse.

## History

The most important information leading to a diagnosis of physical abuse is obtained through the medical history. While perpetrators of child physical abuse and their victims come from all socioeconomic classes, certain factors place children at increased risk of physical abuse.[4] Adults who have been abused as children may become perpetrators of abuse as adults, although this is generally not the case.[5]

### Physical Indicators of Child Abuse

- Bruises on uncommonly injured body surfaces
- Blunt-instrument marks or burns
- Human hand marks or bite marks
- Multiple injuries at different stages of healing
- Evidence of poor care or failure to thrive
- Circumferential immersion burns
- Unexplained retinal hemorrhages

Certain "red flags" in the medical history should raise the possibility of a diagnosis of child abuse.[6] In many cases, injuries to children who cannot yet talk are not witnessed and may be attributed by the caregiver to another person, either a child or an adult.

Children are commonly injured accidentally, and a history of age-appropriate injury, not witnessed, should not by itself raise the suspicion of child abuse. However, injury resulting from inappropriate supervision may raise the issue of neglect, a form of child abuse. When the patient's injuries are attributed to another child, the other child's developmental ability must be considered. A complicated and challenging scenario arises when the caregiver accuses an adult from whom the caregiver is divorced or separated as the perpetrator. In this case, the injury must be evaluated in the context of the history obtained from all those involved and from the physical examination.

The history of a child suspected to be abused should be elicited in a non-accusatory manner. When possible, separate interviews should be held for the caregiver(s) and the child. The interviewer should inform the caregiver of the concern about abuse and the steps to be taken in the evaluation, including assurance regarding the child's safety and the possibility of a referral to the local child protective services agency. When the medical evaluation is inconsistent with the history provided by the child's caregiver, physical abuse should be seriously considered.

## Physical Examination

Young children are commonly injured accidentally in the course of daily activities and play. However, the patterns of injuries seen in children who are physically abused differ from injuries seen in children who are hurt accidentally. The physical manifestations of nonaccidental trauma are varied and most commonly involve the skin, bone, or central nervous system. Nonaccidental trauma may affect any organ system and mimic signs of accidental trauma or other disease processes. The "Physical Indicators of Child Abuse" section of this chapter presents patterns of physical findings that strongly suggest a diagnosis of physical abuse.

The skin is the most commonly injured organ system and the easiest to examine. The location of bruises can sometimes be suggestive of accidental versus nonaccidental trauma. Children commonly fall and scrape or bruise the skin covering anterior parts of the body such as the shins, knees, hands, elbows, nose, periorbital area, and forehead. Unexplained injuries to protected parts of the body such as the buttocks, thighs, torso, frenulum, ears, and neck are suggestive of child abuse. The likelihood of having accidental bruises is a function of a child's behavior and developmental ability. Bruises are rare in infants who do not cruise or walk.[7] The shape or pattern of injury may also suggest inflicted trauma. Bruises in the shapes of handprints, belt buckles, cord loops, or encirclements represent child physical abuse.[7]

The dating of bruises by color is advocated by medical textbooks and older literature on child abuse. The age of a bruise and the historical

143

timing of an injury may have important legal implications for determining a perpetrator's identity. Determining the bruise's age by its color is a subjective step that does not take into account the individual patient's skin tone, the bruise's location (whether overlying soft tissue or bone), the patient's relative nutritional state, or other indeterminate factors. When judging the age of a bruise, the physician may be better off making a rough estimate of the injury's date—within a day if the bruise is erythematous, or older than a day if yellow or brown shades are present.[8] The presence of bruises that have various ages may signify multiple episodes of injury caused by ongoing physical abuse.

Children may be abused by burning, which can result in disfiguring or fatal injuries. Cigarette burns leave centimeter-sized circular marks on the skin. Scald marks on the hands, feet, or buttocks that have a glove, sock, or circular appearance and spare the intertriginous areas are caused by deliberate immersion of the child in a sink or bathtub of hot water. It may be difficult to distinguish between an injury caused by scalding liquid thrown at the child from a burn resulting when a child accidentally tips a hot pan from a stove. The presence of excessive splash burns or of scalds on areas of the body not likely to get wet when a child spills a container of hot liquid suggests an inflicted injury.[9]

The physical examination should proceed carefully with inspection and palpation of all body surfaces. Specifically, all bruises and burns should be noted and described in terms of location, size, shape, and color. Areas of tenderness may represent occult trauma and should be evaluated radiologically. Careful measurements should be taken and photographed. Photographs should include the patient's name, date of photograph, and a measurement scale. It should be noted if bruises resemble a particular instrument pattern (for example: belt buckle, cord).

Careful attention should be paid to the oral cavity, groin, and scalp for signs of occult trauma. The funduscopic examination is an often-overlooked part of the evaluation when physical abuse is suspected. Retinal hemorrhages are highly suspicious for abuse resulting from "shaken-baby syndrome."[10] Infants who are forcibly shaken may present with unexplained injuries, seizures, or a decreased level of consciousness. Nonspecific symptoms such as vomiting, irritability, or abnormal respiration may be manifestations of abusive head injury. The diagnosis is easily overlooked and should be considered if facial or scalp bruises are present. In addition, the presence of xanthochromic cerebrospinal fluid may indicate an old intracranial bleed.[11]

## Radiologic Evaluation

The skeletal system may be injured in situations of child abuse or as a result of everyday activities. All fractures must be interpreted in the context of the child's developmental ability and the history of injury. For example, a transverse long-bone fracture in a three-month-old child is highly suspicious for physical abuse but may be unremarkable in an eight-year-old child. While any type of fracture can be the result of child abuse, certain fractures are much more specific for nonaccidental trauma. Fractures involving parts of the skeletal system or caused by mechanisms of injury unlikely to be from accidental trauma should be viewed with suspicion.

Uncommon fractures with a high specificity for being caused by nonaccidental trauma include metaphyseal "corner or bucket-handle" lesions, posterior rib fractures, scapular fractures, spinous process fractures, and sternal fractures. Fractures with moderate specificity for nonaccidental trauma include multiple fractures, especially bilateral, fractures of different ages, epiphyseal separations, vertebral body fractures and subluxations, digital fractures, and complex skull fractures. Common fractures with low specificity for abuse include clavicular fractures, long-bone shaft fractures, and linear skull fractures.

A complete skeletal survey is indicated in children younger than two years when physical abuse is suspected. Radiographs in a skeletal survey should minimally include single anteroposterior (AP) views of each extremity and the pelvis, as well as AP and lateral views of the chest and skull.[13] Any abnormality seen should be viewed with at least two projections. A single "babygram" radiograph of the patient is diagnostically inadequate and should be avoided. The degree of healing seen on plain radiographs of fractures may also be useful for giving the injury an approximate age.

Specialized imaging may play a limited role in the evaluation of children with suspected physical abuse. Skeletal scintigraphy may be indicated when there is a high degree of suspicion for nonaccidental trauma but occult fractures are not seen on plain radiographs. A computed tomographic study of the head should be obtained in all children with suspected central nervous system injury.

## Differential Diagnosis and Laboratory Evaluation

Evaluating suspected child abuse is a challenging task, and an incorrect diagnosis of child abuse can be as devastating to a family as the impact of missing a diagnosis of abuse can be to a child. A brief list of the many medical conditions that may mimic child abuse follows:

- Hematologic
  - Hemophilia
  - Idiopathic thrombocytopenic purpura
  - Von Willebrand disease
  - Henoch-Schönlein purpura
- Dermatologic
  - Phytophotodermatitis
  - Mongolian spots
  - Vascular malformations
  - Subcutaneous fat necrosis
- Infectious
  - Bullous impetigo
  - Staphylococcal scalded skin syndrome
  - Petechia or purpura from systemic bacterial or viral infections
- Metabolic congenital
  - Osteogenesis imperfect
  - Ehlers-Danlos syndrome
  - Rickets
- Insensitivity to pain disorders
- Accidental trauma
  - Toddler's fracture
  - Stress fracture

Several of these disorders may be distinguished from nonaccidental trauma by the other physical signs of the syndrome or by a natural history of the skin lesion that differs from that expected for an inflicted injury. Children with a history of easy bruising should receive a bleeding disorder screen consisting of a complete blood count, prothrombin time, partial thromboplastin time, and bleeding time. If the physician is still uncertain about the etiology of a finding suggestive of child abuse, referral to a subspecialist is indicated. It is important to remember that children with conditions whose presentation may mimic child abuse may also be victims of physical abuse.

## Management of Suspected Child Abuse

All 50 states have child-protection ordinances mandating that professionals who come in contact with children report cases of suspected abuse to the local child protective services agency. Making a report indicates that child abuse or neglect is a serious diagnostic consideration, not a definitive diagnosis. Each jurisdiction varies in terms of what constitutes abuse and the reporting mechanism. Physicians who care for children should familiarize themselves with the child protection statutes in the area in which they practice. The law requires reporting all cases of suspected, but not necessarily proven, abuse. Physicians who report their suspicions in good faith are protected from lawsuits. Information elicited during the course of a child abuse evaluation may potentially be used in a legal proceeding against the alleged perpetrator. Documentation in the medical record should be done with great care, because the record may become evidence in a criminal prosecution.

The physician caring for a child suspected of being physically abused must also make a determination, often in cooperation with the child protective services agency, regarding the safe disposition of the child. If the child cannot safely be sent home with a caregiver, the child may need to be admitted temporarily to a hospital and, in extreme cases, emergency custody of the child must be taken. Physical abuse in a child may indicate that other members of the household, particularly the mother, are also victims of domestic violence.[15] The appropriate evaluation and safety of other family members must also be considered.

The evaluation of a child suspected of being physically abused is a common and serious problem for any physician who cares for children. A history inconsistent with the medical evaluation and certain patterns of physical findings should alert the examining physician to the possibility of child abuse. In addition to the traditional roles of diagnosis and treatment, the physician also has the responsibilities of evidence collection, alerting the child protective services agency and protecting the child.

*—David M. Pressel, M.D., Ph.D.*

Dr. Pressel is assistant professor of pediatrics and a pediatric hospitalist at Temple University School of Medicine and Temple University

Children's Medical Center, Philadelphia. Dr. Pressel received his medical degree from Washington University School of Medicine, St. Louis, where he also obtained a doctorate degree in neuroscience. He served a residency in pediatrics at St. Louis Children's Hospital.

## References

1.  Caffey J. Multiple fractures in the long bones of infants suffering from chronic subdural hematomas. *Am J Roentgenol* 1946;56:163.

2.  Kempe CH, Silverman FN, Steele BF, Droegemueller W, Silver HK. The battered-child syndrome. *JAMA* 1962;181:17–24.

3.  Wang CT, Daro D. *Current trends in child abuse reporting and fatalities: the results of the 1997 annual fifty state survey.* Chicago: Center on Child Abuse Prevention Research, National Committee for Prevention of Child Abuse, 1997. Available at http://www.childabuse.org/50data97.html. Accessed July 7, 1999.

4.  Christian CW. Etiology and prevention of abuse: family and individual factors. In: Ludwig S, Kornberg AE, eds. *Child abuse: a medical reference. 2d ed.* New York: Churchill Livingstone, 1992:39–47.

5.  Kaufman J, Zigler E. Do abused children become abusive parents? *Am J Orthopsychiatry* 1987;57: 186–92.

6.  Schmitt BD. The child with nonaccidental trauma. In: Kempe CH, Helfer RE, eds. *The battered child. 3d ed.* Chicago: University of Chicago Press, 1980: 128–46.

7.  Sugar NF, Taylor JA, Feldman KW. Bruises in infants and toddlers. *Arch Pediatr Adolesc Med* 1999;153:399–403.

8.  Schwartz AJ, Ricci LR. How accurately can bruises be aged in abused children? Literature review and synthesis. *Pediatrics* 1996;97:254–7.

9.  Feldman KW. Child abuse by burning. In: Kempe CH, Helfer RE, eds. *The battered child. 3d ed.* Chicago: University of Chicago Press, 1980:147–62.

10. Riffenburgh RS, Sathyavagiswaran L. Ocular findings at autopsy of child abuse victims. *Ophthalmology* 1991;98:1519–24.

11. Jenny C, Hymel KP, Ritzen A, Reinert SE, Hay TC. Analysis of missed cases of abusive head trauma. *JAMA* 1999;281:621–6 [published erratum appears in *JAMA* 1999;282:29].

12. Kleinman PK. Skeletal trauma: general considerations. In: Kleinman PK, ed. *Diagnostic imaging of child abuse.* Baltimore: Williams and Wilkins, 1987:8–25.

13. American College of Radiology Standard Web site. *ACR standard for skeletal surveys in children.* Available at: http://www.acr.org/cgi-bin/fr?tmpl:standards,pdf:diag/skeletal.pdf. Accessed March 21, 2000.

14. Wardinsky TD. Genetic and congenital defect conditions that mimic child abuse. *J Fam Pract* 1995; 41:377–83.

15. McGibben L, De Vos E, Newberger EH. Victimization of mothers of abused children: a controlled study. *Pediatrics* 1989;84:531–5.

Chapter 16

# Abusive Head Trauma (Shaken Baby Syndrome)

Abusive head trauma/inflicted traumatic brain injury, or AHT (also called shaken baby/shaken impact syndrome or SBS), is a form of inflicted head trauma.

AHT can be caused by direct blows to the head, dropping or throwing a child, or shaking a child. Head trauma is the leading cause of death in child abuse cases in the United States.

## How These Injuries Happen

Unlike other forms of inflicted head trauma, abusive head trauma results from injuries caused by someone vigorously shaking a child. Because the anatomy of infants puts them at particular risk for injury from this kind of action, the vast majority of victims are infants younger than one year old. The average age of victims is between three and eight months, although these injuries are occasionally seen in children up to four years old.

The perpetrators in these cases are most often parents or caregivers. Common triggers are frustration or stress when the child is crying. Unfortunately, the shaking may have the desired effect: although at first the baby cries more, he or she may stop crying as the brain is damaged.

"Abusive Head Trauma (Shaken Baby Syndrome)," June 2008, reprinted with permission from www.kidshealth.org. Copyright © 2008 The Nemours Foundation. This information was provided by KidsHealth, one of the largest resources online for medically reviewed health information written for parents, kids, and teens. For more articles like this one, visit www.KidsHealth.org or www.TeensHealth.org.

Approximately 60% of identified victims of shaking injury are male, and children of families who live at or below the poverty level are at an increased risk for these injuries as well as any type of child abuse. It is estimated that the perpetrators in 65% to 90% of cases are males—usually either the baby's father or the mother's boyfriend, often someone in his early twenties.

When someone forcefully shakes a baby, the child's head rotates about the neck uncontrollably because infants' neck muscles aren't well developed and provide little support for their heads. This violent movement pitches the infant's brain back and forth within the skull, sometimes rupturing blood vessels and nerves throughout the brain and tearing the brain tissue. The brain may strike the inside of the skull, causing bruising and bleeding to the brain.

The damage can be even greater when a shaking episode ends with an impact (hitting a wall or a crib mattress, for example), because the forces of acceleration and deceleration associated with an impact are so strong. After the shaking, swelling in the brain can cause enormous pressure within the skull, compressing blood vessels and increasing overall injury to its delicate structure.

Normal interaction with a child, like bouncing the baby on a knee, will not cause these injuries, although it's important to never shake a baby under any circumstances because gentle shaking can rapidly escalate.

## What Are the Effects?

AHT often causes irreversible damage. In the worst cases, children die due to their injuries.

Children who survive may have:

- partial or total blindness,
- hearing loss,
- seizures,
- developmental delays,
- impaired intellect,
- speech and learning difficulties,
- problems with memory and attention,
- severe mental retardation, or
- cerebral palsy.

Even in milder cases, in which babies look normal immediately after the shaking, they may eventually develop one or more of these problems. Sometimes the first sign of a problem isn't noticed until the child enters the school system and exhibits behavioral problems or learning difficulties. But by that time, it's more difficult to link these problems to a shaking incident from several years before.

## Signs and Symptoms

In any abusive head trauma case, the duration and force of the shaking, the number of episodes, and whether impact is involved all affect the severity of the infant's injuries. In the most violent cases, children may arrive at the emergency room unconscious, suffering seizures, or in shock. But in many cases, infants may never be brought to medical attention if they don't exhibit such severe symptoms.

In less severe cases, a child who has been shaken may experience:

- lethargy,
- irritability,
- vomiting,
- poor sucking or swallowing,
- decreased appetite,
- lack of smiling or vocalizing,
- rigidity,
- seizures,
- difficulty breathing,
- altered consciousness,
- unequal pupil size,
- an inability to lift the head, or
- an inability to focus the eyes or track movement.

## Diagnosis

Many cases of AHT are brought in for medical care as "silent injuries." In other words, parents or caregivers don't often provide a history that the child has had abusive head trauma or a shaking injury, so doctors don't know to look for subtle or physical signs. This can sometimes result in children having injuries that aren't identified in the medical system.

And again, in many cases, babies who don't have severe symptoms may never be brought to a doctor. Many of the less severe symptoms such as vomiting or irritability may resolve and can have many non-abusive causes.

Unfortunately, unless a doctor has reason to suspect child abuse, mild cases (in which the infant seems lethargic, fussy, or perhaps isn't feeding well) are often misdiagnosed as a viral illness or colic. Without a diagnosis of child abuse and any resulting intervention with the parents or caregivers, these children may be shaken again, worsening any brain injury or damage.

If shaken baby syndrome is suspected, doctors may look for:

- hemorrhages in the retinas of the eyes;

- skull fractures;

- swelling of the brain;

- subdural hematomas (blood collections pressing on the surface of the brain);

- rib and long bone (bones in the arms and legs) fractures;

- bruises around the head, neck, or chest.

## The Child's Development and Education

What makes AHT so devastating is that it often involves a total brain injury. For example, a child whose vision is severely impaired won't be able to learn through observation, which decreases the child's overall ability to learn.

The development of language, vision, balance, and motor coordination, all of which occur to varying degrees after birth, are particularly likely to be affected in any child who has AHT. Such impairment can require rigorous physical and occupational therapy to help the child acquire skills that would have developed on their own had the brain injury not occurred.

As they get older, kids who were shaken as babies may require special education and continued therapy to help with language development and daily living skills, such as dressing themselves.

Before age three years, a child can receive speech or physical therapy through the Department of Public Health/Early Intervention. Federal law requires that each state provide these services for children who have developmental disabilities as a result of being abused.

Some schools are also increasingly providing information and developmental assessments for kids under the age of three years. Parents can turn to a variety of rehabilitation and other therapists for early intervention services for children after abusive head trauma. Developmental assessments can assist in improving education outcomes as well as the overall well-being of the child. After a child who's been diagnosed with abusive head trauma turns three years old, it's the school district's responsibility to provide additional special educational services.

## *Preventing AHT*

Abusive head trauma is 100% preventable. A key aspect of prevention is increasing awareness of the potential dangers of shaking.

Finding ways to alleviate the parent or caregiver's stress at the critical moments when a baby is crying can significantly reduce the risk to the child. Some hospital-based programs have helped new parents identify and prevent shaking injuries and understand how to respond when infants cry.

The National Center on Shaken Baby Syndrome offers a prevention program, the Period of Purple Crying, which seeks to help parents and other caregivers understand crying in normal infants. By defining and describing the sometimes inconsolable infant crying that can sometimes cause stress, anger, and frustration in parents and caregivers, the program hopes to educate and empower people to prevent AHT.

One method that may help is author Dr. Harvey Karp's "five S's":

1. Shushing (using "white noise" or rhythmic sounds that mimic the constant whir of noise in the womb, with things like vacuum cleaners, hair dryers, clothes dryers, a running tub, or a white noise compact disc [CD]).

2. Side/stomach positioning (placing the baby on the left side— to help digestion—or on the belly while holding him or her, then putting the sleeping baby in the crib or bassinet on his or her back).

3. Sucking (letting the baby breastfeed or bottle-feed, or giving the baby a pacifier or finger to suck on).

4. Swaddling (wrapping the baby up snugly in a blanket to help him or her feel more secure).

5.  **S**winging gently (rocking in a chair, using an infant swing, or taking a car ride to help duplicate the constant motion the baby felt in the womb).

If a baby in your care won't stop crying, you can also try the following:

- Make sure the baby's basic needs are met (for example, he or she isn't hungry and doesn't need to be changed).

- Check for signs of illness, like fever or swollen gums.

- Rock or walk with the baby.

- Sing or talk to the baby.

- Offer the baby a pacifier or a noisy toy.

- Take the baby for a ride in a stroller or strapped into a child safety seat in the car.

- Hold the baby close against your body and breathe calmly and slowly.

- Call a friend or relative for support or to take care of the baby while you take a break.

- If nothing else works, put the baby on his or her back in the crib, close the door, and check on the baby in ten minutes.

- Call your doctor if nothing seems to be helping your infant, in case there is a medical reason for the fussiness.

To prevent potential AHT, parents and caregivers of infants need to learn how to respond to their own stress. It's important to talk to anyone caring for your baby about the dangers of shaking and how it can be prevented.

Chapter 17

# Munchausen by Proxy Syndrome

**Munchausen by proxy syndrome (MBPS)** is a relatively uncommon condition that involves the exaggeration or fabrication of illnesses or symptoms by a primary caretaker. One of the most harmful forms of child abuse, MBPS was named after Baron von Munchausen, an 18th century German dignitary known for telling outlandish stories.

## About MBPS

In MBPS, an individual—usually a mother—deliberately makes another person (most often his or her own preschool child) sick or convinces others that the person is sick. The parent or caregiver misleads others into thinking that the child has medical problems by lying and reporting fictitious episodes. He or she may exaggerate, fabricate, or induce symptoms. As a result, doctors usually order tests, try different types of medications, and may even hospitalize the child or perform surgery to determine the cause.

Typically, the perpetrator feels satisfied by gaining the attention and sympathy of doctors, nurses, and others who come into contact

"Munchausen by Proxy Syndrome," December 2008, reprinted with permission from www.kidshealth.org. Copyright © 2008 The Nemours Foundation. This information was provided by KidsHealth, one of the largest resources online for medically reviewed health information written for parents, kids, and teens. For more articles like this one, visit www.KidsHealth.org or www.TeensHealth.org.

with him or her and the child. Some experts believe that it isn't just the attention that's gained from the "illness" of the child that drives this behavior, but also the satisfaction in being able to deceive individuals that they consider to be more important and powerful than themselves.

Because the parent or caregiver appears to be so caring and attentive, often no one suspects any wrongdoing. A perplexing aspect of the syndrome is the ability of the parent or caregiver to fool and manipulate doctors. Frequently, the perpetrator is familiar with the medical profession and is very good at fooling the doctors. Even the most experienced doctors can miss the meaning of the inconsistencies in the child's symptoms. It's not unusual for medical personnel to overlook the possibility of MBPS because it goes against the belief that a parent or caregiver would never deliberately hurt his or her child.

Children who are subject to MBPS are typically preschool age, although there have been reported cases in kids up to 16 years old, and there are equal numbers of boys and girls. About 98% of the perpetrators are female.

Diagnosis is very difficult, but would involve some of the following:

- A child who has multiple medical problems that don't respond to treatment or that follow a persistent and puzzling course

- Physical or laboratory findings that are highly unusual, don't correspond with the child's medical history, or are physically or clinically impossible

- Short-term symptoms that tend to stop when the perpetrator isn't around

- A parent or caregiver who isn't reassured by "good news" when test results find no medical problems, but continues to believe that the child is ill

- A parent or caregiver who appears to be medically knowledgeable or fascinated with medical details or appears to enjoy the hospital environment

- A parent or caregiver who's unusually calm in the face of serious difficulties with the child's health

- A parent or caregiver who's highly supportive and encouraging of the doctor, or one who is angry and demands further intervention, more procedures, second opinions, or transfers to more sophisticated facilities

## Causes of MBPS

In some cases, the parents or caregivers themselves were abused, both physically and sexually, as children. They may have come from families in which being sick was a way to get love. The parent's or caregiver's own personal needs overcome his or her ability to see the child as a person with feelings and rights, possibly because the parent or caregiver may have grown up being treated like he or she wasn't a person with rights or feelings.

Other theories say that Munchausen by proxy syndrome is a cry for help on the part of the parent or caregiver, who may be experiencing anxiety or depression or have feelings of inadequacy as a parent or caregiver of a young child. Some may feel a sense of acknowledgement when the doctor confirms their caregiving skills. Or, the parent or caregiver may just enjoy the attention that the sick child—and, therefore, he or she—gets.

The suspected person may also have symptoms similar to the child's own medical problems or an illness history that's puzzling and unusual. He or she frequently has an emotionally distant relationship with a spouse, who often fails to visit the seriously ill child or have contact with doctors.

## What Happens to the Child?

In the most severe instances, parents or caregivers with MBPS may go to great lengths to make their children sick. When cameras were placed in some children's hospital rooms, some perpetrators were filmed switching medications, injecting kids with urine to cause an infection, or placing drops of blood in urine specimens.

Some perpetrators aggravate an existing problem, such as manipulating a wound so that it doesn't heal. One parent discovered that scrubbing the child's skin with oven cleaner would cause a baffling, long-lasting rash.

Whatever the course, the child's symptoms—whether created or faked—don't happen when the parent isn't present, and they usually go away during periods of separation from the parent. When confronted, the parent usually denies knowing how the illness occurred.

According to experts, common conditions and symptoms that are created or faked by parents or caregivers with MBPS include: failure to thrive, allergies, asthma, vomiting, diarrhea, seizures, and infections.

The long-term prognosis for these children depends on the degree of damage created by the perpetrator and the amount of time it takes to recognize and diagnose MBPS. Some extreme cases have been reported in which children developed destructive skeletal changes, limps, mental retardation, brain damage, and blindness from symptoms caused by the parent or caregiver. Often, these children require multiple surgeries, each with the risk for future medical problems.

If the child lives to be old enough to comprehend what's happening, the psychological damage can be significant. The child may come to feel that he or she will only be loved when ill and may, therefore, help the parent try to deceive doctors, using self-abuse to avoid being abandoned. And so, some victims of MBPS later become perpetrators themselves.

## Getting Help for the Child

If Munchausen by proxy syndrome is suspected, health care providers are required by law to report their concerns. However, after a parent or caregiver is charged, the child's symptoms may increase as the person who is accused attempts to prove the presence of the illness. If the parent or caregiver repeatedly denies the charges, the child should be removed from the home and legal action should be taken on the child's behalf.

In some cases, the parent or caregiver may deny the charges and move to another location, only to continue the behavior. Even if the child is returned to the perpetrator's custody while protective services are still involved, the child may continue to be a victim of abuse. For these reasons, it's always advised that these cases be resolved quickly.

## Getting Help for the Parent or Caregiver

Most often, abusive Munchausen by proxy syndrome cases are resolved in one of three ways:

1. The perpetrator is apprehended.

2. The perpetrator moves on to a younger child when the original victim gets old enough to "tell."

3. The child dies.

To get help, the parent or caregiver must admit to the abuse and seek psychological treatment. But if the perpetrator doesn't admit to the wrongdoing, psychological treatment has little chance of remedying the situation. Psychotherapy depends on truth, and MBPS perpetrators generally live in denial.

Chapter 18

# Corporal Punishment and Child Abuse

## Chapter Contents

## Section 18.1

# *Link between Spanking and Physical Abuse*

"UNC Study Shows Link between Spanking and Physical Abuse," August 19, 2008. © 2008 University of North Carolina Medical Center News Office. Reprinted with permission.

Spanking has been, and still is, a common method of child discipline used by American parents. But mothers who report that they or their partner spanked their child in the past year are nearly three times more likely to state that they also used harsher forms of punishment than those who say their child was not spanked, according to a new study led by the Injury Prevention Research Center at the University of North Carolina (UNC) at Chapel Hill. Such punishments included behaviors considered physically abusive by the researchers, such as beating, burning, kicking, hitting with an object somewhere other than the buttocks, or shaking a child less than two years old.

"In addition, increases in the frequency of spanking are associated with increased odds of abuse, and mothers who report spanking on the buttocks with an object—such as a belt or a switch—are nine times more likely to report abuse, compared to mothers who report no spanking with an object," said Adam J. Zolotor, M.D., the study's lead author and an assistant professor in the department of family medicine in the UNC School of Medicine. The study was published on the website of the *American Journal of Preventive Medicine* on Tuesday (August 19, 2008) and was scheduled for publication in the print version of the journal on September 17, 2008.

Although some surveys show evidence of a modest decline in spanking over the last 30 years, recent surveys show that up to 90 percent of children between the ages of three and five years are spanked by their parents at least occasionally.

Zolotor and his co-authors conducted an anonymous telephone survey on parenting of a probability sample of 1,435 mothers in North Carolina and South Carolina in 2002. Forty-five percent of the mothers reported that they or their partner had spanked their child in the previous 12 months and 25 percent reported spanking with an object on the buttocks. Four percent reported using harsher forms of punishment that met the study's definition of physical abuse.

Statistical analyses of the survey data found that while any spanking was associated with increased risk of abuse, spanking with an object was strongly associated with abuse. Only two percent of the mothers who reported no spanking reported use of physically abusive punishment. In comparison, six percent of mothers who reported spanking and 12 percent of mothers who reported spanking with an object also reported abusive punishment.

"This study demonstrated for the first time that parents who report spanking children with an object and parents who frequently spank children are much more likely to report other harsh punishment acts consistent with physical abuse," Zolotor said. The study concluded that efforts to reduce spanking, especially with an object, through media, educational, and legislative means may reduce physical child abuse.

The American Academy of Pediatrics states that "striking a child with an object is unacceptable and may be dangerous." Zolotor said the study supports this policy statement by underscoring that while spanking increases the likelihood of physical abuse, frequent spanking and spanking with an object are far more likely to lead to abuse. He said this may be due to the limited effectiveness of discipline when parents have few other tools for discipline (such as positive reinforcement and time-out).

# Section 18.2

## *Corporal Punishment in Schools*

Excerpted from "Plain Talk about Spanking (2009 Edition)," by Jordan Riak, Produced and distributed by Parents and Teachers Against Violence in Education (PTAVE), P.O. Box 1033, Alamo, CA 94507. The complete text of this booklet is available at http://nospank.net/pt2009.pdf.

### *Spanking at School*

The disciplinary hitting of students in the United States typically involves battering the buttocks with a flat board called a paddle. At the time of this writing, the practice is legal in 21 states. It should be understood that paddling is not the only method used to inflict pain on students. Forced exercise and denial of use of the bathroom, for instance, are commonly used as forms of corporal punishment. But paddling, because it is specifically prescribed and so blatant, serves to overshadow and thereby give cover to less obvious forms of abuse.

Corporal punishment is deemed by its users and defenders as being in the children's best interests and essential to the smooth functioning of the school. Were that true, schools that are the most punitive would be the highest-performing, children who are routinely punished would be the best behaved, and teachers' colleges would teach paddling. In fact, school systems with the highest rates of corporal punishment are the worst performing, children who are the most punished are the most troubled and difficult to manage, and there is not one accredited college in the United States that instructs future educators in the proper method for hitting children. Documented research shows a correlation between school corporal punishment and certain negative social outcomes. States that have the highest rates of school paddling also have the lowest graduation rates, the highest rates of teen pregnancy, the highest incarceration rates and the highest murder rates. (For further information, see "Correlation between high rates of corporal punishment in public schools and social pathologies," 2002, online at http://www.nospank.net/corrrelationstudy.htm.)

The use of corporal punishment in schools also has a demoralizing effect on teachers who don't condone the practice. They have difficulty working alongside paddlers. Their survival in such an environment depends on their willingness to remain silent about what they witness. They know that paddlers feel threatened by their very presence. It's not unusual for a paddling school to degenerate to a level where it is nothing more than a magnet and safe haven for incompetent teachers, including some who are dangerously unfit to be left in charge of children. Teachers who favor a power-based management style, including the use of corporal punishment, sometimes rise to positions of authority where they set a bad example for everyone under their control and influence. A teacher recounts this experience when he applied for a position in such a place:

> The interview began with the director asking me how I felt about corporal punishment. I told him that I disapproved of it and that I couldn't and wouldn't do it. He replied, 'Well, since that's the way you feel, you're of no use to us here,' and the interview was over."

School corporal punishment has disappeared nearly everywhere in the developed world. Not one country in Europe permits it, and abolition is spreading at a rapid pace among developing nations. Virtually nowhere is there any movement within governments or among educators to reverse this trend and return to the old ways. Only one country on record temporarily revoked its prohibition against hitting students: Germany during the Nazi era. Meanwhile, approximately 1/4 million beatings are inflicted on students in schools of the United States every year. Typical injuries resulting from spanking can be viewed online at http://www.nospank.net/violatn.htm.

What should enlightened, responsible parents do about corporal punishment in their schools? If you knew that a school bus had bald tires and faulty brakes, you would not let your child ride that bus, and you would demand that your school authorities correct the problem immediately. If you knew that the air ducts in your school were contaminated with asbestos and the classrooms were painted with lead-based paint, you'd remove your child immediately and alert other parents to the danger. Corporal punishment is no different. It is very dangerous, and all sensible people in the community should unite in opposition to it.

# Chapter 19

# *Emotional Abuse of Children*

## *What is emotional abuse?*

Emotional abuse of a child is commonly defined as a pattern of behavior by parents or caregivers that can seriously interfere with a child's cognitive, emotional, psychological, or social development. Emotional abuse of a child—also referred to as psychological maltreatment—can include the following:

- **Ignoring:** Either physically or psychologically, the parent or caregiver is not present to respond to the child. He or she may not look at the child and may not call the child by name.

- **Rejecting:** This is an active refusal to respond to a child's needs (for example: refusing to touch a child, denying the needs of a child, ridiculing a child).

- **Isolating:** The parent or caregiver consistently prevents the child from having normal social interactions with peers, family members, and adults. This also may include confining the child or limiting the child's freedom of movement.

- **Exploiting or corrupting:** In this kind of abuse, a child is taught, encouraged, or forced to develop inappropriate or illegal

"Emotional Abuse Fact Sheet," © 2007 American Humane Association (www.americanhumane.org). Reprinted with permission.

behaviors. It may involve self-destructive or antisocial acts of the parent or caregiver, such as teaching a child how to steal or forcing a child into prostitution.

- **Verbally assaulting:** This involves constantly belittling, shaming, ridiculing, or verbally threatening the child.

- **Terrorizing:** Here, the parent or caregiver threatens or bullies the child and creates a climate of fear for the child. Terrorizing can include placing the child or the child's loved one (such as a sibling, pet, or toy) in a dangerous or chaotic situation, or placing rigid or unrealistic expectations on the child with threats of harm if they are not met.

- **Neglecting the child:** This abuse may include educational neglect, where a parent or caregiver fails or refuses to provide the child with necessary educational services; mental health neglect, where the parent or caregiver denies or ignores a child's need for treatment for psychological problems; or medical neglect, where a parent or caregiver denies or ignores a child's need for treatment for medical problems.

While the definition of emotional abuse is often complex and imprecise, professionals agree that, for most parents, occasional negative attitudes or actions are not considered emotional abuse. Even the best of parents have occasions when they have momentarily lost control and said hurtful things to their children, failed to give them the attention they wanted, or unintentionally scared them.

What is truly harmful, according to James Garbarino, a national expert on emotional abuse, is the persistent, chronic pattern that "erodes and corrodes a child." (1994). Many experts concur that emotional abuse is typically not an isolated incident.

### *Why does it happen?*

Emotional abuse can, and does, happen in all types of families, regardless of their background. Most parents want the best for their children. However, some parents may emotionally and psychologically harm their children because of stress, poor parenting skills, social isolation, lack of available resources, or inappropriate expectations of their children. They may emotionally abuse their children because the parents or caregivers were emotionally abused themselves as children.

170

## What are the effects of emotional abuse?

Douglas Besharov states in *Recognizing Child Abuse: A Guide for the Concerned,* "Emotional abuse is an assault on the child's psyche, just as physical abuse is an assault on the child's body" (1990). Children who are constantly ignored, shamed, terrorized, or humiliated suffer at least as much, if not more, than if they are physically assaulted. Danya Glaser (2002) finds that emotional abuse can be "more strongly predictive of subsequent impairments in the children's development than the severity of physical abuse."

An infant who is severely deprived of basic emotional nurturance, even though physically well cared for, can fail to thrive and can eventually die. Babies with less severe emotional deprivation can grow into anxious and insecure children who are slow to develop and who have low self-esteem.

Although the visible signs of emotional abuse in children can be difficult to detect, the hidden scars of this type of abuse manifest in numerous behavioral ways, including insecurity, poor self-esteem, destructive behavior, angry acts (such as fire setting and animal cruelty), withdrawal, poor development of basic skills, alcohol or drug abuse, suicide, difficulty forming relationships, and unstable job histories.

Emotionally abused children often grow up thinking that they are deficient in some way. A continuing tragedy of emotional abuse is that when these children become parents they may continue the cycle with their own children.

## Identifying and Preventing Emotional Abuse

Some children may experience emotional abuse only, without ever experiencing another form of abuse. However, emotional abuse typically is associated with and results from other types of abuse and neglect, which makes it a significant risk factor in all child abuse and neglect cases. Brassard, Germain, and Hart (1987, as cited in Pecora et al., 2000) assert that emotional abuse is "inherent in all forms of child maltreatment."

Emotional abuse that exists independently of other forms of abuse is the most difficult form of child abuse to identify and stop. This is because child protective services must have demonstrable evidence that harm to a child has been done before they can intervene. And, since emotional abuse doesn't result in physical evidence, such as bruising or malnutrition, it can be very hard to diagnose.

Researchers have developed diagnostic tools to help professionals who work with children and families identify and treat emotional abuse. Professionals are taught to identify risk factors for emotional abuse, ask appropriate questions about a family's history and the family's present behaviors, and provide appropriate resources (such as financial resources, mental health services, or parenting classes) to help parents and caregivers create safe, stable environments for their children and themselves.

## What You Can Do

All children need acceptance, love, encouragement, discipline, consistency, stability, and positive attention. What can you do when you feel your behavior toward your child is not embodying these qualities but is bordering on emotional abuse? Here are some suggestions:

• Never be afraid to apologize to your child. If you lose your temper and say something in anger that wasn't meant to be said, apologize. Children need to know that adults can admit when they are wrong.

• Don't call your child names or attach labels to your child. Names such as "Stupid" or "Lazy," or phrases like "good for nothing," "You'll never amount to anything," "If you could only be more like your brother," and "You can never do anything right," tear at a child's self-esteem. A child deserves respect.

• Address the behavior that needs correcting and use appropriate discipline techniques, such as time-outs or natural consequences. Be sure to discuss the child's behavior and the reason for the discipline, both before and immediately after you discipline. Discipline should be provided to correct your child's behavior, rather than to punish or humiliate him or her.

• Compliment your child when he or she accomplishes even a small task, or when you see good behavior.

• Walk away from a situation when you feel you are losing control. Isolate yourself in another room for a few minutes (after first making sure the child is safe), count to ten before you say anything, ask for help from another adult, or take a few deep breaths before reacting.

• Get help. Support is available for families at risk of emotional abuse through local child protection services agencies, community centers, churches, physicians, mental health facilities, and schools.

## References

Besharov, D. J. (1990). *Recognizing child abuse: A guide for the concerned*. New York: The Free Press.

Garbarino, J., and Garbarino, A. (1994). *Emotional maltreatment of children*. Chicago: National Committee to Prevent Child Abuse, 2nd Ed.

Glaser, D. (2002, June). Emotional abuse and neglect (psychological maltreatment): A conceptual framework. *Child Abuse & Neglect*, 26, 697–714.

Pecora, P., Whittaker, J., Maluccio, A., and Barth, R. (2000). *The child welfare challenge*. New York: Aldine de Gruyter.

## Resources

Dubowitz, H., and DePanfilis, D. (Eds.). (2000). *Handbook for child protection practice*. Thousand Oaks, CA: Sage Publications, Inc.

Feild, T., and Winterfeld, A. (2003). Guidelines on abuse—Emotional abuse. *Tough problems, tough choices: Guidelines for needs-based service planning in child welfare*. Englewood, CO: American Humane and Casey Outcomes and Decision-Making Project.

Chapter 20

# Harassment and Abuse in Youth Sports

The age-old notion that children's participation in organized sports should be fun, contribute to physical and emotional development, and enhance social skills has been swept aside in what's become an increasingly hostile environment that's ultra-competitive, high-pressured, and often encourages and rewards a do-anything-it-takes-to-win approach. Parents and volunteer coaches, the most important role models in a young athlete's life, pay lip service to the importance of good sportsmanship and simply doing the best they can. But, it has become all too clear through their actions that what the scoreboard says at the conclusion of the game is what it is really all about. Adults, in their roles as coaches, league administrators, and spectators, are often inflicting their misguided motives and ideals on youth sports and, in the process, depriving youngsters of what should be a fun-filled experience.

Youth sports have become a hotbed of chaos, violence, and meanspiritedness. Physical and emotional abuse of children, rampant cheating, and total disrespect for opponents are but a few of the unacceptable behaviors being tolerated. These disgraceful behaviors have polluted the youth sports landscape, poisoned the fun, distorted child development, and left behind countless children with broken hearts, crushed dreams, and shattered psyches.

Text in this chapter is excerpted from "Recommendations for Communities," © 2003 National Alliance for Youth Sports. Reprinted with permission. Reviewed in March 2009 by Dr. David A. Cooke, MD, FACP.

175

The following incidents have taken place: Two women assaulted a mother following a youth baseball championship game in Utah that left her unconscious; a youth baseball coach for children ages 12 and 13 was taken into custody in Wisconsin on accusations that he grabbed and wrestled an umpire to the ground; a baseball coach in New Jersey was fined $1,000 and sentenced to five days in the sheriff's work program for assaulting one of his 13-year-old players during a practice; more than 30 adults brawled at the conclusion of an under-14 soccer tournament game in Los Angeles that led to three parents being arrested; a youth league baseball coach in Cleveland was thrown out of a game following a profane outburst that led sheriff's deputies to cite him for disorderly conduct; in Tennessee a 16-year-old was charged with attempted second-degree murder after he used an aluminum bat to bash the head of a pitcher who struck him out during a youth baseball game; an umpire and parent were called into police headquarters after exchanging blows at a baseball game among grade schoolers in New Jersey; a soccer dad was arrested after taking a swing at the father of an opposing player at a game in Indiana; a parent was arrested in Florida on charges he hit a Little League umpire and cut one of his truck tires after a game; in Michigan, a parent had a complaint filed against him by another parent accusing him of yelling obscenities and threatening a child on the opposing team; and in Ohio, a youth soccer player fractured a goalie's cheekbone with a kick to the face at the end of a game that left the player unconscious, along with injuries to his eyes, nose, jaw, and teeth.

These are just a few examples of the many incidents that are taking place in big cities and small towns across the country. Sadly, there are thousands of other incidents of physical and emotional abuse of children that go unnoticed, or are simply ignored due to misguided adults who fail to distinguish the difference between sports at the professional and collegiate levels with those of children playing in youth leagues across the country. A coach or parent's unkind words or actions on the playing field won't make the headlines of the local newspaper or that evening's television newscast, but that doesn't mean the damage to the youngster is any less severe.

A youth sports study conducted by the Minnesota Amateur Sports Commission (MASC) found that:

- 45.3% of the youngsters surveyed said they had been called names, yelled at, or insulted while participating in sports;

- 21% said they had been pressured to play with an injury;

- 17.5% said they had been hit, kicked, or slapped while participating in sports;

- 8.2% said they had been pressured to intentionally harm others while playing sports;

- 8% said they had been called names with sexual connotations while participating in sports; and,

- 3.4% said they had been pressured into sex or sexual touching.

Children can learn many positive attributes through their sports participation that they can carry with them the rest of their life. Unfortunately, the same holds true for negative aspects as well. If children are told that it is okay to cheat in sports in order to win, then the message they're hearing is that it is all right to cheat in everyday life. If they see that violence is used to settle disputes on the playing field, then that is likely an option they will choose when they encounter a difficult problem later in life. It is a vicious cycle, and every child who is instilled with these attitudes is one more person that's being sent out into the world with the negative tools to contribute to the moral decay of our society.

In an article entitled *Kids Speak Out: Violence in Youth Sports* that appeared in the August, 2001 issue of *Sports Illustrated For Kids*, 57 percent of the more than 3,000 responses said there was too much violence in youth sports; and 74 percent said they have seen out-of-control adults at their games. Thirty-six percent of the children cited embarrassment as the top emotion they felt when witnessing bad adult behavior, followed by disappointment (25%), anger (23%), and fear (16%). In response to what kind of bad behavior they had seen, 37 percent said parents yelling at kids, 27 percent said parents yelling at coaches or officials, 25 percent said coaches yelling at officials or kids, and four percent said violence by adults. When children were asked, what is the best way to get parents to behave, 48 percent said the kids should tell their parents to relax, 36 percent said parents should be banned from games if they cannot control themselves, and 15 percent said they should have parents sign a code of conduct.

In May of 2001, Survey USA polled 500 parents in Indianapolis, Indiana on their views on violence in youth sports. The survey found that 55 percent of the parents polled said they have seen parents engage in verbal disputes at youth sporting events; 21 percent of the parents said they've witnessed a physical altercation between other parents at the youth sporting event; and 73 percent believe that parents who become physically or verbally abusive during games should be banned from youth sports. A similar study was conducted by Survey USA in a five-county region in South Florida in 1999 that found that 82 percent felt that parents are too aggressive in youth sports; 56 percent said they have seen aggressive parents in youth sports; and 72 percent believe aggressive parents should be banned from youth sports.

One of the primary weaknesses found in many organized youth sports programs is that no policies typically exist to deal with basic problems that often surface. In fact, even when policies are in place, they often are outdated or simply don't focus on the well-being of children, and consequently they end up fueling problems rather than alleviating them.

Furthermore, when a large number of adults are thrown together in a youth sports setting, they're each going to be bringing their own morals, attitudes, and beliefs to the games. Consequently, the chances of conflict arising are quite high. The potential for these problems to surface is even greater when no type of program or training exists to inform coaches, parents, officials, and administrators of their roles and responsibilities and the expected behavior; as well as if no policies are in place to deal with basic issues that are sure to emerge at some point during the season.

Again, consider that the problems that are prevalent in youth sports today concerning violent behavior, verbal abuse, and the mistreatment of children, would not be tolerated in our school systems. So, why are they accepted in youth sports?

## Changing the Culture in Your Community

Throughout the country, approximately 2.5 million volunteers fill vital roles as coaches and administrators in youth sports. These individuals are well-meaning, and more often than not have the best of intentions when they assume these positions. Unfortunately, a large number have never been sufficiently trained in all of the key areas that encompass their responsibilities. This often leads to implementing policies and making decisions that don't serve the best interests of the children who are participating. Consequently, an abundance of youth sports programs currently exist that actually are exposing children to needless risks—both physically and emotionally.

Throughout the more than half-century existence of organized youth sports in this country, programs have continually been conducted in which few, if any, individuals are held accountable for what transpires on the playing field. Programs that operate in a mode in which education and accountability are not an integral part of the process are asking for trouble in the form of needless and time-consuming litigation; exposing itself to a greater chance on on-field violence; and causing irreparable harm to countless children.

So, how do leaders in the community go about getting all the adults involved in the program to bond together and work toward a common goal? If there's a firm belief entrenched throughout the community regarding the importance of positive sports in a child's life, then the framework is already in place to achieve top-quality programming.

The positive attributes that are often associated with sports include fun, fitness, skill building, teamwork, learning to follow rules, enhanced social skills, commitment, discipline, and so forth. Obviously, we expect children to gain these same benefits from attending school. Furthermore, when children go to school we want it to be fun so that kids will enjoy learning and have a deep-rooted interest in wanting to continue the learning process for years to come. The same goes for sports. We also want kids to grow self-confident and build their self-esteem by achieving varying levels of success in school. Again, the same goes for sports, it all fits. In fact, it can safely be said that youth sports is an extension of the child's education, where they can continue to learn and develop each of these important aspects basic to positive and productive human growth and development.

If the operational philosophy is adopted whereby the primary goal is to generate outcomes in sports programs that match the expectations of our school system, then great strides can be made in the overall delivery and effectiveness of sports programs.

Changing the culture of children's sports is not as difficult as it may seem at first glance. There are several resources and educational tools readily available that can enhance a community's youth sports programming, and help redirect its focus to ensure that youngsters reap the many benefits that are available when programs are conducted with the best interests of children as the primary objective.

Chapter 21

# Children Who Bully

Bullying among children is aggressive behavior that is intentional and that involves an imbalance of power or strength. Typically, it is repeated over time. Bullying can take many forms such as hitting or punching (physical bullying); teasing or name-calling (verbal bullying); intimidation through gestures or social exclusion (nonverbal bullying or emotional bullying); and sending insulting messages by e-mail (cyberbullying).

There is no one single cause of bullying among children. Rather, individual, family, peer, school, and community factors can place a child or youth at risk for bullying his or her peers.

### Characteristics of Children Who Bully

Children who bully their peers regularly (those who admit to bullying more than occasionally) tend to have these characteristics:

- Be impulsive, hot-headed, dominant
- Be easily frustrated
- Lack empathy

---

This chapter includes text from "Children Who Bully," Health Resources and Services Administration (HRSA), 2004; "Warning Signs That a Child Is Being Bullied," HRSA, 2004; and, "Myths about Bullying," HRSA, 2004. Reviewed in March 2009 by Dr. David A. Cooke, MD, FACP.

- Have difficulty following rules
- View violence in a positive way

Boys who bully tend to be physically stronger than other children.

### Family Risk Factors for Bullying

Children who bully are more likely than their non-bullying peers to live in homes where there is:

- a lack of warmth and involvement on the part of parents;
- overly-permissive parenting (including a lack of limits for children's behavior);
- a lack of supervision by parents;
- harsh, physical discipline; and
- a model for bullying behavior.

### Peer Risk Factors for Bullying

Children and youth who bully are more likely to have friends who bully and who have positive attitudes toward violence.

### Bullying and Other Violent or Antisocial Behaviors

Research shows that bullying can be a sign of other serious antisocial or violent behavior. Children and youth who frequently bully their peers are more likely than others to do the following:

- Get into frequent fights
- Be injured in a fight
- Vandalize property
- Steal property
- Drink alcohol
- Smoke
- Be truant from school
- Drop out of school
- Carry a weapon

Research also shows that:

- children who bully are more likely to report that they own guns for risky reasons, such as to gain respect or frighten others; and

- boys who were identified as bullies in middle school were four times as likely as their non bullying peers to have more than one criminal conviction by age 24.

## Warning Signs That a Child Is Being Bullied

Many children, particularly boys and older children, do not tell their parents or adults at school about being bullied. It is important that adults are vigilant to possible signs of bullying.

### Warning Signs

Possible warning signs that a child is being bullied include the following:

- Comes home with torn, damaged, or missing pieces of clothing, books, or other belongings

- Has unexplained cuts, bruises, and scratches

- Has few, if any friends, with whom he or she spends time

- Seems afraid of going to school, walking to and from school, riding the school bus, or taking part in organized activities with peers (such as clubs)

- Takes a long, "illogical" route when walking to or from school

- Has lost interest in school work or suddenly begins to do poorly in school

- Appears sad, moody, teary, or depressed when he or she comes home

- Complains frequently of headaches, stomachaches, or other physical ailments

- Has trouble sleeping or has frequent bad dreams

- Experiences a loss of appetite

- Appears anxious and suffers from low self-esteem

## Myths about Bullying

### Bullying Is the Same Thing as Conflict

Wrong. Bullying is aggressive behavior that involves an imbalance of power or strength. Often, bullying is repeated over time.

Conflict involves antagonism among two or more people. Whereas any two people can have a conflict (or a disagreement or a fight), bullying only occurs where there is a power imbalance—where one child has a hard time defending himself or herself. Why is the difference between bullying and conflict important? Conflict resolution or mediation strategies are sometimes misused to solve bullying problems. These strategies can send the message that both children are "partly right and partly wrong," or that, "We need to work out the conflict between you." These messages are not appropriate messages in cases of bullying (or in any situation where someone is being victimized). The appropriate message to the child who is bullied should be, "Bullying is wrong and no one deserves to be bullied. We are going to do everything we can to stop it."

What does work? Research suggests that the best way to deal with bullying is through comprehensive programs that focus on changing the climate of a school and the social norms of the group.

### Most Bullying Is Physical—Hitting, Shoving, Kicking

Physical bullying may be what first comes to mind when adults think about bullying. However, the most common form of bullying—both for boys and girls—is verbal bullying (for example: name-calling, rumor-spreading). It is also common for youth to bully each other through social isolation (such as shunning or leaving a child out on purpose).

### Bullying Isn't Serious—It's Just a Matter of "Kids Being Kids"

Bullying can be extremely serious. Bullying can affect the mental well-being, academic work, and physical health of children who are targeted. Children who are bullied are more likely than other children to have lower self-esteem, and higher rates of depression, loneliness, anxiety, and suicidal thoughts. They also are more likely to want to avoid attending school and have higher school absenteeism rates. Recent research on the health-related effects of bullying indicates that victims of frequent bullying are more likely to experience

184

headaches, sleeping problems, and stomach ailments. Some emotional scars can be long-lasting. Research suggests that adults who were bullied as children are more likely than their non-bullied peers to be depressed and have low self-esteem as adults.

Children who bully are more likely than other children to be engaged in other antisocial, violent, or troubling behaviors. Bullying can negatively affect children who observe bullying going on around them—even if they aren't targeted themselves.

### Bullying Doesn't Happen at My Child's School

Bullying is more common at some schools than others, however it can happen anywhere children and youth gather. Studies show that between 15%–25% of United States' students are bullied with some frequency ("sometimes or more often") while 15%–20% admit that they bully others with some frequency within a school term. The best way to find out about bullying at your child's school is to ask children and youth, themselves. One good way to do this is by administering an anonymous survey about where bullying occurs, when it occurs, and how often it occurs.

### Bullying Is Mostly a Problem in Urban Schools

Bullying occurs in rural, suburban, and urban communities, and among children of every income level, race, and geographic region.

### Bullying Is More Likely to Happen on the Bus Than at School

Although bullying does happen on the bus, most surveys indicate that bullying is more likely to occur on school grounds. Common locations for bullying include playgrounds, the classroom, the cafeteria, bathrooms, and hallways. A student survey can help determine where the hotspots are in any particular school.

### Children and Youth Who Are Bullied Will Usually Tell an Adult

Adults are often unaware of bullying—in part because many children and youth don't report it. Most studies find that only 25%–50% of bullied children talk to an adult about the bullying. Boys and older children are less likely than girls and younger children to tell adults about bullying. Why are children reluctant to report bullying? They may fear retaliation by children doing the bullying. They also may fear that adults won't take their concerns seriously or will deal inappropriately with the bullying situation.

### Children and Youth Who Bully Are Mostly Loners with Few Social Skills

Children who bully usually do not lack friends. In fact, some research finds that they have larger friendship networks than other children. Importantly, they usually have at least a small group of friends who support and encourage their bullying behavior. Bullies also generally have more leadership skills than victims of bullying or children not involved in bullying.

### Bullied Kids Need to Learn How to Deal with Bullying on Their Own

Some children have the confidence and skills to stop bullying when it happens, but many do not. Moreover, children shouldn't be expected to deal with bullying on their own. Bullying is a form of victimization or peer abuse. Just as society does not expect victims of other types of abuse (for example, child maltreatment or domestic abuse) to "deal with it on their own," we should not expect this from victims of bullying. Adults have critical roles to play in helping to stop bullying, as do other children who witness or observe bullying.

### Most Children and Youth Who Observe Bullying Don't Want to Get Involved

The good news is that most children and youth think that bullying is "not cool" and feel that they should do something if they see it happen. In a study of tweens, (Brown, Birch, and Kancherla, 2005), 56% said that they usually either say or do something to try to stop bullying that they observe or tell someone who could help. These children and youth play a critical role in helping stop bullying in schools and communities.

# Chapter 22

# *Youth Violence*

Youth violence refers to harmful behaviors that can start early and continue into young adulthood. The young person can be a victim, an offender, or a witness to the violence.

Youth violence includes various behaviors. Some violent acts—such as bullying, slapping, or hitting—can cause more emotional harm than physical harm. Others, such as robbery, assault, or rape, can lead to serious injury or even death.

### *Why is youth violence a public health problem?*

Youth violence is widespread in the United States (U.S.). It is the second leading cause of death for young people between the ages of 10 and 24.[1]

- In the U.S., 5,686 young people age 10 to 24 were murdered—an average of 16 each day—in 2005.[1]

- Over 720,000 violence-related injuries in young people age 10 to 24 were treated in U.S. emergency rooms in 2006.[1]

- In a 2005 nationwide survey, 36% of high school students reported being in a physical fight during the past 12 months.[2]

- Nearly 7% of high school students in 2005 reported taking a gun, knife, or club to school in the 30 days before the survey.[2]

"Understanding Youth Violence," Centers for Disease Control and Prevention (CDC), 2008.

- An estimated 30% of kids between 6th and 10th grade report being involved in bullying.[3]

### How does youth violence affect health?

Deaths resulting from youth violence are only part of the problem. Many young people seek medical care for violence-related injuries. These injuries can include cuts, bruises, broken bones, and gunshot wounds. Some injuries, like gunshot wounds, can lead to lasting disabilities.

Violence can also affect the health of communities. It can increase health care costs, decrease property values, and disrupt social services.[4] The cost of youth violence exceeds $158 billion each year.[5]

### Who is at risk for youth violence?

A number of factors can increase the risk of a youth engaging in violence. However, the presence of these factors does not always mean that a young person will become an offender.

Risk factors for youth violence include the following:

- Prior history of violence
- Drug, alcohol, or tobacco use
- Association with delinquent peers
- Poor family functioning
- Poor grades in school
- Poverty in the community

Note: This is only a partial list of risk factors.

### How can we prevent youth violence?

The ultimate goal is to stop youth violence before it starts. Several prevention strategies have been identified.

- Parent- and family-based programs improve family relations. Parents receive training on child development. They also learn skills for talking with their kids and solving problems in nonviolent ways.

- Social-development strategies teach children how to handle tough social situations. They learn how to resolve problems without using violence.

- Mentoring programs pair an adult with a young person. The adult serves as a positive role model and helps guide the young person's behavior.

- Changes can be made to the physical and social environment. These changes address the social and economic causes of violence.

## How do the Centers for Disease Control and Prevention (CDC) approach youth violence prevention?

CDC uses a 4-step approach to address public health problems like youth violence.

*Step 1: Define the Problem*

Before we can prevent youth violence, we need to know how big the problem is, where it is, and whom it affects. CDC learns about a problem by gathering and studying data. These data are critical because they help decision makers send resources where they are needed most.

*Step 2: Identify Risk and Protective Factors*

It is not enough to know that youth violence is affecting a certain group of people in a certain area. We also need to know why. CDC conducts and supports research to answer this question. Then programs can be developed to reduce or get rid of risk factors.

*Step 3: Develop and Test Prevention Strategies*

Using information gathered in research, CDC develops and tests strategies to prevent youth violence.

*Step 4: Ensure Widespread Adoption*

In this final step, CDC shares the best prevention strategies. CDC may also provide funding or technical help so communities can adopt these strategies.

## References

1. Centers for Disease Control and Prevention, National Center for Injury Prevention and Control. Web-based Injury Statistics

Query and Reporting System (WISQARS) [online]. (2008) [cited 2008 April 9]. Available from: http://www.cdc.gov/ncipc/wisqars.

2. Centers for Disease Control and Prevention. Youth risk behavioral surveillance—United States, 2005. *MMWR, Surveillance Summaries* 2006; 55(no. SS-5).

3. Nansel TR, Overpeck M, Pilla RS, Ruan WJ, Simons-Morton B, Scheidt P. Bullying behaviors among US youth: prevalence and association with psychosocial adjustment. *Journal of the American Medical Association* 2001; 285(16):2094–100.

4. Mercy J, Butchart A, Farrington D, Cerdá M. Youth violence. In: Krug E, Dahlberg LL, Mercy JA, Zwi AB, Lozano R, editors. *The World Report on Violence and Health*. Geneva (Switzerland): World Health Organization; 2002, p. 25–56.

5. Children's Safety Network Economics and Data Analysis Resource Center. *State costs of violence perpetrated by youth*. [cited 2006 Jul 31]. Available from: http://www.edarc.org/pubs/tables/youth-viol.htm.

# Chapter 23

# *Youth and Aggression through Technology*

### *How common is electronic aggression?*

Because electronic aggression is fairly new, limited information is available, and those researching the topic have asked different questions about it. Thus, information cannot be readily compared or combined across studies, which limits our ability to make definitive conclusions about the prevalence and impact of electronic aggression.

We know that most youth (65–91%) report little or no involvement in electronic aggression. However, 9% to 35% of young people say they have been the victim of electronic aggression. As with face-to-face bullying, estimates of electronic aggression perpetration are lower than victimization, ranging from 4% to 21%. In some cases, the higher end of the range (21% and 35%) reflects studies that asked about electronic aggression over a longer time period (a year as opposed to two months). In other cases, the higher percentages reflect studies that defined electronic aggression more broadly (spreading rumors, telling lies, or making threats as opposed to just telling lies).

We currently know little about whether certain types of electronic aggression are more common than other forms. A study that looked

Excerpted from "Electronic Media and Youth Violence: A CDC Issue Brief for Educators and Caregivers," Centers for Disease Control and Prevention (CDC), 2008. The complete report is available online at http://www.cdc.gov/violenceprevention/pdf/ EA-brief-a.pdf.

at electronic aggression victimization over the past year, found that making rude or nasty comments was the type of electronic aggression most frequently experienced by victims (32%), followed by rumor spreading (13%), and then by threatening or aggressive comments (14%).

## Who is at risk?

Whether the rates of electronic aggression perpetration and victimization differ for boys and girls is unknown. Research examining differences by sex is limited, and findings are conflicting. Some studies have not found any differences, while others have found that girls perpetrate electronic aggression more frequently than do boys.

There is also little information about whether electronic aggression decreases or increases as young people age. As with other forms of aggression, there is some evidence that electronic aggression is less common in 5th grade than in 8th grade, but is higher in 8th grade than 11th grade, suggesting that electronic aggression may peak around the end of middle school or beginning of high school.

Current studies on electronic aggression have focused primarily on white populations. We have no information on how electronic aggression varies by race or ethnicity.

It is important to note that there is an overlap between victims and perpetrators of electronic aggression. As with many types of violence, those who are victims are also at increased risk for being perpetrators. Across the studies conducted by our panelists between 7% and 14% of surveyed youth reported being both a victim and a perpetrator of electronic aggression.

Although the news media has recently devoted a lot of attention to the potential dangers of technology, face-to-face verbal and physical aggression are still far more common than electronic aggression. Verbal bullying is the type of bullying most often experienced by young people, followed by physical bullying, and then by electronic aggression. However, electronic aggression is becoming more common. In 2000, 6% of internet users ages 10–17 said they had been the victim of online harassment, defined as threats or other offensive behavior [not sexual solicitation] sent online to someone or posted online. By 2005, this percentage had increased to 9%. As technology becomes more affordable and sophisticated, rates of electronic aggression are likely to continue to increase, especially if appropriate prevention and intervention policies and practices are not put into place.

## What is the relationship between victims and perpetrators of electronic aggression?

Electronic technology allows adolescents to hide their identity, either by sending or posting messages anonymously, by using a false name, or by assuming someone else's on-screen identity. So, unlike the aggression or bullying that occurs in the school yard, victims and perpetrators of electronic aggression may not know the person with whom they are interacting. Between 13% and 46% of young people who were victims of electronic aggression, report not knowing the identity of their harasser. Similarly, 22% of young people who admit they perpetrate electronic aggression report they do not know the identity of their victim. In the school yard, the victim can respond to the bully or try to get a teacher or peer to help. In contrast, in the electronic world, a victim is often alone when responding to aggressive e-mails or text messages, and his or her only defense may be to turn off the computer, cell phone, or personal digital assistant (PDA). If the electronic aggression takes the form of posting of a message or an embarrassing picture of the victim on a public website, the victim may have no defense.

As for the victims and perpetrators who are not anonymous, in one study, almost half of the victims (47%) said the perpetrator was another student at school. In addition, aggression between siblings is no longer limited to the backseat of the car: 12% of victims reported their brother or sister was the perpetrator, and 10% of perpetrators reported being electronically aggressive toward a sibling.

## Do certain types of electronic technology pose a greater risk for victimization?

The news media often carry stories about young people victimized on social networking websites. Young people do experience electronic aggression in chat rooms: 25% of victims of electronic aggression said the victimization happened in a chat room and 23% said it happened on a website. However, instant messaging appears to be the most common way electronic aggression is perpetrated. Fifty-six percent of perpetrators of electronic aggression and 67% of victims said the aggression they experienced or perpetrated was through instant messaging. Victims also report experiencing electronic aggression through e-mail (25%) and text messages (16%).

The way electronic aggression is perpetrated (through instant messaging, the posting of pictures on a website, sending an e-mail) is also related to the relationship between the victim and the perpetrator.

Victims are significantly more likely to report receiving an aggressive instant message when they know the perpetrator from in-person situations (64% of victims), than they are if they only know the perpetrator online (34%). Young people who are victimized by people they only know online are significantly more likely than those victimized by people they know from in-person situations to be victimized through e-mail (18% versus 5%), chat rooms (18% versus 4%), and online gaming websites (14% versus 0%).

In terms of frequency, electronic aggression perpetrated by young people who know each other in-person appears to be more similar to face-to-face bullying than does aggression perpetrated by young people who only know each other online. For example, like in-person bullying, electronic aggression between young people who know each other in-person is more likely to consist of a series of incidents. Fifty-nine percent of the incidents perpetrated by young people who knew each other in-person involved a series of incidents by the same harasser, compared to 27% of incidents perpetrated by online-only contacts. In addition, 59% of the incidents perpetrated by young people who knew each other in-person involved sending or posting messages for others to see, versus 18% of those perpetrated by young people the victims only knew online.

### What problems are associated with being a victim of electronic aggression?

We are just beginning to look at the impact of being a victim of electronic aggression. At this point, we do not have information that shows that being a victim of electronic aggression causes a young person to have problems. However, the information we do have suggests that, as with young people who experience face-to-face aggression, those who are victims of electronic aggression are more likely to have some difficulties than those who are not victimized.

For example, young people who are victims of internet harassment are significantly more likely than those who have not been victimized to use alcohol and other drugs, receive school detention or suspension, skip school, or experience in-person victimization. Victims of internet harassment are also more likely than non-victims to have poor parental monitoring and to have weak emotional bonds with their caregiver. Although these difficulties could be the result of electronic victimization, they could also be factors that increase the risk of electronic victimization (but do not result from it), or they could be related to something else entirely. At this point, the risk factors for victimization through technology and the impact of victimization need further study.

Some research does show that the level of emotional distress experienced by a victim is related to the relationship between the victim and perpetrator and the frequency of the aggression. Young people who were bullied by the same person both online and off-line were more likely to report being distressed by the incident (46%) than were those who reported being bullied by different people online and off-line (15%), and those who did not know who was harassing them online (18%). Victims who were harassed by online peers and did not know their perpetrator in off-line settings also experienced distress, but they were more likely to experience distress if the harassment was perpetrated by the same person repeatedly (as opposed to a single incident), if the harasser was aged 18 or older, or if the harasser asked for a picture.

Finally, distress may not be limited to the young person who is victimized. Caregivers who are aware that their adolescent has been a victim of electronic aggression can also experience distress. Caregivers report that sometimes they are even more fearful, frustrated, and angry about the incidents of electronic aggression than are the young victims.

## *What are the problems associated with being a perpetrator of electronic aggression?*

Consistent with the discussion of victimization, we have limited information about what increases or decreases the chance that an adolescent will become a perpetrator of electronic aggression. One study suggests that young people who say they are connected to their school, perceive their school as trusting, fair, and pleasant, and believe their friends are trustworthy, caring, and helpful, are less likely to report being perpetrators of electronic, physical, and verbal aggression. We also have some evidence that perpetrators of electronic aggression are more likely to engage in other risky behaviors. For example, like perpetrators of other forms of aggression, perpetrators of electronic aggression are more likely to believe that bullying peers and encouraging others to bully peers are acceptable behaviors. Additionally, young people who report perpetrating electronic aggression are more likely to also report perpetrating face-to-face aggression.

## *Is electronic aggression just an extension of school yard bullying?*

Are the kids who are victims of electronic aggression the same kids who are victims of face-to-face aggression at school? Is electronic aggression just an extension of school yard bullying? The information we currently have suggests that the answer to the first question is maybe, and the answer to the second question is no. One study found that 65% of young people who reported being a victim of electronic aggression were not victimized at school. Conversely, another study found considerable overlap between electronic aggression and in-person bullying, either as victims or perpetrators. The study found few young people (6%) who were victims or perpetrators of electronic bullying were not bullied in-person.

Evidence that electronic aggression is not just an extension of school yard bullying comes from information from young people who are home-schooled. If electronic aggression was just an extension of school yard bullying, the rates of electronic aggression would be lower for those who are home-schooled than for those who attend public or private school. However, the rates of internet harassment for young people who are home-schooled and the rates for those who attend public and private schools are fairly similar.

The vast majority of electronic aggression appears to be experienced and perpetrated away from school grounds. Discussions with middle and high school students suggest that most electronic aggression occurs away from school property and outside of school hours, with the exception of electronic aggression perpetrated by text messaging using cell phones. Schools appear to be a less common setting because of the amount of structured activities during the school day and because of the limited access to technology during the school day for activities other than school work. Additionally, because other teens are less likely to be, for instance, on social-networking websites during school hours, the draw to such websites during the day is limited. Even when electronic aggression does occur at school, victimized students report that they are very reluctant to seek help because, in many cases, they would have to disclose that they violated school policies that often prohibit specific types of technology use (cell phones, social networking websites) during the school day.

Whether electronic aggression occurs at home or at school, it has implications for the school and needs further exploration. As was previously mentioned, young people who were harassed online were more likely to get a detention or be suspended, to skip school, and to experience emotional distress than those who were not harassed. In addition, young people who receive rude or nasty comments via text messaging are significantly more likely to report feeling unsafe at school.

## *What can we do?*

A common response to the problem of electronic aggression is to use blocking software to prevent young people from accessing certain websites. There are several limitations with this type of response, especially when the blocking software is the only option that is pursued. First, young people are also victimized via cell-phone text messaging, and blocking software will not prevent this type of victimization. Second, middle and high school students have indicated that blocking software at school is limited because many students can navigate their way around this software and because most students do not attempt to access social networking websites during the school day. Students can also access sites that may be blocked on home and school computers from another location. Finally, blocking software may limit some of the benefits young people experience from new technology including social networking websites. For instance, the growth of internet and cellular technology allows young people to have access to greater amounts of information, to stay connected with family and established friends, and to connect and learn from people worldwide. Additionally, some young people report that they feel better about themselves online than they do in the real world and feel it is easier to be accepted online. Thus, while blocking software may be one important tool that caregivers and schools choose to use, the panel emphasized the need for comprehensive solutions. For example, a combination of blocking software, educational classes about appropriate electronic behavior for students and parents, and regular communication between adults and young people about their experiences with technology would be preferable to any one of these strategies in isolation.

# Chapter 24

# *Teen Dating Abuse*

Dating violence is a type of intimate partner violence. It occurs between two people in a close relationship. There are three common types of dating violence.

- **Physical:** This occurs when a partner is pinched, hit, shoved, or kicked.

- **Emotional:** This means threatening a partner or harming his or her sense of self-worth. Examples include name calling, teasing, threats, bullying, or keeping him or her away from friends and family.

- **Sexual violence:** This is forcing a partner to engage in a sex act when he or she does not or cannot consent.

Unhealthy relationships can start early and last a lifetime. Dating violence often starts with teasing and name calling. These behaviors are often thought to be a normal part of a relationship. But these behaviors can lead to more serious violence like physical assault and rape.

## *Why is dating violence a public health problem?*

Dating violence is a serious problem in the United States. Many teens do not report it because they are afraid to tell friends and family.

"Understanding Teen Dating Violence," Centers for Disease Control and Prevention (CDC), 2008.

- 72% of 8th and 9th graders reportedly date.[1]
- One in four adolescents reports verbal, physical, emotional, or sexual abuse from a dating partner each year. [1, 2]
- About 10% of students nationwide report being physically hurt by a boyfriend or girlfriend in the past 12 months.[3]

### How does dating violence affect health?

Dating violence has a negative effect on health throughout life. Teens who are victims are more likely to do poorly in school. They may engage in unhealthy behaviors, like drug and alcohol use. The anger and stress that victims feel may lead to eating disorders and depression. Some teens even think about or attempt suicide. Victims may also carry the patterns of violence into future relationships.[4] Physically abused teens are three times more likely than their non-abused peers to experience violence during college.

### Who is at risk for dating violence?

Studies show that people who harm their dating partners are more depressed, have lower self-esteem, and are more aggressive than peers. Other warning signs for dating violence include the following:

- Use of threats or violence to solve problems
- Alcohol or drug use
- Inability to manage anger or frustration
- Poor social skills
- Association with violent friends
- Problems at school
- Lack of parental supervision, support, or discipline
- Witnessing abuse at home

### How can we prevent dating violence?

The ultimate goal is to stop dating violence before it starts. Strategies that promote healthy relationships are vital. During the pre-teen and teen years, young people are learning skills they need to form positive relationships with others. This is an ideal time to promote healthy relationships and prevent patterns of dating violence that can last into adulthood.

Prevention programs change the attitudes and behaviors linked with dating violence. One example is Safe Dates, a school-based program that is designed to change social norms and improve problem-solving skills.

## References

1. Foshee VA, Linder GF, Bauman KE, et al. The Safe Dates project: theoretical basis, evaluation design, and selected baseline findings. *American Journal of Preventive Medicine* 1996;12(Suppl 2):39–47.

2. Avery-Leaf S, Cascardi M, O'Leary KD, Cano A. Efficacy of a dating violence prevention program on attitudes justifying aggression. *Journal of Adolescent Health* 1997;21:11–7.

3. Centers for Disease Control and Prevention: Youth Risk Behavioral Surveillance—United States, 2007, *MMWR* 2008;57 (No.SS#4).

4. Smith PH, White JW, Holland LJ. A longitudinal perspective on dating violence among adolescent and college-age women. *American Journal of Public Health*. 2003.;93(7):1104–9.

## For More Information

**Choose Respect Initiative**
Website: http://www.chooserespect.org

**National Domestic Violence Hotline**
P.O. Box 161810
Austin, TX 78716
Toll-Free Hotline: 800-799-SAFE (7233)
Toll-Free TTY: 800-787-3224
Phone: 512-794-1133
Website: http://www.ndvh.org

**Rape, Abuse & Incest National Network (RAINN)**
2000 L Street, NW, Suite 406
Washington, DC 20036
National Sexual Assault Hotline Toll-Free: 800-656-HOPE (4673)
Phone: 202-544-3064
Fax: 202-544-3556

Website: http://www.rainn.org
E-mail: info@rainn.org

## *National Sexual Violence Resource Center*

123 N. Enola Drive
Enola, PA 17025
Toll-Free: 877-739-3895
Phone: 717-909-0710
Fax: 717-909-0714
TTY: 717-909-0715
Website: http://www.nsvrc.org
E-mail: resources@nsvrc.org

# Part Three


# Sexual Abuse of Children

# Chapter 25

# *Child Sexual Abuse*

## Sexual Violence: Facts at a Glance

### *Children and Youth*

In a nationally representative survey of children 17 years or younger:[1]

- 60.4% of female and 69.2% of male victims were first raped before age 18.

- 25.5% of females were first raped before age 12, and 34.9% were first raped between the ages of 12–17.

- 41.0% of males were first raped before age 12, and 27.9% were first raped between the ages of 12–17.

- A 2005 survey of high school students found that 10.8% of girls and 4.2% of boys from grades 9–12 were forced to have sexual intercourse at some time in their lives.[2]

- Among high school students, 9.3% of Black students, 7.8% of Hispanic students, and 6.9% of White students reported that

---

This chapter begins with excerpts from the following documents produced by the Centers for Disease Control and Prevention (CDC): "Sexual Violence: Facts at a Glance," 2008, and "Understanding Sexual Violence," 2007. The chapter also includes "Commonly Asked Questions about Child Sexual Abuse," © 2008 Stop It Now! (www.stopitnow). Reprinted with permission.

they were forced to have sexual intercourse at some time in their lives.[2]

## Understanding Sexual Violence

Sexual violence (SV) refers to sexual activity where consent is not obtained or freely given. Anyone can experience SV, but most victims are female. The person responsible for the violence is typically male and is usually someone known to the victim. The person can be, but is not limited to, a friend, coworker, neighbor, or family member.

There are many types of SV. Not all include physical contact between the victim and the perpetrator (person who harms someone else). Examples include sexual harassment, threats, intimidation, peeping, and taking nude photos. Other SV, including unwanted touching and rape, does include physical contact.

### *How does sexual violence affect health?*

SV can impact health in many ways. Some ways are serious and can lead to long-term health problems. These include chronic pain, headaches, stomach problems, and sexually transmitted diseases. In addition, rape results in about 32,000 pregnancies each year.

SV can have an emotional impact as well. Victims often are fearful and anxious. They may replay the attack over and over in their minds. They may have problems with trust and be wary of becoming involved with others. The anger and stress that victims feel may lead to eating disorders and depression. Some even think about or attempt suicide.

SV is also linked to negative health behaviors. For example, victims are more likely to smoke, abuse alcohol, use drugs, and engage in risky sexual activity.

## Commonly Asked Questions about Child Sexual Abuse

### *What is considered child sexual abuse?*

If you are not exactly sure what sexual abuse is, you're not alone. All sexual activity between an adult and a child is sexual abuse. Sexual touching between children can also be sexual abuse.

Sexual abuse between children is often defined as when there is a significant age difference (usually three or more years) between the children, or if the children are very different developmentally or size-wise. Sexual abuse does not have to involve penetration, force, pain, or even touching. If an adult engages in any sexual behavior (looking, showing, or touching) with a child to meet the adult's interest or sexual needs, it is sexual abuse.

*Child Sexual Abuse Includes Harmful Contact and Non-Contact Behaviors*

Abusive physical contact or touching includes:

* touching a child's genitals or private parts for sexual purposes;
* making a child touch someone else's genitals or play sexual games;
* putting objects or body parts (like fingers, tongue or penis) inside the vagina, in the mouth or in the anus of a child for sexual purposes.

Non-contact sexual abuse includes:

* showing pornography to a child;
* deliberately exposing an adult's genitals to a child;
* photographing a child in sexual poses;
* encouraging a child to watch or hear sexual acts;
* inappropriately watching a child undress or use the bathroom.

**Sexually abusive images of children and the internet:** As well as the activities described, there is also the serious and growing problem of people making and downloading sexual images of children on the internet. To view sexually abusive images of children is to participate in the abuse of a child, and may cause someone to consider sexual interactions with children as acceptable.

## Is there a typical profile of someone who sexually abuses children?

No. You cannot pick out a sex offender in a crowd. People who may sexually abuse children are fathers, mothers, step-parents, grandparents, uncles, aunts, and cousins. They are neighbors, baby sitters, religious leaders, teachers, and coaches. They come from all classes, racial and religious backgrounds, and may be homosexual or heterosexual. Most of those we know about who sexually abuse children are men, but some are women.

Some people who abuse children have adult sexual relationships and are not solely, or even mainly, sexually interested in children. More than a third of those who engage in sexual activity with children are under the age of 18 themselves. In many of these instances, the abusive child may not understand that his or her sexual actions toward another child are harmful.

It's important to remember that many terms used to describe people who sexually abuse children, like "pedophile" or "sexual predators," are often misused according to their clinical or legal definition. And, media stereotypes of "child predators" and "monsters" may actually make it more difficult for us to recognize or acknowledge inappropriate behaviors in those people we know.

## What is the impact of child sexual abuse?

Increased likelihood of depression, substance abuse, sexually transmitted disease, promiscuous behavior, criminal behavior, and difficulties in adult relationships have all been associated with victims of child sexual abuse. One study found that 80% of children who have been sexually abused have some symptoms of posttraumatic stress disorder (PTSD).

In addition to the emotional costs, one study found that sexually violent acts against children in the United States (U.S.) (ages 0–14) cost $71 billion every year, or 61% of the cost of all violent crime for this age group. A single year of regular mental health counseling for the existing 45 million adult survivors of sexual abuse in the U.S. would cost more than $200 billion.

## Is child sexual abuse really such a big problem?

Yes. As many as one in three girls and one in seven boys will be sexually abused at some point in their childhood, according to most reliable studies of child sexual abuse in the United States. That means in a kindergarten class of 20 children, at least four are likely to be sexually abused before they graduate from high school.

Surveys of U.S. adults consistently show that more than one in five adults were sexually abused during childhood. That means that there are potentially 45 million adults now living in the U.S. who were sexually abused as children.

## Are children who get sexually abused more likely to become sexually abusive as teens or adults?

No. The vast majority of sexual abuse victims live their lives without ever sexually abusing others.

Some people who sexually abuse children were victims of abuse or neglect as children. And having been abused as a child does heighten the risk for becoming someone who sexually abuses children. It's not an excuse, just a fact. But many childhood experiences besides sexual abuse are associated with sexually harmful behavior in youth, including exposure to violence, lack of emotional connection early in life, and physical abuse. Acknowledging and addressing the distress these children have already faced is a good way to begin ending this abusive cycle. Experts and parents agree that with specialized treatment these children can heal.

### What stops us from seeing abuse?

It's very disturbing to imagine that someone you know could be sexually harming a child. Without certain proof of abuse, it's so much easier to dismiss such thoughts or to think you're overreacting. You may also be worried about the possible consequences of taking action, especially if the concern involves someone you or your family depends on for financial, emotional or social support. One of the common thoughts parents have is: "My child would have told me if they were being abused and they haven't, so it can't be happening."

For those reasons, people often wait until after a child has been abused before they take action. Many people have lived through the discovery that someone close to them was abusing a child. Looking back, they wonder how they missed the signs. But when something is so difficult to think about, it's only human to find ways of denying it to ourselves. Common misunderstandings about sexual abuse often contribute to that denial. When adults trust their gut feelings and speak up, they can prevent child sexual abuse from happening.

### Does treatment of adults who have sexually abused children really work?

Yes. Experts agree that with successful completion of specialized treatment, people who sexually abuse children can learn how to control their actions and become part of the solution of keeping children safe.

Child sexual abuse is a crime and must be dealt with first through the child protection and criminal justice systems. But to prevent future abuse, it's in our best interest as a society to provide the best treatment available to every abuser who wants to change. It's also in our best interest as a society to build a system that really supports offenders in their recovery so that they have a chance to contribute positively to society. When people who abuse are firmly supported and held accountable by their friends and families, they are more likely to complete their treatment programs and live productive, abuse-free lives.

### *Are adults convicted of child sex offenses more likely to re-offend than people convicted of other crimes?*

No. Contrary to what most people think, crime statistics show that adults convicted of child sex offenses are much less likely to re-offend than those convicted of any other major crime. Even without treatment, recidivism rates for those convicted of sexually abusing a child are estimated to be about 15–20%. With treatment, many studies show an additional reduction in recidivism by as much as a 33% to as low as 12%.

### *What should I do if I know a child has been abused?*

Believe the child—children are rarely mistaken about what happened. One of the most important things a parent or adult can do when a child tells about sexual abuse is to respond to the child in a calm and matter-of-fact manner. Take a deep breath. Let the child know that no matter what happened or what he or she says, you will still love him or her.

If the child has been abused, take the time to reassure the child that he or she has done nothing wrong. Let the child know that you will do whatever you can to keep him or her safe. Let the child know you are someone he or she can safely talk to about this issue. Listen carefully to the responses without suggesting answers. It may be useful to practice with someone else first and get support to help keep your own emotions in check. Recognize that confusion, guilt, and shame about abuse can make the conversation difficult, both for you and for the child. Acknowledge the child's discomfort and offer praise for their courage to talk about a confusing experience. Remember that if it's difficult for you to discuss your concerns, it is likely to be much more difficult for the child.

Next, get help. The sexual abuse of children is against the law. It is important to seek professional help and not confront this alone. By taking action you may reduce the risk of others in your community or family from being sexually abused. Healing from child sexual abuse is possible with specialized treatment and support. There are resources throughout the country that can help a family through this difficult situation.

Reporting the abuse to authorities is an upsetting prospect for many families. Yet, filing a report can be a first step to accessing support services. Children who are abused and their families need help to recover from their trauma. Anyone who is harming a child sexually also needs help and support to stop the behavior.

### What should I do if I am concerned that a child or teen may sexually abuse another child?

Act now, if you are worried that your son or daughter or another child may be sexually harming another child.

Get help from a professional therapist immediately and develop a family safety plan to address the concerning behaviors. By taking action, you will reduce the risk that other children in your community or family will be sexually abused. And, prompt intervention can get a child with sexual behavior problems the treatment he or she needs to grow into a productive member of our community. Healing from child sexual abuse is possible with treatment and support. There are resources throughout the country that can help a family through this difficult situation.

### Can therapy help a child who has been sexually abused recover?

Yes. The lives of children who have been sexually abused are forever changed. But many adults have healed from childhood sexual abuse and are living caring and productive lives.

Some children may be ready to talk about their abuse and deal with it soon after it happens. Others may need to move more slowly, gradually testing the safety of addressing the issues that arise. Children do best with a combination of love from caregivers, and support from a counselor who has special training to work with children who have experienced sexual trauma. Children and youth frequently respond best to specialized, sex-specific treatment when it is offered early and with the support of trusted adults.

Since child sexual abuse affects all members of a family or group, everyone including the adults is likely to need support. There are resources throughout the country that can help a child and its family through this difficult situation.

## References

1.  Basile KC, Chen J, Lynberg MC, Saltzman LE. Prevalence and characteristics of sexual violence victimization. *Violence and Victims* 2007;22(4): 437–448.

2. Centers for Disease Control and Prevention. Youth Risk Behavior Surveillance—United States. 2005. Surveillance Summaries, 2006. *MMWR* 2006;55:SS-5.

# Chapter 26

# *Warning Signs of Child Sexual Abuse*

## Warning Signs

"Warning sign" is really just another way of saying "opportunity for prevention"—a chance for caring adults to recognize possible risk and to take action to protect children. Read the behavioral descriptions that follow. Some are serious violations. But many may suggest that a child may be at risk or an adult, adolescent, or child is struggling to control potentially harmful impulses.

Remember, the most effective prevention takes place before there's a child victim to heal.

## Warning Signs in Children and Adolescents of Possible Child Sexual Abuse

Any one sign doesn't mean that a child was sexually abused, but the presence of several suggests that you begin asking questions and consider seeking help. Keep in mind that some of these signs can emerge at other times of stress such as:

---

This chapter includes the following information from Stop It Now!: "Warning Signs," "Warning Signs in Children and Adolescents of Possible Child Sexual Abuse," "Age-Appropriate Sexual Behavior," "Behaviors to Watch for When Adults Are with Children," "Signs That an Adult May Be At-Risk to Harm a Child," and "Signs That a Child or Teen May Be At-Risk to Harm Another Child," © 2008 Stop It Now! (www.stopitnow). Reprinted with permission.

- during a divorce,
- death of a family member or pet,
- problems at school or with friends, and
- other anxiety-inducing or traumatic events.

### Behavior You May See in a Child or Adolescent

- Has nightmares or other sleep problems without an explanation
- Seems distracted or distant at odd times
- Has a sudden change in eating habits (refuses to eat, loses or drastically increases appetite, has trouble swallowing)
- Sudden mood swings: rage, fear, insecurity, or withdrawal
- Leaves "clues" that seem likely to provoke a discussion about sexual issues
- Writes, draws, plays, or dreams of sexual or frightening images
- Develops new or unusual fear of certain people or places
- Refuses to talk about a secret shared with an adult or older child
- Talks about a new older friend
- Suddenly has money, toys, or other gifts without reason
- Thinks of self or body as repulsive, dirty, or bad
- Exhibits adult-like sexual behaviors, language, and knowledge

*Signs More Typical of Younger Children*

- An older child behaving like a younger child (such as bed-wetting or thumb sucking)
- Has new words for private body parts
- Resists removing clothes at appropriate times (bath, bed, toileting, diapering)
- Asks other children to behave sexually or play sexual games
- Mimics adult-like sexual behaviors with toys or stuffed animal
- Wetting and soiling accidents unrelated to toilet training

*Signs More Typical in Adolescents*

- Self-injury (cutting, burning)
- Inadequate personal hygiene
- Drug and alcohol abuse
- Sexual promiscuity
- Running away from home
- Depression, anxiety
- Suicide attempts
- Fear of intimacy or closeness
- Compulsive eating or dieting

### Physical Warning Signs

Physical signs of sexual abuse are rare. If you see these signs, bring your child to a doctor. Your doctor can help you understand what may be happening and test for sexually transmitted diseases.

- Pain, discoloration, bleeding, or discharges in genitals, anus, or mouth
- Persistent or recurring pain during urination and bowel movements
- Wetting and soiling accidents unrelated to toilet training

## Age-Appropriate Sexual Behavior

It can be hard to acknowledge that all of us, even children, are sexual beings, have sexual feelings, and are curious about sex and sexuality. Children's curiosity can lead to exploring their own and each other's body parts by looking and touching.

They may peek when family members are in the bathroom, or changing clothes, or try to listen outside the bedroom. They may look at magazines, books, videos, and on the internet.

It can be hard to tell the difference between "normal" sexual behaviors and behaviors that are signs that a child may be developing a problem. Sexual play that is more typical or expected in children will more often have the following traits:

- The sexual play is between children who have an ongoing mutually enjoyable play and/or school friendship.

- The sexual play is between children of similar size, age, and social and emotional development.

- It is lighthearted and spontaneous. The children may be giggling and having fun when you discover them.

- When adults set limits (for example, children keep their clothes on at day care), children are able to follow the rules.

### Preschool Age (0–5 Years)

*Common*

- Will have questions and express knowledge relating to:
  - differences in gender, private body parts;
  - hygiene and toileting; and
  - pregnancy and birth.
- Will explore genitals and can experience pleasure.
- Showing and looking at private body parts.

*Uncommon*

- Having knowledge of specific sexual acts or explicit sexual language.
- Engaging in adult-like sexual contact with other children.

### School-Age (6–8 Years)

*Common*

- Will need knowledge and have questions about:
  - physical development, relationships, sexual behavior;
  - menstruation and pregnancy; and
  - personal values.
- Experiment with same-age and same gender children, often during games or role-playing.
- Self stimulation in private is expected to continue.

*Uncommon*

- Adult-like sexual interactions.

- Having knowledge of specific sexual acts.
- Behaving sexually in a public place or through the use of phone or internet technology.

## School-Age (9–12 Years)

Hormonal changes and external influences, such as peers, media, and internet, will increase sexual awareness, feelings, and interest at the onset of puberty.

*Common*

- Will need knowledge and have questions about:
  - sexual materials and information;
  - relationships and sexual behavior;
  - using sexual words and discussing sexual acts and personal values, particularly with peers.
- Increased experimentation with sexual behaviors and romantic relationships.
- Self stimulation in private is expected to continue.

*Uncommon*

- Regularly occurring adult-like sexual behavior.
- Behaving sexually in a public place.

## Adolescence (13–16 Years)

*Common*

- Will need information and have questions about:
  - decision making,
  - social relationships and sexual customs,
  - personal values and consequences of sexual behavior.
- Self stimulation in private is expected to continue.
- Girls will begin menstruation; boys will begin to produce sperm.
- Sexual experimentation between adolescents of the same age and gender is common.

- Voyeuristic behaviors are common in this age group.
- First sexual intercourse will occur for approximately one-third of teens.

*Uncommon*

- Masturbation in a public place.
- Sexual interest directed toward much younger children.

(Adapted with permission from Wurtele, S.K. and Miller-Perrin, C.L. *Preventing Sexual Abuse.* University of Nebraska Press. Lincoln, NE. 1992.)

## Behaviors to Watch for When Adults Are with Children

We all have personal likes and things that make us uncomfortable. "Personal space" is the private area of control inside an imaginary line or boundary that defines each person as separate.

Ideally, that boundary helps us stay in charge of our own personal space. It helps keep out the things that make us uncomfortable—unsafe and unwanted feelings, words, images, and physical contact. Solid social rules strengthen the boundary. Behaviors that routinely disrespect or ignore boundaries make children vulnerable to abuse.

Do you know an adult or older child who doesn't seem to understand what's acceptable when it comes to:

### Personal Space

- Makes others uncomfortable by ignoring social, emotional, or physical boundaries or limits.
- Refuses to let a child set any of his or her own limits; or uses teasing or belittling language to keep a child from setting a limit.
- Insists on hugging, touching, kissing, tickling, wrestling with, or holding a child, even when the child does not want this physical contact or attention.
- Frequently walks in on children or teens in the bathroom.

### Relationships with Children

- Turns to a child for emotional or physical comfort by sharing personal or private information or activities, normally shared with adults.

- Has secret interactions with teens or children (for example, games, sharing drugs, alcohol, or sexual material) or spends excessive time e-mailing, text messaging, or calling children or youth.

- Insists on or manages to spend uninterrupted time alone with a child.

- Seems "too good to be true," for example, frequently baby sits different children for free; takes children on special outings alone; buys children gifts, or gives them money for no apparent reason.

- Allows children or teens to consistently get away with inappropriate behaviors.

### *Sexual Conversation or Behavior*

- Frequently points out sexual images or tells dirty or suggestive jokes with children present.

- Exposes a child to adult sexual interactions or images without apparent concern.

- Is overly interested in the sexuality of a particular child or teen (for example, talks repeatedly about the child's developing body or interferes with normal teen dating).

## Signs That an Adult May Be At-Risk to Harm a Child

Someone you care about may be acting in ways that worry or confuse you. The following listed behaviors may indicate a possible risk of sexual abuse to a child, but may also be a way for this adult to ask for help.

Many people with sexual behavior problems believe that others already suspect and often wish someone would ask what's going on or advise them where to call to get help. Remember, you can start a conversation by pointing out harmful impacts on a child without accusing someone of abusive intentions.

Do you have concerns about someone you know in these areas of daily life?

### *Relationships*

- Misses or ignores social cues about others' personal or sexual limits and boundaries.

- Often has a "special" child friend, maybe a different one from year to year.

- Spends most of his or her spare time with children and shows little interest in spending time with someone their own age.

- Encourages silence and secrets in children.

### *Sexual Interactions*

- Links sexuality and aggression in language or behavior, such as sexualized threats or insults, like "whore" or "slut."

- Makes fun of children's body parts, describes children with sexual words like "stud" or "sexy," or talks again and again about the sexual activities of children or teens.

- Masturbates so often that it gets in the way of important day-to-day activities.

- Has an interest in sexual fantasies involving children and seems unclear about what's appropriate with children.

- Looks at child pornography or downloads or views internet pornography and is not willing to show whether children are involved.

- Asks adult partners to dress or act like a child or teen during sexual activity.

### *Personal Safety and Responsibility*

- Has been known to make poor decisions while misusing drugs or alcohol.

- Justifies behavior, defends poor choices or harmful acts; blames others to refuse responsibility for behaviors.

- Minimizes hurtful or harmful behaviors when confronted; denies harmfulness of actions or words despite a clear negative impact.

## Signs That a Child or Teen May Be At-Risk to Harm Another Child

More than a third of all sexual abuse of children is committed by someone under the age of 18. Children, particularly younger children, may take part in inappropriate interactions without understanding how it might be hurtful to others. For this reason, it may be more helpful to talk about a child's sexually "harmful" behavior rather than sexually "abusive" behavior.

Do you know a child or adolescent who is:

### *Confused about Social Rules and Interactions*

- May experience typical gestures of friendliness or affection as sexual.

- Explores his or her own natural sexual curiosity with younger children or those of differing size, status, ability, or power.

- Seeks out the company of younger children and spends an unusual amount of time with them rather than with peers.

- Takes younger children to "secret" places or hideaways or plays "special" games with them (for example, playing doctor, undressing or touching games, and so forth).

- Insists on physical contact with a child when the child resists the attention.

### *Anxious, Depressed, or Seeming to Need Help*

- Tells you they do not want to be alone with a child, or group of children, or becomes anxious about being with a particular young person.

- Was physically, sexually, or emotionally abused and has not been offered adequate resources and support for recovery.

- Seems to be crying for help, for example behaves as if they want to be caught; leaves "clues," or acts in ways that seem likely to provoke a discussion about sexual issues.

### *Impulsively Sexual or Aggressive*

- Links sexuality and aggression in language or behavior (makes sexual threats or insults).

- Unable to control inappropriate sexual behaviors involving another child after being told to stop.

- Engages in sexually harassing behavior.

- Shares alcohol, drugs, or sexual material with younger children or teens.

4

- Views sexual images of children on the internet or elsewhere.

- Forces sexual interaction, including direct contact and non-contact (like exposing genitals) on another adolescent or child.

## What You Can Do If You See Warning Signs

- Create a safety plan. Don't wait for proof of child sexual abuse.

- Look for patterns of behavior that make children less safe. Keep track of behaviors that concern you.

- Review the "Let's Talk Guidebooks" available at http://www.stopitnow.com/guidebooks.

## For More Information

***Stop It Now!***
351 Pleasant Street, Suite B-319
Northampton, MA 01060
Toll-Free Helpline: 888-PREVENT (773-8368)
Phone: 413-587-3500
Fax: 413-587-3505
Website: http:www.stopitnow.com

Stop It Now! has an online help center at http://GetHelp.StopItNow.org and offers other resources and guidance for responding to specific situations.

# Chapter 27

# *Incest: Sexual Abuse within the Family*

## *What is incest?*

Incest is any sexual contact between a child or adolescent and a person who is closely related or perceived to be related, including stepparents and live-in partners of parents. The person initiating contact is usually a parent or step-parent, most often male. Incest perpetrators also include siblings, cousins, mothers, uncles, aunts, or grandparents. The activity may happen once or many times over a period of years. Such activity is illegal.

## *What are some characteristics of families in which incest occurs?*

Families in which incest occurs often appear no different than other families. However, secrecy, isolation, and psychological stress are major parts of family life. Children in these families commonly feel guilty about the abuse they suffer, not understanding that it comes from choices made by the adult abuser.

Abusers come from all races, religious groups, income levels, professions, and age groups. They may enjoy good reputations in their communities and seem quite normal. In reality abusers are emotionally distressed, isolated, and immature. They have false or distorted

"Incest: Sexual Abuse within the Family," © Texas Association Against Sexual Assault (www.taasa.org). Reprinted with permission.

ideas about sexuality and often believe that there is nothing wrong with their abusive behavior.

Some abusers, particularly male abusers, tend to think that they have a right to control the family and behave in a forceful manner. Other abusers get power by appearing helpless and needy, pressuring their victims to take care of their needs and feel sorry for them.

A non-abusive mother in the family usually gives her children the feeling that she is unable to influence what happens in the family. She may be overworked and ill much of the time, depressed, economically dependent, or cut off from social contacts outside the family. She may be an unacknowledged victim of sexual assault herself.

### What should a person do who suspects that a child is being victimized?

Anyone who suspects that a child is being abused in any way should report those suspicions to child protective services (CPS) or a local law enforcement agency.

## Possible Signs That a Child May Have Been Victimized

Young children may exhibit one or more of the following behaviors:

- reverting to bed-wetting, clinging, or whining
- sexual knowledge, behavior, or language unusual for their age
- withdrawal from other people
- frequent genital or bowel movement problems
- unexplained gagging or vomiting
- loss of appetite
- agitation, hyperactivity, irritability, or aggressiveness
- seducing or acting out sex acts with other children

Signs of abuse in older children may include the following:

- skipping school, change in school performance
- eating disorders
- depression, anxiety, or mood swings
- poor self-image or self-hatred

- substance abuse
- running away or fear of going home
- repeated physical complaints such as infections, cramping, or abdominal pains
- dizziness, gagging, and severe headaches
- self-destructive or mutilating behaviors such as cutting, burning, and suicide attempts
- seductive or promiscuous behavior and/or prostitution

### What problems might incest create for children?

When "protector" and "abuser" are the same person, the child learns that it is not safe to trust. Inability to trust others is a major problem for incest survivors.

Abused children usually believe that their abuse is the result of something they did or that they deserve to be abused for some reason. They may also believe that all families are like theirs—that children are commonly abused by older family members and forced to keep the abuse a secret.

It is often difficult for abused children to get help. Telling the family "secret" opens the family to outside pressures and increases a child's feelings of not being safe. Children may not believe that anything will be done once the abuse is revealed or that too much will be done and they will be blamed for the disruption in their family. They may hope that the abuse will simply end.

### How do abused children handle their abuse?

Incest creates much mental and physical stress for victimized children. They are forced to develop unusual methods of maintaining a small sense of security and control during abusive situations, including:

- separating themselves from the experience by blanking out, or by being somewhere else in their minds during the abuse;
- making certain parts of their bodies numb or deadened to pain, or creating pain to distract them from the pain of the abuse (biting their lips or holding their breath);
- using alcohol or drugs to numb themselves to emotional and physical pain during or after the abuse;

- pretending to be asleep during the abuse and making their bodies go limp.

## *How does incest affect the lives of incest survivors?*

Incest experiences may lead children to form negative opinions about themselves, resulting in serious depression, guilt, and feelings of powerlessness. Self-destructive behaviors, that include involvement in victimizing relationships, may result.

Incest victims may learn that their role in relationships is to give to others without expecting to be nurtured in return. Their sexuality is used in a way that may make them fearful of being touched.

Many victims have negative feelings about their bodies, perform poorly in school because they are unable to concentrate, or get into trouble due to fighting or other antisocial behaviors. During adolescence they may become more and more isolated socially and emotionally.

Incest victims often take sexuality to one extreme or the other—withdrawing from voluntary sexual activity because it creates anxiety or other painful feelings, or becoming highly sexually active because it is the only way they know to get affection or to feel in control. Male incest survivors may reject "maleness" because their abuser was male, or go out of their way to demonstrate their own "maleness" in order to feel in control of their lives.

Incest victims may feel that they make poor judgments about other people. They are likely to have little, if any experience with forming good relationships.

Some children may respond sexually to the abuse as a way of getting relief from the tension it creates. This may cause increased feelings of guilt and confusion.

## *How can incest survivors help themselves?*

Many incest survivors overcome their abuse and live rewarding lives, but the healing process may be long and difficult. Professional counseling is usually necessary.

Incest survivors can learn to make good decisions about relationships. They can learn to feel better about their bodies by developing a sense of ownership and control over them. They can learn to distinguish between touching which is caring and touching which merely uses their bodies. They can learn to be assertive and establish personal boundaries in relationships.

## *For More Information*

### *Rape, Abuse & Incest National Network (RAINN)*
2000 L Street, NW, Suite 406
Washington, DC 20036
Toll-Free: 800-656-HOPE (4673)
Phone: 202-544-3064
Fax: 202-544-3556
Website: http://www.rainn.org
E-mail: info@rainn.org

### *Texas Association Against Sexual Assault (TAASA)*
6200 La Calma, Suite 110
Austin, Texas 78752
Phone: 512-474-7190
Fax: 512-474-6490
Website: http://www.taasa.org

# Chapter 28

# *Sexual Abuse by Educators and School Staff*

In a single day, the following stories made the news: A special education teacher in Indiana was arrested for molesting a 16-year-old girl. A high school band director in California admitted to having sex with a 17-year-old boy. A former teacher and bus driver in North Dakota was arrested for sexually abusing a 6-year-old girl for more than a year.

The vast majority of the three million teachers in the U.S. are caring, dedicated professionals who recoil at such abuse. Still, the headlines illustrate an alarming truth: One out of five girls and nearly one out of ten boys will be sexually abused by a school employee at some point during their academic careers.

The victims represent all grade levels, ethnicity, family incomes and geographic regions, yet research indicates female students and students of color are disproportionately targeted. The effects of abuse are devastating; targeted students are more likely to skip school, are less likely to participate in class, and often experience emotional and developmental trauma.

Abusers are almost always men and often are popular among students and other school staff. They're typically teachers or coaches, but can be teacher's aides, bus drivers, volunteers, counselors, or principals.

In the past five years, schools have sanctioned at least 2,750 educators for sexual misconduct with minors. Experts say this is just the

Text in this chapter is from "The ABCs of Sexual Misconduct," reprinted with permission from Teaching Tolerance (www.tolerance.org), a Project of the Southern Poverty Law Center, © 2007.

tip of the iceberg. A majority of sexually abusive educators never get reported, and many who are reported simply get shuffled to another school. Most perpetrators abuse more than one student.

## Facts about Misconduct

### What Is Sexual Misconduct?

Over the course of four years, researcher Charol Shakeshaft examined reports of educator sexual misconduct and abuse. She determined that "sexual conduct" between school employees and students typically comes in the following three forms:

- Visual: such as showing sexually explicit photographs to students, or exposing one's genitals

- Verbal: such as commenting on a student's body parts or making sexually explicit jokes

- Physical: from fondling or touching, to molestation and rape

Because these acts can be very upsetting, people often choose to use euphemisms when discussing them. In everyday discussions, the terms "sexual abuse," "sexual misconduct," and "sexual harassment" often are used interchangeably. That is the case in this publication.

Legally, however, the terms have distinct meanings:

### Sexual Abuse

According to federal law, sexual conduct meets the threshold of sexual abuse when the perpetrator knowingly:

- "causes another person to engage in a sexual act by threatening or placing that other person in fear;" or,

- "engages in a sexual act with another person if that other person is a) incapable of appraising the nature of the conduct, or b) physically incapable of declining participation in, or communicating unwillingness to engage in, that sexual act."

### Sexual Harassment

Sexual harassment is a form of sex discrimination prohibited by Title IX. According to the U.S. Department of Education, the law recognizes two types of sexual harassment:

- *Quid pro quo* harassment: This occurs "when a school employee causes a student to believe that he or she must submit to unwelcome sexual conduct in order to participate in a school program or activity. It can also occur when an employee causes a student to believe that the employee will make an educational decision based on whether or not the student submits to unwelcome sexual conduct."

- Hostile environment: This occurs "when unwelcome sexually harassing conduct is so severe, persistent or pervasive that it affects a student's ability to participate in, or benefit from, an education program or activity, or creates an intimidating, threatening, or abusive educational environment."

### *Sexual Misconduct*

Legally, sexual misconduct applies to a broader category of acts that fail to meet the threshold of abuse or harassment. Commonly, however, sexual misconduct is used in press reports and non-legal documents as an umbrella term for acts of sexual abuse or harassment.

### *Who Are the Abusers?*

Out of the three million teachers in the United States, only a tiny fraction will attempt to sexually abuse a student in their care. Those who do usually fall into one of two categories: adults who enter the teaching profession to obtain greater access to children, with the intent to abuse them; and adults who convince themselves that they are in love with, or in a consensual relationship with, their student targets.

### *Some Myths about Sexual Misconduct in Schools*

- Myth: It's easy to spot an abusive educator. Fact: Many abusive educators are outgoing, personable and popular among students and other teachers.

- Myth: Targeted students are always shy, awkward, or come from broken homes. Fact: While it's true that social isolation increases a student's vulnerability to sexual abuse, there is no one mold for victims. Some education professionals have ignored warning signs, thinking a student is too popular to be abused.

- Myth: A large percentage of abusers are women. Fact: Watching the news during the past year, a viewer might get the impression

Child Abuse Sourcebook, Second Edition

that most school sex offenses happen at the hands of female teachers. In reality, most studies show that 80–96% of abusive educators are male. Yet, when the abuser is a woman, it more frequently generates sensational headlines.

- Myth: Abuse by female teachers isn't a big deal if the victim is male. Fact: As Charol Shakeshaft writes, "males have been socialized to believe they should be flattered or appreciative of sexual interest from a female." Abusive female teachers turn into jokes for late-night comedians. In truth, boys experience emotional and psychological damage just as much as girls.

## The Warning Signs

Robert Shoop, author of *Sexual Exploitation in Schools*, offers practical advice for recognizing sexual misconduct and ways to overcome common obstacles to reporting.

No teacher or administrator wants to have to ask, "Did I miss something?" or, "Should I have known something was wrong?" or, "Could I have prevented this tragedy?" However, I think it is very important that every teacher asks, "Could there be someone in my school who is molesting children?"

After a teacher is arrested and convicted of child abuse, his or her fellow teachers consistently express amazement that this happened in their school. Many teachers still can't believe that a teacher in their school could sexually abuse students. They believe that if such abuse happens, it happens elsewhere—that it is so rare and idiosyncratic, it does not warrant attention.

Research shows us this belief is naïve. Following are some of the early warning signs of abuse, and the major obstacles that prevent many teachers from reporting them.

### Early Warning Signs

Threshold behaviors are the easiest warning signs to overlook. These behaviors occur in the early stages of an abusive teacher's grooming of his or her victim. If caught in these activities, a teacher often comes up with an explanation that might sound reasonable. However, threshold behaviors are red flags that should prompt further investigation.

Some of these threshold behaviors include the following:

**Overly affectionate behaviors:** These would include excessive hugging or touching. An example can be seen in a recent court case.

Colleagues of a teacher who was convicted of having sexual relations with several elementary students commented, "I had some qualms about how affectionate he was with his students, but he is old enough to be their grandfather."

**Inappropriate, non-education related contact:** In some cases, it was common knowledge that students frequently met at teachers' houses to have parties or watch movies. In one case, a student was frequently signed out of class to go to a teacher's room for non-instructional purposes. In another, a student was frequently seen driving a teacher's car in the evenings and on weekends. Abusive teachers have given students flowers, sent them cards, and bought them gifts.

**Sexual harassment:** Teachers who engage in sexual teasing, telling sexual jokes, touching a student's hair or body, frequent or prolonged hugging, or other harassing behaviors are guilty of sexual harassment. Some teachers who eventually sexually molest students begin by making less overt gestures. Schools must have a zero-tolerance policy for sexual harassment.

## Overcoming Roadblocks

Even if teachers observe early warning signs, they may be hesitant to report. What are the common roadblocks, and how can we push past them?

**Cognitive dissonance:** This psychological term describes the stressful situation of holding two conflicting thoughts at the same time. The fact that most teachers are ethical and honorable makes it difficult for them to believe that one of their own is a child molester. Many colleges of education neglect the topic of teacher sexual abuse of children, and school districts seldom conduct in-service training sessions on this topic. This perpetuates the perception that sexual misconduct seldom occurs.

**Fear of making false accusations:** Many teachers are fearful of making a mistake that could destroy a colleague's career. Perhaps because teachers fear false complaints against themselves, they tend to give colleagues the benefit of the doubt. In reality, the vast majority of abuse goes unreported—there are very few documented cases of false accusations.

**Fear of being sued:** Some teachers fail to report their suspicions, and some administrators hesitate to begin an investigation, because they fear the accused teacher will charge them with defamation of character or wrongful discharge. Teachers and other staff members must be committed to err on the side of protecting the child, rather than protecting the school from litigation.

**Stereotyping:** Sometimes, teachers will stifle their suspicion because the teacher and/or student in question doesn't fit a certain stereotype. However, teachers who molest do not wear trench coats and hang around playgrounds. They often are highly respected by their colleagues, admired by the community, and adored by their students. These people often are married with children. In addition, students who are victims come from all grade levels, family backgrounds, and personality types.

**Misguided loyalty:** For far too long, school districts have allowed teachers suspected of inappropriate behaviors to resign. Many school boards and administrators are so concerned about their district's reputation that they want the problem to just go away. Not only does this behavior contribute to the under-reporting of teacher sexual abuse of students, it allows the molester to move to another district and continue to prey on children.

## Five Things Teachers Can Do

**Pay attention:** It is critical that educators at all levels acknowledge that teacher-to-student sexual abuse is a serious problem. Educators must continuously scan the environment for information. All rumors, whispers, and sometimes-oblique complaints must be taken seriously.

**Solicit help from parents:** A parent asking their child "how was school today?" and receiving the reply, "fine," will not have elicited helpful information about what is going on in school. Many parents think that teachers molest only high school students. Parents must begin an early conversation about what is happening at school. They must monitor e-mails, text messages, phone calls, internet social networking sites, blogs, greeting cards, and yearbooks.

**Trust your gut, and ask questions:** Sometimes there is no way for anyone to know that abuse is taking place. In many cases, however, the signs are there, but they go unnoticed. Seeing early warning signs of teacher-to-student sexual abuse requires that you trust your intuition. If you are uncomfortable by a teacher's behavior, or if something seems out of place or unusual, you should heighten your scrutiny and ask questions.

**Follow school policies:** Advocate for school and district policies that define sexual misconduct and provide necessary tools for reporting suspicious behavior.

**Understand state laws:** Some form of child abuse discovery and reporting law exists in every state. Everyone in the education profession is a mandatory reporter and has a legal duty to protect students and report suspected abuse.

## Chapter 29

# *Children and Adolescents Who Sexually Abuse Other Children*

As parents and caregivers, we want to do all we can to protect our children, while giving them the freedom they need to develop and become healthy adults. Sometimes, the world can feel full of risks, many of them obvious, and others more confusing. In order to strike the right balance between protection and independence for our children, we adults need the best possible information.

This chapter is for everyone involved in bringing up children. It explains that some children do sexually abuse other children, describes how we can recognize the warning signs, and outlines some actions we adults can take to prevent sexual abuse.

### *Do children sexually abuse other children?*

Most people already are aware of the risk of sexual abuse that some adults present to our children. There is growing understanding that the vast majority of children who are sexually abused, are abused by someone they know, and often trust. Unfortunately, very few adults recognize that children and adolescents also can present a risk to other children. In fact, over a third of all sexual abuse of children is committed by someone under the age of 18.

This can be a difficult issue to address, partly because it is often challenging for adults to think of the children or adolescents we know

---

"Do Children Sexually Abuse Other Children?" © 2008 Stop It Now! (www.stopitnow). Reprinted with permission.

as capable of sexually abusing others. Also, it is not always easy to tell the difference between natural sexual curiosity and potentially abusive behaviors. Children, particularly younger children, may engage in inappropriate interactions without understanding the hurtful impact it has on others. For this reason, it may be more helpful to talk about a child's sexually harmful behavior rather than sexually abusive behavior.

It is essential that all adults have the information needed to recognize potentially harmful activities at an early stage and to seek help so the behaviors can be stopped. Every adult who cares about children has an opportunity, as both teacher and role model, to show children how to interact without harming others, either while they are still children, or later, as adults. Adults have the added responsibility of ensuring that all children who have been involved in a harmful sexual situation, whatever their role, are given the help they need to live healthy, productive lives.

### What is healthy sexual development?

Most adults understand that children pass through different stages of development as they grow. Sometimes, adults have more difficulty acknowledging that, from birth, children are sexual beings. Like other areas of a child's development, it is normal for children's awareness and curiosity about their own sexual feelings to change as they pass from infancy into childhood, and then through puberty to adolescence.

Each child is an individual and will develop in his or her own way. However, there is a generally accepted range of behaviors linked to children's changing age and developmental stages. These behaviors may include exploration with other children of similar power or stature—by virtue of age, size, ability, or social status. Sometimes, it can be difficult to tell the difference between sexual exploration that is appropriate to a developmental stage and interactions that are warning signs of harmful behavior.

Occasionally, adults may need to set limits when children engage in behaviors we consider inappropriate, even if the children may be unaware of potential harm. This is a chance to talk with them about keeping themselves and others safe, and to let them know that you are someone they can talk to when they have questions. Adults can help children be comfortable with their sexual development and understand appropriate sexual boundaries, for example, adults can model appropriate, respectful behavior.

Children with disabilities or developmental challenges benefit from special attention to their safety. Depending on the nature of their disability, they may develop at different rates, which can make them more vulnerable to being abused. They may also inadvertently harm another child without understanding the hurtful impact of their actions. For example, children with disabilities sometimes behave sexually in ways that are out of step with their age. Particular care may be needed to help children understand their sexual development and to ensure that these children and their caregivers can communicate effectively about any questions or worries they have.

It is important to recognize that, while people from various backgrounds have different expectations about what is acceptable behavior for children, sexual abuse is present across all ethnic groups, cultures, and religious beliefs

## What is sexually harmful behavior?

Sexually harmful behavior by children and young people may range from experimentation that has gone too far to serious sexual assault.

It is important for adults to recognize that many children will engage in some forms of sexual exploration with children of a similar age, size, social status, or power. Sometimes a child or young person may engage in sexual play with a much younger or more vulnerable child, or use force, tricks, or bribery to involve someone in sexual activity. While such manipulation may be a cause for concern, it is critical to realize that manipulation may not, in itself, indicate a tendency toward sexual aggression. Professional help and advice is needed to determine the best way to support a child in managing any concerning impulses.

Keep the following in mind:

- Children as young as four or five may unknowingly engage in sexually harmful behavior, although more often those who sexually harm children are adolescents.

- Usually, but not always, the child or young person causing the harm is older than the victim.

- Often the child being harmed is uncomfortable or confused about what is happening, but may feel that he or she is willingly involved or to blame for being in the situation.

- Many times, one or both children do not understand that the behavior is harmful.

## What about sexually abusive images of children—child pornography?

There is a growing problem of sexual images of children being available for viewing and downloading on the internet. Adults need to supervise children's use of the internet, provide children with clear information about our expectations, and teach them how to make safe choices.

We must educate young people about the following risks:

- Viewing abusive images of children may make harmful sexual interactions with children seem normal or acceptable.

- Viewing sexually abusive images of children hurts those children and others by creating a demand for additional images.

- Downloading child pornography is a criminal offense.

Adults must also remain aware of the risks of developing technology and of how to access resources when a child does engage in harmful online activities. Social networking sites, text messaging, and photo capable cell phones are just a few examples of evolving methods of communication that attract young people, but also can create unanticipated vulnerabilities.

## Why do some children sexually harm others?

The reasons children sexually harm others are complicated, varied, and not always obvious. Some of them may have been emotionally, sexually, or physically abused themselves, while others may have witnessed physical or emotional violence at home. Some may have come in contact with sexually explicit movies, video games, or materials that are confusing to them. In some instances, a child or adolescent may act on a passing impulse with no harmful intent, but may still cause harm to themselves or to other children.

Whatever the reason, without help, some sexually abusing youth will go on to abuse children as adults. It is important to seek advice and help promptly whenever there is any concern or question about a child or adolescent.

## How do we recognize the warning signs of sexually harmful behavior?

One of the most difficult discoveries a parent can make is to learn that your child may have sexually harmed or abused another child.

Denial, shock, and anger are common reactions. Because a quick and sensitive response can help diminish the harmful effects on the whole family, it is important to get professional advice about what to do as soon as you become aware of warning signs.

The good news is that positive, supportive help for the child or young person and his or her family can make a real difference. Evidence shows that the earlier children get help, the more able they are to learn the skills they need to control their behavior. If you are in this situation, remember that you are not alone. Many other parents who have been through similar experiences found that by taking action the child and family got the help they needed and were able to avoid future abuse. The first step is to recognize the value of talking it over with someone else.

## *What are warning signs of sexually harmful or abusive behavior?*

Behaviors that may indicate increased risk include the following:

- Regularly minimizing, justifying, or denying the impact of inappropriate behaviors on others

- Making others uncomfortable by consistently missing or ignoring social cues about others' personal or sexual limits and boundaries

- Preferring to spend time with younger children rather than peers

- Insisting on physical contact with a child even when that child resists

- Responding sexually to typical gestures of friendliness or affection

- Reluctance to be alone with a particular child; becoming anxious when a particular child is coming to visit

- Offering alcohol, drugs, sexual material, or inappropriate privileges to younger child

Stronger indicators of risk for abusive behavior include these:

- Linking sexuality and aggression in language or behavior; engaging in sexually harassing behavior online or in person; and forcing any sexual interaction

241

- Turning to younger or less powerful children rather than peers to explore natural sexual curiosity

- The inability to control inappropriate sexual behaviors involving another child after being told to stop

- Taking younger children to secret places or hideaways to play special undressing or touching games

While any single behavior may suggest that a child needs help, these behaviors do not, in themselves, indicate that a child is likely to engage in ongoing, sexually-harmful behaviors.

### Why don't children tell?

There are many reasons why children may find it very difficult to tell anyone that they are being abused, whether by an adult or by another child. Most children do not tell anyone about sexual abuse before they become adults themselves. Some common reasons why children do not tell include these:

- Children may not understand that the behavior is inappropriate or harmful.

- Sometimes they want to protect the other child or youth, whom they may care about, or they do not want to upset the adults with troubling information.

- Children may feel guilty or that they are to blame for the interaction.

- A child may hope that if he or she is good enough, the harmful behavior will stop on its own.

- Children may feel obligated to remain silent, having received a combination of gifts, treats, and threats about what will happen if they say no or tell someone. Threats may include physical harm to the victim, a relative, a pet, or breakup of the family.

- Children may feel embarrassment about what is happening or fear that they will not be believed.

- Sometimes, a child may be confused by suggestions that they enjoyed the sexual interaction and wanted it to happen.

- The child who is harmed may be confused about his or her feelings and be persuaded that what is happening is okay or that everyone is doing it, particularly if another child or adolescent initiates the sexual behaviors.

- Very young or disabled children may not have the words or means of communication to let people know what is going on.

For these reasons, maintaining open communications—talking with and listening carefully to children—is an important part of preventing child sexual abuse. Because children often find it so hard to tell us in words, it is important to be alert to the behavioral warning signs that they may be being abused, and then act to learn more.

## What are the signs that a child or young person may be being sexually abused?

Do you notice some of the following behaviors in a child you know?

- Nightmares, sleep problems, extreme fears without an obvious explanation
- Sudden or unexplained personality changes; seems withdrawn, angry, moody, clingy, checked-out, or shows significant changes in eating habits
- An older child behaving like a younger child, for example, bedwetting or thumb-sucking
- Develops fear of particular places or resists being alone with particular child or young person for unknown reasons
- Shows resistance to routine bathing, toileting, or removing clothes even in appropriate situations
- Play, writing, drawings, or dreams include sexual or frightening images
- Refuses to talk about a secret he or she has with an adult or older child
- Stomach aches or illness, often with no identifiable reason
- Leaves clues that seem likely to provoke a discussion about sexual issues
- Uses new or adult words for body parts; engages in adult-like sexual activities with toys, objects, or other children
- Develops special relationship with older friend that may include unexplained money, gifts, or privileges

- Intentionally harming himself or herself, for example, drug or alcohol use, cutting, burning, running away, sexual promiscuity

- Physical symptoms, such as unexplained soreness, pain, or bruises around genitals or mouth; sexually transmitted disease; or pregnancy

### *How can we protect our children?*

There are many things adults can do to prevent the sexual abuse of children: setting clear standards for what is considered appropriate, respectful behavior; staying alert for situations where those expectations are broken; and speaking up promptly to address any concerns are the cornerstones of any effective effort to protect children.

Communication is key. Talking to children about their activities, hopes, and anxieties on a daily basis increases the likelihood that a child, who is worried about his or her own behavior, will be able to tell someone. The sooner adults recognize potentially concerning situations, the better protected children will be.

### *What are some things that adults can do to help prevent sexually harmful behavior between children?*

1. **Set and respect physical boundaries:** Make sure that all members of the family have rights to privacy in dressing, bathing, sleeping, and other personal activities. As adults we are responsible for modeling the boundaries we want our children to honor. Even young children should be respected and their preferences accommodated when possible.

2. **Encourage children to also respect themselves and others:** Much of what young people see in the adult world ignores or even ridicules the importance of treating others respectfully and of demanding the same for oneself. Highly sexualized images in advertising, music lyrics, video games, and films can sometimes make it difficult for adolescents—or even young children—to distinguish between innocent experimentation and sexually harmful behaviors. Teach children to value respectful interactions—including sexual interactions. Create environments at home and in your social groups where children will see that emotionally or sexually aggressive

behaviors are not tolerated and that hurtful behaviors are challenged.

3. **Demonstrate to children that it is all right to say no and that they need to accept no from others:** Teach children when it is okay to say no—for example when they do not want to play, or be tickled, hugged, or kissed. Help them understand what is considered acceptable and unacceptable behavior. Encourage them to always speak up if someone acts in a way that makes them uncomfortable, even if they were unable to object or to say no at the time. Teach children that they must listen to and accept others' limits as well.

4. **Stay aware of how children are interacting with one another:** Be alert to the warning signs that your child, or another child or young person, may be acting in ways that make it difficult for other children to set a limit, or in ways that are sexually aggressive or abusive. Seek information and help as soon as you feel uncomfortable. Don't keep it a secret.

5. **Talk with children, and listen to what they have to say:** Adults and adolescents who sexually abuse children usually rely on secrecy. They often try to silence children and to build trust with adults, counting on them to be silent if they are confused. The first step to breaking through this secrecy is to develop an open and trusting relationship with your children. This means listening carefully to their fears and concerns and letting them know they should not worry about telling you anything. It is important to talk with them about sexuality, offer accurate answers to their questions, and to be comfortable using correct terms for parts of the body.

6. **Set clear guidelines and keep a careful eye on children's internet and video game use and the television shows and movies they watch:** Explain to children the risks associated with using the internet, restrict access to sites that are not age-appropriate, and ask them to tell you if they receive messages or e-mails containing suggestive or sexually explicit material. Keep your computer in a public place so you can easily monitor their use. Check that television shows, films, and videos are age-appropriate. Watch programs with children and use what they see as teachable moments to share information and values. Make agreements with other adults that

the guidelines of a visiting child's parents or guardians will be respected during play dates or visits.

7.   **Take sensible precautions about whom you choose to take care of your children:** Be thoughtful about whom you choose to care for your children. Find out as much as you can about baby sitters and don't leave your child with anyone you have doubts about. If your child is unhappy about spending time with a particular person, talk to the child about his or her concerns.

8.   **Regularly remind children of other trusted adults whom they can talk to:** Sometimes the child or young person whose behavior concerns us is a close family member or the son or daughter of a friend. In those situations, it may be especially painful for us, as parents and caregivers, to admit what may be happening. It may be even harder for a child to tell that someone the family cares about is harming her or him. An adult outside the immediate family is often in a better position to acknowledge concerns and to take protective actions.

### *What can you do if you suspect your child is sexually harming another child or thinking about doing so?*

It is very disturbing to suspect that your child, or a child you know, may be sexually harming someone. It is so much easier to dismiss such thoughts or to think you're overreacting. You may also be worried about the possible consequences of taking action.

Help is available. It is much better to talk over the situation with someone than to discover later that you were right to be concerned and did nothing.

Remember, you are not alone. Every year thousands of people grapple with situations where someone in their family or circle of friends is suspected of inappropriate sexual behavior.

1.   **Act quickly:** Action is prevention. If you are worried that your son or daughter may be sexually harming another child, or if you suspect that your child is being abused, act now. Get help from a professional therapist immediately and develop a safety plan addressing the concerning behaviors. Prompt intervention also can get the sexually abusing youth the treatment needed to stop abusing and to grow up as a safe member of our community.

2.  **Stay steady:** When speaking to children about your concerns, remember to stay calm and ask simple and direct questions. Listen carefully to the responses without suggesting answers. It may be useful to practice with someone else first and get support to help keep your own emotions in check. Recognize that confusion, guilt, and shame about abuse can make the conversation difficult, both for you and for the child. Acknowledge the child's discomfort and offer praise for his or her courage to talk about a confusing experience. Remember that if it's difficult for you to discuss your concerns, it is likely to be much more difficult for the child.

3.  **Get support for everyone:** Whatever is revealed, reassure them that you love them and that you are committed to helping them. Children will look to adults for reassurance that they will be all right. Keep reminding yourself that healing for everyone is possible. Children and adolescents frequently respond best to specialized, sex-specific treatment when it is offered early and with the support of trusted adults. Sexual abuse affects all members of a family or group. The entire family, including the adults, are likely to need support.

4.  **Be prepared to report:** Reporting the abuse to authorities is an upsetting prospect for many families. Yet, filing a report can be a first step to accessing support services. Children who are abused and their families need help to recover from their trauma. Anyone who is harming a child sexually also needs help and support to stop the behavior. Sometimes, in the most serious cases and depending upon the age of the child or adolescent, reporting may result in legal consequences. Although this can be a difficult process for everyone involved, when combined with specialized treatment, it may be the best way to prevent further harm and even harsher future consequences.

5.  **Make use of valuable lessons learned.** If you have been involved in helping a child cope with harmful sexual behaviors, your experience and knowledge about abuse and treatment may be extremely valuable to others. The opportunity to prevent sexual abuse does not end with the discovery of abuse. Use the lessons you have learned to educate others about prevention and to support other families facing similar concerns.

## Take Action

If you are unsure or worried about the behavior of someone you know (whether they are an adult or a child), we have information that can help you consider your possible next steps. With guidance, adults can learn about sexual abuse; identify specialized treatment options for themselves or someone they care about; develop a safety plan; find language for an effective conversation when they have concerns, and learn how to report those concerns to authorities when appropriate.

## Prevention, Treatment, and Recovery Resources

### Association for the Treatment of Sexual Abusers (ATSA)
4900 SW Griffith Drive, Suite 274
Beaverton, OR 97005
Phone: 503-643-1023
Fax: 503-643-5084
Website: http://www.atsa.com
E-mail: atsa@atsa.com

A national organization developing and disseminating professional standards and practices in the field of sex offender research, evaluation, and treatment. Call or e-mail for a referral to a local treatment provider.

### Child Molestation Research and Prevention Institute
1401 Peachtree Street, Suite 120
Atlanta, GA 30309
Phone: 404-872-5152
Website: http://www.childmolestationprevention.org

Online directory for sex-specific therapists for evaluation and treatment. Extensive reading lists for parents of children with sexual behavior problems and parents of victims, for professionals, adults with sexual behavior concerns, adults molested as children and their partners.

### National Center on Sexual Behavior of Youth
940 N.E. 13th St., 3B-3406
Oklahoma City, OK 73104
Phone: 405-271-8858
Fax: 405-271-2510
Website: http://www.ncsby.org

Information concerning sexual development and youth with sexual behavior problems.

## National Center for Victims of Crime (NCVC)
2000 M St., NW, Suite 480
Washington, DC 20036
Toll-Free: 800-FYI-CALL (394-2255)
Toll-Free TDD: 800-211-7996
Phone: 202-467-8700
Fax: 202-467-8701
Website: http://www.ncvc.org
E-mail: webmaster@ncvc.org or gethelp@ncvc.org

An information and referral center for victims. Through its database of over 30,000 organizations, NCVC refers callers to services including crisis intervention, research information, assistance with the criminal justice process, counseling, support groups, and referrals to local attorneys in victim-related cases.

## Safer Society Foundation
P.O. Box 340
Brandon, VT 05733-0340
Phone: 802-247-3132
Fax: 802-247-4233
Website: http://www.safersociety.org

Call for a referral to a local treatment provider for a child, adolescent or adult with sexual behavior concerns. Also provides publications for youth or adults with sexual behavior problems, their families, survivors, treatment providers, and mandated reporters.

## Stop It Now!
351 Pleasant St., Suite 319
Northampton, MA 01060
Toll-Free Helpline: 888-PREVENT (773-8368)
Phone: 413-587-3500
Website: http://www.stopitnow.org
E-mail: helpline@stopitnow.org

In collaboration with a network of community-based programs, Stop It Now! reaches out to adults who are concerned about their own or others' sexualized behavior toward children. They provide support, information, and resources that enable individuals and families to keep children safe and create healthier communities.

# Chapter 30

# *Online Exploitation and Abuse of Children and Youth*

Increasingly, the internet is used to facilitate the sexual exploitation of children through child pornography and enticement offenses. This activity is a growing threat to the safety of children in the United States and, indeed, throughout the world.

## *Child Pornography and Sexual Solicitation of Children by Predators Continue to Proliferate Online*

Despite all of the hard work undertaken by federal, state, and local law enforcement, the scope of these dangers facing our children is immense. The growth in the overall reported instances of child sexual exploitation has been tremendous since 1998. The size and the speed of the increases is staggering: from 1998 to 2005, the annual reports to the CyberTipline rose by 1,452%.

Two types of dangers to children are especially problematic. First, the threat of sexual predators contacting children online, with the hope of luring them to meet in person, has been amply demonstrated by academic studies as well as recent investigative journalism reports. A youth internet safety survey conducted between August 1999 and January 2000 found that approximately one in five children per year receives an unwanted sexual solicitation online. One in thirty-three children per year receives an aggressive sexual solicitation—one in

---

Text in this chapter is excerpted from "Project Safe Childhood: Part II," U.S. Department of Justice, May 2006.

which a solicitor asks to meet them somewhere, calls them on the telephone, or sends mail, money, or gifts. And one in four per year has an unwanted exposure to sexually explicit material. Meanwhile, only 25% of the youth who encountered a sexual solicitation told a parent. Only a fraction of all episodes were reported to authorities, such as a law enforcement agency, an internet service provider, or a hotline. According to a recent media report, at any given time, 50,000 predators are on the internet prowling for children. These figures make clear that the threat of online enticement of children is immense.

Second, the victimization of children through the production and distribution of child pornography is equally troubling, and on the rise. It was estimated, even in 2003, that more than 20,000 images of child pornography are posted on the internet each week. The National Center for Missing and Exploited Children's (NCMEC) CyberTipline logged a 39% increase in reports of the possession, creation, or distribution of child pornography in 2004. The gravity of these increases is more dramatically demonstrated by comparing the actual number of reports in 1998 to those logged in 2004, rather than merely reciting percentage increases. In 1998, the CyberTipline received 3,267 reports of child pornography. In 2004, the CyberTipline received 106,119 of these reports, marking more than a 30-fold increase in child pornography reports in a six year period. Judging simply by crime statistics, it is clear that the internet is helping to fuel an epidemic of child pornography.

Not only is there an increase in the volume of pornographic images, there is also an escalation in the severity of the abuse depicted, with the images found today more frequently involving younger children—including toddlers and even infants—and despicable acts such as penetration of infants. And technology lends itself to the dissemination of more graphic images via the web, with its easy access, low cost, and apparent anonymity.

Experts agree that the escalation in both the prevalence and severity of child pornography is driven at least in part by advances in computer technology and increased access to the internet. According to a recent study, 78.6% of Americans go online, and almost two-thirds of Americans use the internet at home. While it is impossible to determine exactly how many people are looking at child pornography, experts attribute the escalation in the quantity of child pornography being created and distributed to the growth of the internet, and the concomitant ease with which child predators can now buy, sell, and swap images. The resulting sense of community among child predators is in turn helping to embolden those who may have had misgivings about a sexual interest in children, and it is thus driving a market for new images with fresh faces. Before the internet, it was difficult and risky for child exploiters to go out and find other child exploiters with whom to share images, which left the child pornography industry relegated to small black markets in underground bookstores or secret mailings. Today, the internet has provided these pedophiles with an accessible, convenient, and anonymous means for interacting with their community and obtaining illicit material. The internet has thus taken down borders that at one time served as a deterrent to child pornographers.

## These Escalating Trends Present a Serious Risk to Our Society

The harm caused by enticement offenses is beyond question. Sexual abuse is a serious crime that deeply affects any victim, especially children, and it has dramatic secondary effects on our society. The looming danger of our children being preyed upon by pedophiles in chat rooms or through social networking sites is, in short, among the gravest threats facing children today.

The impact of child pornography on victims, and on society as a whole, is far less appreciated today than the threat of enticement offenses. Child pornography images are not just pictures, akin to any number of other images legally available on the internet. Most images of child pornography depict victims—children—who have been exploited and abused. These images are permanent visual records of child sexual abuse. For this reason, the very term commonly used to describe these terrible images—child pornography—does not adequately convey the horrors these images depict. A more accurate term would be "images of child sexual abuse," because the very production of the images necessarily involves the sexual abuse of a child. And the child is re-victimized each time they are viewed.

The nation should be alarmed at the fact that child pornography is being produced, possessed, and distributed in record numbers. According to a 2005 study entitled "Child-Pornography Possessors Arrested in Internet-Related Crimes: Findings from the National Juvenile Online Victimization Study," which studied defendants arrested and charged with possession of child pornography between July 2000 and June 2001:

- More than 80% of arrested [child pornography] possessors had images of prepubescent children, and 80% had images of minors being sexually penetrated. Approximately one in five (21%) arrested [child pornography] possessors had images of children enduring bondage, sadistic sex, and other sexual violence. More than one in three (39%) [child pornography] possessors had videos depicting child pornography with motion and sound.

- Although their identities are often unknown, many of the children in these graphic images were sexually victimized and assaulted. Those who possess these pictures—for sexual gratification, curiosity, as a means of profit, or for other reasons—are adding to the burdens of these young victims, whose trauma may be increased by knowing their pictures are circulating globally on the internet with no hope of permanent removal or could be entered into circulation in the future.

Child pornography victimizes children in a very real and dramatic way. Of course, no child can consent to being sexually exploited through the production of sexually explicit images. Each time the image is viewed or distributed, the child is again victimized. In addition to the obvious physical injuries that a child can suffer due to sexual abuse, the emotional and psychological trauma is devastating, and lasting. Many child victims suffer from depression, withdrawal, anger, and other conditions that often continue into adulthood. They experience feelings of guilt and responsibility for the abuse, a sense of powerlessness, and feelings of worthlessness.

Thus, for the sole fact of the victimization and damage that child pornography visits upon children, possession of child pornography is a heinous crime that must be stamped out. But that is only half of the story of the pernicious effect of child pornography. Possession of child pornography is a serious crime for four additional reasons.

1. The exchange of child pornography by and between child exploiters validates and encourages them in their beliefs and behaviors.

2. The greater availability of child pornography has led to the production, receipt, and distribution of more shocking, graphic images, which are increasingly involving younger children and infants.

3. The compulsion to collect child pornography images may lead to a compulsion to molest children, or may be indicative of a propensity to molest children.

4. Child pornography is frequently used by molesters as an affirmative tool, either to silence their victims, to blackmail them
into further exploitation, or to entice other children.

## A Call to Arms

The measures taken to this point have not served to dramatically
lessen the number of incidents of child exploitation. Indeed, all of the
evidence leads to the conclusion that the exploitation of children is a
burgeoning problem. The explosion in the production and trafficking
of child pornography, in particular, represents nothing short of an
epidemic confronting our country. Although law enforcement efforts
alone cannot solve this problem, investigative agencies and prosecutors must redouble their efforts and allocate resources to ensure an
adequate response.

Attorney General Gonzales called on all Americans to join the cause:
"I am...calling on all responsible Americans and corporate citizens—
down to every last parent, teacher, and minister—to educate themselves about the problem and see how they can help out. Together, we
can make our homes and our neighborhoods safer for our sons and
for our daughters."

# Chapter 31

# *Female Genital Mutilation*

## *Key Facts*

- Female genital mutilation (FGM) includes procedures that intentionally alter or injure female genital organs for non-medical reasons.

- An estimated 100 to 140 million girls and women worldwide are currently living with the consequences of FGM.

- In Africa, about three million girls are at risk for FGM annually.

- The procedure has no health benefits for girls and women.

- Procedures can cause severe bleeding and problems urinating, and later, potential childbirth complications and newborn deaths.

- It is mostly carried out on young girls sometime between infancy and age 15 years.

- FGM is internationally recognized as a violation of the human rights of girls and women.

Female genital mutilation (FGM) comprises all procedures that involve partial or total removal of the external female genitalia, or other injury to the female genital organs for non-medical reasons.

"Female Genital Mutilation," May 2008, http://www.who.int/mediacentre/factsheets/fs241/en/index.html. © 2008 World Health Organization. Reprinted with permission.

The practice is mostly carried out by traditional circumcisers, who often play other central roles in communities, such as attending childbirths. Increasingly, however, FGM is being performed by medically trained personnel.

FGM is recognized internationally as a violation of the human rights of girls and women. It reflects deep-rooted inequality between the sexes, and constitutes an extreme form of discrimination against women. It is nearly always carried out on minors and is a violation of the rights of children. The practice also violates a person's rights to health, security, and physical integrity; the right to be free from torture and cruel, inhuman, or degrading treatment; and the right to life when the procedure results in death.

## Procedures

Female genital mutilation is classified into four major types:

1. Clitoridectomy: partial or total removal of the clitoris (a small, sensitive and erectile part of the female genitals) and, rarely, the prepuce (the fold of skin surrounding the clitoris) as well.

2. Excision: partial or total removal of the clitoris and the labia minora, with or without excision of the labia majora (the labia are "the lips" that surround the vagina).

3. Infibulation: narrowing of the vaginal opening through the creation of a covering seal. The seal is formed by cutting and repositioning the inner, and sometimes outer, labia, with or without removal of the clitoris.

4. Other: all other harmful procedures to the female genitalia for non-medical purposes, for example: pricking, piercing, incising, scraping, and cauterizing the genital area.

## Health Consequences

FGM has no health benefits, and it harms girls and women in many ways. It involves removing and damaging healthy and normal female genital tissue, and interferes with the natural functions of girls' and women's bodies.

Immediate complications can include severe pain, shock, hemorrhage (bleeding), tetanus or sepsis (bacterial infection), urine retention, open sores in the genital region, and injury to nearby genital tissue.

Long-term consequences can include:

- recurrent bladder and urinary tract infections;
- cysts;
- infertility;
- the need for later surgeries. (For example, the FGM procedure that seals or narrows a vaginal opening (type 3) is surgically changed to allow for sexual intercourse and childbirth, and sometimes stitched close again afterwards); and,
- an increased risk of childbirth complications and newborn deaths.

## *Who is at risk?*

Procedures are mostly carried out on young girls sometime between infancy and age 15, and occasionally on adult women. In Africa, about three million girls are at risk for FGM annually.

Between 100 to 140 million girls and women worldwide are living with the consequences of FGM. In Africa, about 92 million girls age 10 years and above are estimated to have undergone FGM.

The practice is most common in the western, eastern, and northeastern regions of Africa, in some countries in Asia and the Middle East, and among certain immigrant communities in North America and Europe.

## *Causes*

The causes of female genital mutilation include a mix of cultural, religious, and social factors within families and communities.

- Where FGM is a social convention, the social pressure to conform to what others do and have been doing is a strong motivation to perpetuate the practice.

- FGM is often considered a necessary part of raising a girl properly, and a way to prepare her for adulthood and marriage.

- FGM is often motivated by beliefs about what is considered proper sexual behavior, linking procedures to premarital virginity and marital fidelity. FGM is believed by some to reduce a woman's libido and help her resist "illicit" sexual acts. When a vaginal opening is covered or narrowed (type 3), for example, a woman is physically hindered from premarital sex. Afterwards, a painful procedure is needed to reopen the closure to enable sexual intercourse.

- FGM is associated with cultural ideals of femininity and modesty, which include the notion that girls are "clean" and "beautiful" after removal of body parts that are considered "male" or "unclean."

- Though no religious scripts prescribe the practice, practitioners often believe the practice has religious support.

- Religious leaders take varying positions with regard to FGM: some promote it, some consider it irrelevant to religion, and others contribute to its elimination.

- Local structures of power and authority, such as community leaders, religious leaders, circumcisers, and even some medical personnel can contribute to upholding the practice.

- In most societies, FGM is considered a cultural tradition, which is often used as an argument for its continuation.

- In some societies, recent adoption of the practice is linked to copying the traditions of neighboring groups. Sometimes it has started as part of a wider religious or traditional revival movement.

- In some societies, FGM is being practiced by new groups when they move into areas where the local population practice FGM.

## International Response

In 1997, the World Health Organization (WHO) issued a joint statement with the United Nations Children's Fund (UNICEF) and the United Nations Population Fund (UNFPA) against the practice of FGM. A new statement, with wider United Nations support, was then issued in February 2008 to support increased advocacy for the abandonment of FGM.

The 2008 statement documents new evidence collected over the past decade about the practice. It highlights the increased recognition of the human rights and legal dimensions of the problem and provides current data on the frequency and scope of FGM. It also summarizes research about why FGM continues, how to stop it, and its damaging effects on the health of women, girls, and newborn babies.

Since 1997, great efforts have been made to counteract FGM, through research, work within communities, and changes in public policy. Progress at both international and local levels includes:

- wider international involvement to stop FGM;

- the development of international monitoring bodies and resolutions that condemn the practice;
- revised legal frameworks and growing political support to end FGM; and
- in some countries, decreasing practice of FGM, and an increasing number of women and men in practicing communities who declare their support to end it.

Research shows that, if practicing communities themselves decide to abandon FGM, the practice can be eliminated very rapidly.

## WHO Response

WHO efforts to eliminate female genital mutilation focus on:

- advocacy: developing publications and advocacy tools for international, regional, and local efforts to end FGM within a generation;
- research: generating knowledge about the causes and consequences of the practice, how to eliminate it, and how to care for those who have experienced FGM;
- guidance for health systems: developing training materials and guidelines for health professionals to help them treat and counsel women who have undergone procedures.

WHO is particularly concerned about the increasing trend for medically trained personnel to perform FGM. WHO strongly urges health professionals not to perform such procedures.

## For More Information

**WHO Media Centre**
World Health Organization
Avenue Appia 20
1211 Geneva 27
Switzerland
Telephone: +41 22 791 2222
Website: http://www.who.int/mediacentre/en/
E-mail: mediainquiries@who.int

# Part Four

# Intervention and Treatments for Child Maltreatment

# Chapter 32

# *Helping Children Who Are Experiencing Abuse or Neglect*

Every adult involved in the life of a child plays a critical role in helping maintain that child's safety. It is important to recognize your vital role and learn how to help protect the children in your life from abuse and neglect.

If you suspect that a child is a victim of abuse or neglect and you are unsure whether the child's situation has been reported to child protective services (CPS), you should report your concerns to your local CPS agency.

### *What happens once a report is made?*

After receiving a report of child abuse or neglect, CPS will use that information, along with any previous history of involvement with the family, in order to determine the best course of action. If CPS determines that the report does not meet the legal standards of child abuse or neglect, or there is not enough evidence or information to investigate the report, CPS will usually refer the family to another agency that will provide the family with appropriate services (such as counseling, parenting skills classes, substance abuse programs). Alternatively, the information you share might lead CPS to begin a family assessment or investigation. Depending on the laws in your state and your relationship with the child, you may have the opportunity to communicate with a CPS worker regarding the child's progress. Educators and school personnel, in particular, are an excellent resource and may be asked to share additional information to help determine the facts of a case and develop a treatment plan for the child and family.

Any party discussing a child abuse case must adhere to the principles of confidentiality, since details of a case may be shared only with appropriate parties as designated by law. This protection by the law protects both the child and family from rumors, judgments, and stereotyping that may further isolate and alienate them, and thus negatively affect intervention efforts.

### Should you still have contact with the family?

Depending on the nature of your relationship with the child or family, you might continue to have regular contact with the family after a report has been made. Please know that you are just as important to the family's recovery as you are to the child's. Appropriate interactions with parents who are suspected of child abuse or neglect will have a positive influence on the family's ability to recover. The following are guidelines for interacting with the child's family:

- Be objective and supportive. Remember that most parents want to be good parents but may need additional help, encouragement, and guidance.

- Be an active listener. Do not blame, accuse, or make judgments about family members or their situations.

- Offer your support in any way in which you feel comfortable. Families in these situations can greatly benefit from social support, which could include anything from baby sitting to carpooling to just offering to listen.

- Limit your conversations to the activities that involve you. It is not your responsibility to investigate suspected child abuse or neglect.

- Address the family in a manner that is consistent with your role or relationship with the family. If you are an educator, be professional and objective. If you are a friend, family member, or neighbor, be friendly, helpful, supportive, and understanding. Do not allow yourself to be placed in an adversarial role if the parents become defensive, argumentative, accusatory, or upset.

- Encourage parents and provide them with information about educational programs on parenting, job skills, and child development; programs and activities for children; and counseling, alcohol, drug abuse, or adult education and enrichment programs, if this seems appropriate given the nature of your relationship. (You can even offer to join them and take advantage of the opportunity to learn new skills.)

Remember, families experiencing abuse or neglect issues are often under a great deal of stress in multiple areas of their lives. Your interaction, involvement, or support can be an important stress reducer for the child and for the parents.

The following tips can help you develop a nurturing relationship with any child who may be suffering from negative self-esteem or who is being abused or neglected. Children need positive adult role models; therefore, your warmth, empathy, and interest can help a child see adults in positive, supportive, and caring roles.

### Listen

- Be an approachable, patient, and supportive listener. Listen without being critical or negative toward the child or the child's parents.

- Show that you understand and believe what the child says, even if it is difficult. Make sure to not blame, punish, or accuse the child of doing anything wrong.

- Let the child know that you are there for him or her to talk to openly, should he or she wish to do so. Leaving an open line of communication is much more beneficial to the child than pressuring him or her to self-disclose or reveal his or her experiences of abuse or neglect before he or she is ready to talk about it.

### Empathize

- Validate the child's feelings, emotions, and experiences. Do not belittle or minimize the child's feelings; he or she has those feelings for a reason.

- Affirm the child's decision to confide in you. Tell the child that he or she is doing the right thing by talking to an adult whom he or she trusts. Let the child know that you are there for him or her and want to help keep him or her safe.

- Assure the child often that he or she is not to blame. Child victims may believe that the abuse or neglect is their fault.

- Don't overreact. Stay calm. Fear and anger are normal reactions, but you may frighten the child and prevent him or her from confiding in you in the future if you become agitated.

- Do not talk negatively about the abuser in front of the child. Remember that child victims of abuse may be very loyal to their abusers, especially if the abuser is a parent. Despite the pain they may feel as a result of the abuse, many children still love their parents and want to be loved and wanted by them.

*Be a Positive Role Model*

- Provide a lot of positive feedback and reinforcement to help build the child's self-esteem. As often as possible, tell the child how he or she positively contributes to your life, the child's family, and the world. Talk about the child's potential and what he or she has to offer, and sincerely tell the child that he or she is good, smart, and kind.

- Help the child learn conflict resolution skills by teaching or modeling them. Children who have been abused or neglected may be unfamiliar with non-violent ways of dealing with conflict.

- When a child acts in ways that seem strange, remember to look for the feelings behind the actions. Children may try to protect themselves from their negative feelings by pretending those feelings do not exist. Also, they may seek your attention through negative behaviors because they do not know how to gain your attention using positive ones. Look for opportunities to encourage and reinforce positive behavior.

*Promote Positive Interaction*

- Do not pity, overly-focus attention on, or treat children who have experienced abuse or neglect differently from others with whom you are involved. Children who have been the victims of abuse or neglect want to be seen as normal and feel like other children.

- Foster the child's relationships with peers by encouraging extra-curricular and school-related activities.

- Help build the child's confidence. Allow children to have possessions of their own (such as a desk or work space, books, backpack, toys) and give them resources and opportunities to be successful at taking care of their responsibilities.

All these acts can reinforce a child's resiliency and sense of well-being. Keep in mind, however, that these acts do not replace informing CPS if you suspect a child is being abused or neglected. Your first responsibility as a trusted adult is to make a report of your concern to CPS if you feel a child's safety is at risk.

## Resources

American Humane Association. (1994). *Twenty years after CAPTA: A portrait of the child protective services system.* Englewood, CO: Author.

Children, Youth, and Families Department, Child Care Services Bureau. (1998). *Reporting child abuse it's everyone's responsibility.* South Deerfield, MA: Channing L. Bete Co., Inc.

Erickson, E. L., McEvaoy, A. W, and Colucci, N. D., Jr. (1979). *Child abuse and neglect: A guidebook for educators and community leaders.* Holmes Beach, FL: Learning Publications, Inc.

National Center on Child Abuse and Neglect. (1992). *The role of educators in the prevention and treatment of child abuse and neglect.* Washington, DC: U.S. Government Printing Office.

## For More Information

***American Humane***
63 Inverness Dr., East
Englewood, CO 80112-5117
Toll-Free: 800-227-4645
Phone: 303-792-9900
Fax: 303-792-5333
Website: http://www.americanhumane.org
E-mail: info@americanhumane.org

Chapter 33

# Legislation Regarding Child Maltreatment

## Chapter Contents

## Section 33.1

## *Child Maltreatment Legislation and Caseworker Practice*

Excerpted from "Working with the Courts in Child Protection
User Manual Series: Chapter 3," Child Welfare Information Gateway,
U.S. Department of Health and Human Services (HHS), 2006.

Children had little legal protection from maltreatment until the early 20th century when addressing child abuse and neglect became a component of the new juvenile court movement. Court practices varied, but generally were inadequate to meet the needs of abused and neglected children and their families. The identification of battered child syndrome in 1962 heightened public interest in child maltreatment and resulted in the passage of legislation in most states to enhance protections for children.

As recently as the late 1970s, it was common that the only people in the courtroom in child maltreatment cases were the caseworker, the judge, and sometimes the parents. Children rarely participated in the process and none of the parties, including child protective services (CPS), had legal representation. Nor were there guardians ad litem (GAL) or court-appointed special advocates (CASAs). The court's role was limited. If it found abuse or neglect, it would place the child in the custody of CPS, and that ended its responsibility. There were no case plans, no court reports, no periodic reviews, no reasonable efforts requirement, and no permanency planning.

Since then, sweeping changes have occurred in the law, CPS practice, and the litigation of child maltreatment cases. Family dynamics and problems (for example, acquired immunodeficiency syndrome [AIDS], homelessness, and substance abuse) have become more complex as well. These changes have increased the frequency of interaction between the courts and CPS dramatically and have transformed the nature of their relationship. Therefore, it is imperative that CPS caseworkers understand the implications of significant legislation on successful outcomes for families.

## The Child Abuse Prevention and Treatment Act

The first federal legislation to address child maltreatment became law in 1974 with the passage of the Child Abuse Prevention and Treatment Act (CAPTA) (P.L. 93-247). In return for federal funding, CAPTA required that states adopt mandatory child abuse reporting laws, ensure the confidentiality of agency records and court proceedings, and appoint a GAL for every child in maltreatment proceedings in juvenile court. CAPTA has been reauthorized periodically and amended by Congress, most recently as part of the Keeping Children and Families Safe Act of 2003 (P.L. 108-36).

The recent amendment to CAPTA changed the confidentiality requirements so that states now are obligated to share confidential information with any agency or individual who has a statutory duty to protect children. This amendment also contains language that allows states flexibility to determine state policies that permit public access to child abuse court proceedings.

## The Individuals with Disabilities Education Act

Originally enacted in 1975, the Individuals with Disabilities Education Act (IDEA) (P.L. 94-142) entitles eligible children to education programs that meet their special needs. An individual education plan (IEP) is developed for eligible children to identify their specific educational needs as well as strategies for meeting them. In its most recent reauthorization, CAPTA contains a provision that requires CPS to refer children under the age of three for evaluation of IDEA eligibility in substantiated cases of abuse or neglect.

## The Indian Child Welfare Act

The Indian Child Welfare Act (ICWA) (P.L. 95-608) of 1978 requires specific protections to Native American children involved in CPS and juvenile court proceedings. If a child is affiliated with a tribal organization, the tribe has the right to intervene in proceedings or to petition to have the case transferred to tribal court.

## The Adoption Assistance and Child Welfare Act

The Adoption Assistance and Child Welfare Act (P.L. 96-272) of 1980 requires that CPS make reasonable efforts to avoid unnecessary removals of children from their homes and to reunify foster children with their families. "Reasonable efforts" means providing a parent with useful resources that enable them to protect the child, to provide a stable home environment, and to promote the child's well-being. If the court finds that reasonable efforts have not been made, CPS funding from federal and state sources may be reduced.

For example, the court also may expect that the following services will be offered to demonstrate reasonable efforts:

- A developmental or medical assessment of the child(ren)
- A child sexual abuse assessment
- A substance abuse assessment and treatment plan for adults with suspected substance abuse
- Domestic violence counseling
- A parenting program
- Emergency benefits for the family such as temporary shelter or groceries voucher
- Enrollment in the Temporary Assistance for Needy Families program
- Vocational rehabilitation services
- Parent and sibling visitation

Additionally, reasonable efforts require that services be available and accessible. Thus, if transportation to substance abuse treatment or weekly urine screens is an issue, the CPS caseworker may want to provide transportation or bus tokens to them.

## The Adoption and Safe Families Act

In 1997, Congress passed the Adoption and Safe Families Act (ASFA) (P.L. 105-89) in response to concerns that many children were remaining in foster care for long periods or experiencing multiple placements. The law requires timely permanency planning for children. Permanency for children involves either reunification with the biological parent, legal guardianship with a relative or caregiver, adoption, or an alternative planned permanent living arrangement. ASFA emphasizes that the child's safety is the paramount concern in any child maltreatment case.

In addition, ASFA addressed the lack of clarity regarding what constituted making "reasonable efforts" to keep families together. The legislation:

274

- restricts the reasonable efforts requirement of attempting to keep families intact by permitting it to be waived under specified circumstances, such as severe or chronic maltreatment or the death of another child in the household due to maltreatment;

- expands the reasonable efforts requirement to make it applicable to CPS efforts to secure permanent homes for children who will not be reunited with their families;

- mandates a permanency hearing to occur no more than 12 months after a child is placed in foster care;

- dictates, with some exceptions, that petitions for termination of parental rights need to be filed for children who have been in foster care for 15 of the previous 22 months;

- includes several provisions to promote, to facilitate, to fund, and to support adoptive placements;

- gives substitute care providers the right to receive notice of court hearings and the opportunity to be heard;

- requires criminal record checks on all substitute care providers; and

- directs that compliance with these provisions and other performance standards be carefully monitored and enforced.

ASFA has a significant impact on caseworker practice, guiding caseworkers through family reunification, the provision of services to the family, and alternative permanent placements, if necessary.

## The Interstate Compact on the Placement of Children

In addition to federal legislation, the Interstate Compact on the Placement of Children (ICPC) also can play an important role in caseworker practice. ICPC is an agreement among all 50 states, the District of Columbia, and the U.S. Virgin Islands regarding placement (for example: kinship care, adoption, foster care) across state lines. The placement must be approved by the ICPC offices of each of the affected states before it can occur.

Due to the special needs of children and/or the lack of an appropriate therapeutic foster care placement, an alternative foster care placement located in a neighboring state may be recommended. This process can be time consuming and can prolong the quest for permanency. Thus, the CPS caseworker will need to contact the State ICPC office imme-diately, follow all ICPC requirements, and pursue timely completion of the ICPC process.

# Section 33.2

# Infant Safe Haven Laws

"Infant Safe Haven Laws," Child Welfare Information Gateway, U.S. Department of Health and Human Services, July 2007.

Many state legislatures have enacted legislation to address infant abandonment and infanticide in response to a reported increase in the abandonment of infants. Beginning in Texas in 1999, "Baby Moses laws" or infant safe haven laws have been enacted as an incentive for mothers in crisis to safely relinquish their babies to designated loca-tions where the babies are protected and provided with medical care until a permanent home is found. Safe haven laws generally allow the parent, or an agent of the parent, to remain anonymous and to be shielded from prosecution for abandonment or neglect in exchange for surrendering the baby to a safe haven.

To date, approximately 47 states and Puerto Rico have enacted safe haven legislation.[1] The focus of these laws is protecting newborns. In approximately 15 states, infants who are 72 hours old or younger may be relinquished to a designated safe haven.[2] Approximately 14 states and Puerto Rico accept infants up to one month old.[3] Other states specify varying age limits in their statutes.[4]

## Who May Leave a Baby at a Safe Haven?

In most states with safe haven laws, either parent may surrender his or her baby to a safe haven. In four states (Georgia, Maryland, Minnesota, and Tennessee), only the mother may relinquish her in-fant.[5] Idaho specifies that only a custodial parent may surrender an infant. In approximately 11 states, an agent of the parent (someone who has the parent's approval) may take a baby to a safe haven for a parent.[6] Six states do not specify the person who may relinquish an infant.[7]

## Safe Haven Providers

The purpose of safe haven laws is to ensure that relinquished infants are left with persons who can provide the immediate care needed for their safety and well-being. To that end, approximately eight states require parents to relinquish their infants to a hospital.[8] Other states designate additional entities as safe haven providers, including emergency medical services, police stations, and fire stations. In four states (Louisiana, Michigan, New Hampshire, and Vermont), emergency medical technicians responding to a 9-1-1 call may accept an infant. In addition, four states (Arizona, New Hampshire, South Carolina, and Vermont) and Puerto Rico allow churches to act as safe havens, but the relinquishing parent must first determine that church personnel are present at the time the infant is left. Generally, anyone on staff at these institutions can receive an infant; however, many states require that staff receiving an infant be trained in emergency medical care.

## Responsibilities of Safe Haven Providers

The safe haven provider is required to accept emergency protective custody of the infant and to provide any immediate medical care that the infant may require. In ten states, when the safe haven receiving the baby is not a hospital, the baby must be transferred to a hospital as soon as possible.[9] The provider is also required to notify the local child welfare department that an infant has been relinquished.

In 21 states, the provider is required to ask the parent for family and medical history information.[10] In 17 states, the provider is required to attempt to give the parent or parents information about the legal repercussions of leaving the infant and information about referral services.[11] In four states (California, Connecticut, Delaware, and North Dakota), a copy of the infant's numbered identification bracelet may be offered to the parent as an aid to linking the parent to the child if reunification is sought at a later date.

## Immunity from Liability for Providers

Safe haven providers are given protection from liability for anything that might happen to the infant while in their care, unless there is evidence of major negligence on the part of the provider.

## Protections for the Parents

In approximately 13 states, anonymity for the parent or agent of the parent is expressly guaranteed in statute.[12] In 28 states and Puerto Rico, the safe haven provider cannot compel the parent or agent of the parent to provide identifying information.[13] In addition, 13 states provide an assurance of confidentiality for any information that is voluntarily provided by the parent.[14]

In addition to the guarantee of anonymity, most states provide protection from criminal liability for parents who safely relinquish their infants. Approximately 30 states and Puerto Rico do not prosecute a parent for child abandonment when a baby is relinquished to a safe haven.[15] In 16 states, safe relinquishment of the infant is an affirmative defense in any prosecution of the parent or his or her agent for any crime against the child, such as abandonment, neglect, or child endangerment.[16]

The privileges of anonymity and immunity will be forfeited in most states if there is evidence of child abuse or neglect.

## Consequences of Relinquishment

Once the safe haven provider has notified the local child welfare department that an infant has been relinquished, the department assumes custody of the infant as an abandoned child. The department has responsibility for placing the infant, usually in a pre-adoptive home, and for petitioning the court for termination of the birth parent's parental rights. Before the baby is placed in a pre-adoptive home, 12 states require the department to request the local law enforcement agency to determine whether the baby has been reported as a missing child.[17] In addition, four states (Illinois, Missouri, Utah, and Wyoming) require the department to check the putative father registry before a termination of parental rights petition can be filed.

Approximately 18 states have procedures in place for a parent to reclaim the infant, usually within a specified time period and before any petition to terminate parental rights has been granted.[18] Five states (Louisiana, Missouri, Montana, South Dakota, and Tennessee) also have provisions for a non-relinquishing father to petition for custody of the child. In 12 states and Puerto Rico, the act of surrendering an infant to a safe haven is presumed to be a relinquishment of parental rights to the child, and no further parental consent is required for the child's adoption.[19]

# References

1.  The word approximately is used to stress the fact that the states frequently amend their laws. This information is current only through July 2007. Alaska, Hawaii, Nebraska, the District of Columbia, American Samoa, Guam, the Northern Mariana Islands, and the Virgin Islands have not yet addressed the issue of abandoned newborns in legislation.

2.  Alabama, Arizona, California, Colorado, Florida, Kentucky, Maryland, Michigan, Minnesota, Mississippi, Ohio, Tennessee, Utah, Washington, and Wisconsin.

3.  Arkansas, Connecticut, Idaho, Louisiana, Maine, Montana, Nevada, New Jersey, Oregon, Pennsylvania, Rhode Island, South Carolina, Vermont, and West Virginia.

4.  Other limits include five days (New York); seven days (Georgia, Illinois, Massachusetts, New Hampshire, North Carolina, and Oklahoma); 14 days (Delaware, Iowa, Virginia, and Wyoming); 45 days (Indiana and Kansas); 60 days (South Dakota and Texas); 90 days (New Mexico); and one year (Missouri and North Dakota).

5.  Maryland and Minnesota do allow the mother to approve another person to deliver the infant on her behalf.

6.  Arizona, Arkansas, Connecticut, Indiana, Iowa, Kentucky, New Jersey, North Dakota, Rhode Island, Utah, and Wyoming.

7.  Delaware, Illinois, Maine, New Mexico, South Carolina, and Vermont.

8.  Connecticut, Delaware, Georgia, Minnesota, North Dakota, Pennsylvania, Utah, and West Virginia.

9.  Florida, Illinois, Kentucky, Louisiana, Maryland, Missouri, Montana, Nevada, New Jersey, and South Carolina.

10. California, Connecticut, Delaware, Iowa, Kentucky, Louisiana, Maine, Massachusetts, Michigan, Minnesota, Montana, North Carolina, North Dakota, Ohio, Oklahoma, South Carolina, South Dakota, Tennessee, Texas, Washington, and Wyoming.

11. Arizona, Connecticut, Delaware, Illinois, Louisiana, Michigan, Minnesota, Montana, New Mexico, North Dakota, Ohio,

Oklahoma, Rhode Island, South Carolina, Tennessee, Washington, and Wisconsin.

12. Arizona, Delaware, Florida, Illinois, Kentucky, Ohio, Oklahoma, Texas, Utah, Washington, West Virginia, Wisconsin, and Wyoming.

13. Arizona, California, Delaware, Idaho, Indiana, Iowa, Louisiana, Massachusetts, Michigan, Minnesota, Montana, Nevada, New Hampshire, New Jersey, New Mexico, North Carolina, North Dakota, Oklahoma, Oregon, Rhode Island, South Carolina, South Dakota, Tennessee, Vermont, Washington, West Virginia, Wisconsin, and Wyoming.

14. California, Connecticut, Delaware, Idaho, Iowa, Maine, Michigan, Montana, Rhode Island, South Carolina, Tennessee, Texas, and Wisconsin.

15. California, Connecticut, Florida, Georgia, Idaho, Illinois, Iowa, Kansas, Kentucky, Louisiana, Maryland, Massachusetts, Minnesota, Missouri, Montana, Nevada, New Mexico, North Carolina, North Dakota, Ohio, Oklahoma, Pennsylvania, Rhode Island, South Carolina, South Dakota, Tennessee, Texas, Vermont, Washington, and Wisconsin.

16. In a state with an affirmative defense provision, a parent or agent of the parent can be charged and prosecuted, but the act of leaving the baby safely at a safe haven can be a defense to such charges. The states with an affirmative defense provision include Alabama, Arizona, Arkansas, Colorado, Delaware, Indiana, Maine, Michigan, Mississippi, New Jersey, New York, Oregon, Utah, Virginia, West Virginia, and Wyoming.

17. California, Delaware, Idaho, Illinois, Kentucky, Louisiana, Montana, New Hampshire, South Carolina, Texas, Utah, and Wyoming.

18. California, Connecticut, Delaware, Florida, Idaho, Illinois, Iowa, Kentucky, Louisiana, Michigan, Montana, Nevada, New Mexico, North Dakota, Ohio, Oklahoma, Tennessee, and Wisconsin.

19. Delaware, Florida, Illinois, Kentucky, Michigan, Missouri, Montana, Nevada, South Carolina, South Dakota, Utah, and Wisconsin.

# Chapter 34

# *Reporting Child Abuse and Neglect*

## *Chapter Contents*

## Section 34.1

# *Reporting Procedures*

Excerpted from "A Coordinated Response to Abuse and Neglect: The Foundation for Practice," Child Welfare Information Gateway, U. S. Department of Health and Human Services (HHS), updated September 18, 2008.

Every state has enacted reporting laws. These laws provide guidance to individuals required to identify and report suspected maltreatment, require investigations by specified agencies to determine if a child was abused, and provide for the delivery of protective services and treatment to maltreated children and their families. Reports of maltreatment required under such laws activate the child protection process.

## *Identification*

The first step in any child protection response system is the identification of possible incidents of child maltreatment. Medical personnel, educators, child care providers, mental health professionals, law enforcement personnel, the clergy, and other professionals are often in a position to observe families and children on an ongoing basis and identify abuse or neglect when they occur. Private citizens, such as family members, friends, and neighbors, also may identify suspected incidents of child maltreatment.

To ensure that community professionals working with children and families recognize possible indicators of child maltreatment, preservice and inservice training must be provided on an ongoing basis. In addition, public awareness campaigns should be planned and implemented to promote understanding of the problem in the community.

## *Reporting*

The next step in responding to child maltreatment is to report the suspected incident. Although there is tremendous variation in the requirements described in state reporting laws, they typically:

- specify selected individuals mandated to report suspected child maltreatment;

- define reportable conditions;

- explain how, when, and to whom reports are to be filed and the information to be contained in the report;

- describe the agencies designated to receive and investigate reports;

- describe the abrogation of certain privileged communication rights (for example, doctor-patient);

- provide immunity from legal liability for reporters; and

- provide penalties for failure to report and false reporting.

**Table 34.1.** Sources of Child Abuse and Neglect Reports in 2000

| Reporter | Percent |
|---|---|
| Education personnel | 16.1 |
| Legal, law enforcement, criminal justice personnel | 15.2 |
| Social services and mental health personnel | 14.4 |
| Medical personnel | 8.3 |
| Child day care and substitute care providers | 2.9 |
| Anonymous or unknown reporters | 13.6 |
| Other relatives | 8.3 |
| Friends and neighbors | 5.9 |
| Parents | 5.9 |
| Alleged victims | 0.9 |
| Alleged perpetrators | 0.1 |
| Other | 9.2 |

Based only on sources of "screened-in" referrals in 2000

## *Procedures for Reporting*

Every state has reporting laws specifying procedures that a mandatory reporter must follow when making a report of suspected child abuse and neglect. Generally, these procedures specify how, where, when, and what to report.

## *How and When to Report*

The majority of states require that reports of child maltreatment be made orally—either by telephone or in person—to the specified authorities. Some states require that a written report follow the oral report, while in other states written reports are filed only upon request, and still other states require written reports only from mandated reporters.

Reports of suspected maltreatment are required by statute to be made immediately to protect children from potentially serious consequences that may be caused by a delay in reporting. While an individual may want to collect additional information before reporting, waiting for proof may place the child in danger.

## *Who Receives the Reports*

Each state designates specific agencies to receive reports of child abuse and neglect. In most states, child protective service (CPS) has the primary responsibility for receiving reports. Other states allow reports to be made to either CPS or law enforcement. Some state laws require that certain forms of maltreatment—such as sexual abuse, child pornography, or severe physical abuse—be reported to law enforcement in addition to CPS. The nature of the relationship of the alleged perpetrator may also affect where reports are made. Most alleged cases of child maltreatment within the family are reportable to CPS. Depending on the state, reports of allegations of abuse or neglect by other caregivers, such as foster parents, daycare providers, teachers, or residential care providers, may need to be filed with a law enforcement office. Additionally, in some states, allegations of abuse in out-of-home care are reported to a centralized investigative body within CPS at the state or regional level.

In most states, statutes also include requirements for cross-system reporting procedures or information sharing among professional entities. Typically, reports are shared among social services agencies, law enforcement, and prosecutors' offices.

## *Reporting Child Abuse and Neglect*

Note: See Chapter 65 for a list of state toll-free telephone numbers for reporting suspected child abuse.

## *Contents of the Report*

Reporting laws describe the information that must be contained in the report. Typically, reports contain the following information:

- Name, age, sex, and address of the child
- Nature and extent of the child's injuries or condition
- Name and address of the parent or other person(s) responsible for the child's care
- Any other information relevant to the investigation

It is essential that reporters provide as much detailed information as possible about:

- the child, the child's condition, and the child's whereabouts;
- the parents and their whereabouts;
- the person alleged to have caused the child's condition and his or her current location;
- the family, including other children in the home; and
- the type and nature of the maltreatment, such as the length of time it has been occurring, whether the maltreatment has increased in severity or frequency, and whether objects or weapons were used.

If the alleged maltreatment occurred in an out-of-home care setting, reporters should provide information about the setting, such as hours of operation; number of other children in the facility, if known; and identification of any others in the facility who may have information about the alleged maltreatment. The more comprehensive the information provided by the reporter the better able CPS staff will be to evaluate the appropriateness of the report for CPS intervention, determine the urgency of the response needed, and prepare for an initial assessment and investigation, if warranted.

While most states allow anonymous reporting, it is preferred that reporters provide their name and contact information. This information will enable a caseworker to ask follow-up questions or obtain clarification. At intake, caseworkers should discuss immunity for reporters, issues of confidentiality, and the extent and nature of follow up with the reporter upon completion of the initial assessment or investigation.

### *Special Issues, Exceptions, and Penalties Related to Reporting*

To encourage reporting of child maltreatment and provide protection for reporters, state statutes include provisions related to privileged communications, immunity for reporters, and penalties for failure to report. The laws also discourage intentionally false reporting through specified penalties.

### Privileged Communications

The law provides special protection to communications in certain relationships. For example, the content of communications between an attorney and client, physician and patient, and clergy and congregant often is protected by a privilege. This means that professionals in such relationships are prohibited from disclosing confidential information communicated to them by their client, patient, or penitent to any unauthorized person. Mandatory child abuse reporting statutes specify when communications are confidential. The attorney-client privilege is most frequently maintained by states. The privilege pertaining to clergy-congregant also is frequently recognized by states. Most states, however, void the physician-patient, mental health professional-patient, and husband-wife privileges in instances of child maltreatment. When a privileged communication is voided, a mandated reporter must report instances of child maltreatment and cooperate in the ensuing investigation.

### Immunity to Reporters

Every state provides immunity from civil or criminal liability for individuals making reports of suspected or known instances of child abuse or neglect. Immunity provisions typically apply both to mandatory reporters and permissive reporters (individuals not required under law to report). These provisions may not prevent the filing of civil lawsuits, but they help prevent, within limitations, an outcome unfavorable to the reporter. Immunity provisions, like other aspects of reporting statutes, vary from state to state. The majority of jurisdictions require that reports be made in good faith. A number of states include a presumption in their statutes that the reporter is acting in good faith. Immunity, therefore, does not extend to reports made maliciously or in bad faith.

## Problems in Reporting

Paradoxically, both underreporting and over-reporting have been cited as problems in the identification of child abuse and neglect.

### Under-Reporting

Numerous professionals admit that during their careers, they have failed to report suspected maltreatment to the appropriate agencies.

One possible reason is that professionals still lack training and knowledge about legal obligations and procedures for reporting. The issue of subjectivity also may account for some of the under-reporting of abuse. Many laws defining child maltreatment are broadly written with ambiguous requirements which may result in professionals lacking guidance and clarity regarding when intervention is required.

One of the biggest obstacles to reporting is personal feelings. Some people do not want to get involved. Others have difficulty reporting a person they suspect is an abuser, especially if they know that person well. Still others may think they can help the family more by working with the child or family themselves. Mandated reporters may believe that their professional relationship with the child will be strained if they report their suspicions of abuse. When a professional has established a relationship with a parent or family prior to recognizing maltreatment, reporting becomes a delicate issue.

Some reporters also may be reluctant to report because they have had negative experiences with CPS or they view social services agencies as overburdened, understaffed, or incompetent. At times, professionals become concerned that nothing will be done if they report or that the investigation and service provision will do more harm than good. Consequently, they choose not to report. This reluctance to report, which can have serious consequences for a child in an unsafe situation, underscores the critical need for ongoing communication and feedback between CPS and mandated reporters. It also underscores the need for CPS to function sensitively and competently in the best interests of the child while creating as little disruption as possible.

Professionals must report regardless of their concerns or previous experiences. The law requires it, and no exemptions are granted to those who have had a bad experience. In addition, while reporting does not guarantee that the situation will improve, not reporting guarantees that, if abuse and neglect exists, the child will continue to be at risk of further and perhaps more serious harm.

### Over-Reporting

Only a portion of reports received and investigated by CPS reflect children who are found to be victims of, or at risk for, maltreatment. While the children and families in these reports may be in need of help or services, they frequently do not meet the legal definition of maltreatment in that family's jurisdiction. This apparent pattern of over-reporting raises several concerns. First, children and families who will not receive child welfare services may be subjected to an intrusive public agency investigation. Second, these reports may divert CPS resources from higher risk cases.

Over-reporting may occur in a community following a serious case of child maltreatment that receives a lot of media attention. There is often a significant increase in the number of reports of suspected child maltreatment made during such times, in part because the community's awareness has been heightened.

# Section 34.2

# *Mandatory Reporting Requirements*

This section includes text from "Mandatory Reporters of Child Abuse and Neglect," and text from "Clergy as Mandatory Reporters of Child Abuse and Neglect," Child Welfare Information Gateway, U.S. Department of Health and Human Services (HHS), 2008.

## *Mandatory Reporters of Child Abuse and Neglect*

All states, the District of Columbia, Puerto Rico, and the U.S. territories of American Samoa, Guam, the Northern Mariana Islands, and the Virgin Islands have statutes identifying persons who are required to report child maltreatment under specific circumstances.

### *Professionals Required to Report*

Approximately 48 states, the District of Columbia, American Samoa, Guam, the Northern Mariana Islands, Puerto Rico, and the U.S. Virgin Islands designate professions whose members are mandated by law to report child maltreatment. The word approximately is used to stress the fact that the states frequently amend their laws. This information is current only through January 2008. Individuals designated as mandatory reporters typically have frequent contact with children. Such individuals may include:

- social workers,
- teachers and other school personnel,

- physicians and other health-care workers,
- mental health professionals,
- childcare providers,
- medical examiners or coroners, and
- law enforcement officers.

Some other professions frequently mandated across the states include commercial film or photograph processors (in 11 states, Guam, and Puerto Rico), substance abuse counselors (in 13 states), and probation or parole officers (in 15 states). Six states (Alaska, Arizona, Arkansas, Connecticut, Illinois, and South Dakota) include domestic violence workers on the list of mandated reporters. Court-appointed special advocates are mandatory reporters in seven states (Arkansas, California, Maine, Montana, Oregon, Virginia, and Wisconsin). Members of the clergy now are required to report in 26 states.

### Reporting by Other Persons

In approximately 18 states and Puerto Rico, any person who suspects child abuse or neglect is required to report. Of these 18 states, 16 states and Puerto Rico specify certain professionals who must report but also require all persons to report suspected abuse or neglect, regardless of profession. New Jersey and Wyoming require all persons to report without specifying any professions. In all other states, territories, and the District of Columbia, any person is permitted to report. These voluntary reporters of abuse are often referred to as permissive reporters.

### Standards for Making a Report

The circumstances under which a mandatory reporter must make a report vary from state to state. Typically, a report must be made when the reporter, in his or her official capacity, suspects or has reasons to believe that a child has been abused or neglected. Another standard frequently used is when the reporter has knowledge of, or observes a child being subjected to, conditions that would reasonably result in harm to the child. Permissive reporters follow the same standards when electing to make a report.

### Privileged Communications

Mandatory reporting statutes also may specify when a communication is privileged. Privileged communications is the statutory recognition of the right to maintain confidential communications between professionals and their clients, patients, or members of the congregation. To enable states to provide protection to maltreated children, the reporting laws in most states and territories restrict this privilege for mandated reporters. All but four states and Puerto Rico currently address the issue of privileged communications within their reporting laws, either affirming the privilege or denying it (not allowing privilege to be grounds for failing to report). For instance:

- physician-patient and husband-wife privileges are the most common to be denied by states;

- attorney-client privilege is most commonly affirmed; and

- clergy-penitent privilege is also widely affirmed, although that privilege is usually limited to confessional communications and, in some states, is denied altogether.

## *Inclusion of the Reporter's Name in the Report*

Most states maintain toll-free telephone numbers for receiving reports of abuse or neglect. Reports may be made anonymously to most of these reporting numbers, but states find it helpful to their investigations to know the identity of reporters. Approximately 16 states, the District of Columbia, American Samoa, Guam, and the Virgin Islands currently require mandatory reporters to provide their names and contact information, either at the time of the initial oral report or as part of a written report. The laws in Connecticut, Delaware, and Washington allow child protection workers to request the name of the reporter. In Wyoming, the reporter does not have to provide his or her identity as part of the written report, but if the person takes and submits photographs or x-rays of the child, his or her name must be provided.

## *Disclosure of the Reporter's Identity*

All jurisdictions have provisions in statute to maintain the confidentiality of abuse and neglect records. The identity of the reporter is specifically protected from disclosure to the alleged perpetrator in 39 states, the District of Columbia, Puerto Rico, American Samoa, Guam, and the Northern Mariana Islands. This protection is maintained even when other information from the report may be disclosed.

Release of the reporter's identity is allowed in some jurisdictions under specific circumstances or to specific departments or officials.

For example, disclosure of the reporter's identity can be ordered by the court when there is a compelling reason to disclose (in California, Mississippi, Oklahoma, Tennessee, Texas, and Guam), or upon a finding that the reporter knowingly made a false report (in Alabama, Arkansas, Connecticut, Kentucky, Louisiana, Minnesota, South Dakota, and Vermont). In some jurisdictions (California, Florida, Minnesota, Tennessee, Vermont, the District of Columbia, and Guam), the reporter can waive confidentiality and give consent to the release of his or her name.

## Clergy as Mandatory Reporters

### *Privileged Communications*

As a doctrine of some faiths, clergy must maintain the confidentiality of pastoral communications. Mandatory reporting statutes in some states specify the circumstances under which a communication is privileged or allowed to remain confidential. Privileged communications may be exempt from the reporting laws. The privilege of maintaining this confidentiality under state law must be provided by statute. Most states do provide the privilege, typically in rules of evidence or civil procedure. If the issue of privilege is not addressed in the reporting laws, it does not mean that privilege is not granted; it may be granted in other parts of state statutes.

This privilege, however, is not absolute. While clergy-penitent privilege is frequently recognized within the reporting laws, it is typically interpreted narrowly in the child abuse or neglect context. The circumstances under which it is allowed vary from state to state, and in some states it is denied altogether. For example, among the states that list clergy as mandated reporters, New Hampshire and West Virginia deny the clergy-penitent privilege in cases of child abuse or neglect. Four of the states that enumerate "any person" as a mandated reporter (North Carolina, Oklahoma, Rhode Island, and Texas) also deny clergy-penitent privilege in child abuse cases.

In states where neither clergy nor any person are enumerated as mandated reporters, it is less clear whether clergy are included as mandated reporters within other broad categories of professionals who work with children. For example, in Virginia and Washington, clergy are not enumerated as mandated reporters, but the clergy-penitent privilege is affirmed within the reporting laws.

Many states and territories include Christian Science practitioners or religious healers among professionals who are mandated to report

**Table 34.2.** States and Clergy as Mandated Reporters of Child Abuse and Neglect

| | Privilege granted but limited to "pastoral communications" | Privilege denied in cases of suspected child abuse or neglect | Privilege not addressed in the reporting laws |
|---|---|---|---|
| Clergy enumerated as mandated reporters | Alabama, Arizona, Arkansas, California, Colorado, Illinois, Louisiana, Maine, Massachusetts, Michigan, Minnesota, Missouri, Montana, Nevada, New Mexico, North Dakota, Ohio, Oregon, Pennsylvania, South Carolina, Vermont, Wisconsin | New Hampshire, West Virginia | Connecticut, Mississippi |
| Clergy not enumerated as mandated reporters but may be included with "any person" designation | Delaware, Florida, Idaho, Kentucky, Maryland, Utah, Wyoming | North Carolina, Oklahoma, Rhode Island, Texas | Indiana, Nebraska, New Jersey, Tennessee, Puerto Rico |
| Neither clergy nor "any person" enumerated as mandated reporters | Virginia, Washington | Not applicable | Alaska, American Samoa, District of Columbia, Georgia, Guam, Hawaii, Iowa, Kansas, New York, Northern Mariana Islands, South Dakota, Virgin Islands |

suspected child maltreatment. In most instances, they appear to be regarded as a type of healthcare provider. Only nine states (Arizona, Arkansas, Louisiana, Massachusetts, Missouri, Montana, Nevada, South Carolina, and Vermont) explicitly include Christian Science practitioners among classes of clergy required to report. The clergy-penitent privilege is also extended to those practitioners by statute.

Table 34.2 summarizes how states have or have not addressed the issue of clergy as mandated reporters (either specifically or as part of a broad category) and/or clergy-penitent privilege (either limiting or denying the privilege) within their reporting laws.

# Section 34.3

# *Penalties for Failure to Report and False Reporting of Child Abuse and Neglect*

Text in this section is from "Penalties for Failure to Report and False Reporting of Child Abuse and Neglect," Child Welfare Information Gateway, U.S. Department of Health and Human Services (HHS), 2007.

Many cases of child abuse and neglect are not reported, even when suspected by professionals. Therefore, nearly every state and U.S. territory imposes penalties, often in the form of a fine or imprisonment, on mandatory reporters who fail to report suspected abuse or neglect as required by law. In addition, to prevent malicious or intentional reporting of cases that are not founded, several states and territories impose penalties against any person who files a report known to be false.

## *Penalties for Failure to Report*

Approximately 46 states, the District of Columbia, American Samoa, Guam, the Northern Mariana Islands, and the Virgin Islands impose penalties on mandatory reporters who knowingly or willfully fail to make a report when they suspect that a child is being abused or neglected. Failure to report is classified as a misdemeanor in 38 states and American Samoa, Guam, and the Virgin Islands. In Arizona, Florida, and Minnesota, misdemeanors are upgraded to felonies for failure to report more serious situations, while in Illinois and Guam, second or subsequent violations are classified as felonies.

Eighteen states and the District of Columbia, Guam, the Northern Mariana Islands, and the Virgin Islands specify in the reporting laws the penalties for failure to report. Upon conviction, a mandated reporter who fails to report can face jail terms ranging from ten days to five years, or fines ranging from $100 to $5,000. In seven states and American Samoa, in addition to any criminal penalties, the reporter may be civilly liable for any damages caused by the failure to report.

## Penalties for False Reporting

Approximately 30 states carry penalties in their reporting laws for any person who willfully or intentionally makes a report of child abuse or neglect that the reporter knows to be false. In 14 states and the Virgin Islands, making false reports is made illegal in other sections of state code.

Thirty-two states and the Virgin Islands classify false reporting as a misdemeanor or similar charge. In Florida, Tennessee, and Texas, false reporting is a felony, while in Arkansas, Illinois, Indiana, Missouri, and Virginia, second or subsequent offenses are upgraded to felonies. In Michigan, false reporting can be either a misdemeanor or a felony, depending on the seriousness of the alleged abuse in the report. No criminal sanctions are imposed in California, Maine, Montana, Minnesota, and Nebraska; however, immunity from civil or criminal action that is provided to reporters of abuse or neglect is not extended to those who make a false report.

Thirteen states and the Virgin Islands specify the penalties for making a false report. Upon conviction, the reporter can face jail terms ranging from thirty days to five years, or fines ranging from $200 to $5,000. Florida imposes the most severe penalties: In addition to a court sentence of five years and $5,000, the department may fine the reporter up to $10,000. In six states (California, Colorado, Idaho, Indiana, Minnesota, and North Dakota), in addition to any criminal penalties, the reporter may be civilly liable for any damages caused by the report.

Chapter 35

# How the Child
# Welfare System Works

The child welfare system is a group of services designed to promote the well-being of children by ensuring safety, achieving permanency, and strengthening families to successfully care for their children. While the primary responsibility for child welfare services rests with the states, the federal government plays a major role in supporting states in the delivery of services through funding of programs and legislative initiatives.

The primary responsibility for implementing federal child and family legislative mandates rests with the Children's Bureau, within the Administration on Children, Youth, and Families (ACYF), Administration for Children and Families (ACF), U.S. Department of Health and Human Services (HHS). The Children's Bureau works with state and local agencies to develop programs that focus on preventing the abuse of children in troubled families, protecting children from abuse, and finding permanent families for those who cannot safely return to their parents.

## The Child Abuse Prevention and Treatment Act

The Child Abuse Prevention and Treatment Act (CAPTA), originally passed in 1974, brought national attention to the need to protect vulnerable children in the United States. CAPTA provides federal

Text in this chapter is from "How the Child Welfare System Works," Child Welfare Information Gateway, U.S. Department of Health and Human Services, April 2008.

funding to states in support of prevention, assessment, investigation, prosecution, and treatment activities as well as grants to public agencies and nonprofit organizations for demonstration programs and projects. Additionally, CAPTA identifies the federal role in supporting research, evaluation, technical assistance, and data collection activities. CAPTA also sets forth a minimum definition of child abuse and neglect. Since it was signed into law, CAPTA has been amended several times. It was most recently amended and reauthorized on June 25, 2003, by the Keeping Children and Families Safe Act of 2003 (P.L. 108-36).

Most families first become involved with their local child welfare system due to a report of suspected child abuse or neglect (sometimes called child maltreatment). Child maltreatment is defined by CAPTA as serious harm (neglect, physical abuse, sexual abuse, and emotional abuse or neglect) caused to children by parents or primary caregivers, such as extended family members or baby sitters. Child maltreatment also can include harm that a caregiver allows to happen or does not prevent from happening to a child. In general, child welfare agencies do not intervene in cases of harm to children caused by acquaintances or strangers. These cases are the responsibility of law enforcement.

The child welfare system is not a single entity. There are many organizations in each community working together to strengthen families and keep children safe. Public agencies, such as departments of social services or child and family services, often contract and collaborate with private child welfare agencies and community-based organizations to provide services to families, such as in-home family preservation services, foster care, residential treatment, mental health care, substance abuse treatment, parenting skills classes, employment assistance, and financial or housing assistance.

Child welfare systems are complex, and their specific procedures vary widely by state. This chapter gives a brief overview of the purposes and functions of child welfare from a national perspective. Child welfare systems typically:

- receive and investigate reports of possible child abuse and neglect;

- provide services to families who need assistance in the protection and care of their children;

- arrange for children to live with foster families when they are not safe at home;

- arrange for adoption or other permanent family connections for children leaving foster care.

## *What happens when possible abuse or neglect is reported?*

Any concerned person can report suspicions of child abuse or neglect. Most reports are made by people who are required by state law to report suspicions of child abuse and neglect—mandatory reporters. As of January 2008, statutes in approximately 18 states and Puerto Rico require any person who suspects child abuse or neglect to report it. Reports of possible child abuse and neglect are generally received by child protective services (CPS) workers and either "screened in" or "screened out." A report is screened in if there is sufficient information to suggest an investigation is warranted. A report may be screened out if there is not enough information on which to follow up or if the situation reported does not meet the state's legal definition of abuse or neglect. In these instances, the worker may refer the person reporting the incident to other community services or law enforcement for additional help.

In 2006, an estimated total of 3.3 million referrals involving six million children were made to CPS agencies. Approximately 61.7 percent were screened in, and more than 38.3 percent were screened out (U.S. Department of Health and Human Services [HHS], 2008).

## *What happens after a report is screened in?*

CPS workers, often called investigators, respond within a particular time period, which may be anywhere from a few hours to a few days, depending on the type of maltreatment alleged, the potential severity of the situation, and requirements under state law. They may speak with the parents and other people in contact with the child, such as doctors, teachers, or childcare providers. They also may speak with the child, alone or in the presence of caregivers, depending on the child's age and level of risk. Children who are believed to be in immediate danger may be moved to a shelter, foster care placement, or a relative's home during the investigation and while court proceedings are pending. An investigator's primary purpose is to determine if the child is safe, if abuse or neglect has occurred, and if there is a risk of it occurring again.

Some jurisdictions now employ an alternative response system. In these jurisdictions, when risk to the children involved is considered to be low, the CPS caseworker may focus on assessing family strengths, resources, and difficulties, and identifying supports and services needed, rather than on gathering evidence to confirm the occurrence of abuse or neglect.

At the end of an investigation, CPS workers typically make one of two findings—unsubstantiated (unfounded), or substantiated (founded). These terms vary from state to state. Typically, a finding of unsubstantiated means there is insufficient evidence for the worker to conclude that a child was abused or neglected, or what happened does not meet the legal definition of child abuse or neglect. A finding of substantiated typically means an incident of child abuse or neglect, as defined by state law, is believed to have occurred. Some states have additional categories, such as unable to determine, that suggest there was not enough evidence to either confirm or refute that abuse or neglect occurred.

The agency will initiate a court action if it determines that the authority of the juvenile court (through a child protection or dependency proceeding) is necessary to keep the child safe. To protect the child, the court can issue temporary orders placing the child in shelter care during the investigation, ordering services, or ordering certain individuals to have no contact with the child. At an adjudicatory hearing, the court hears evidence and decides whether maltreatment occurred and whether the child should be under the continuing jurisdiction of the court. The court then enters a disposition, either at that hearing or at a separate hearing, which may result in the court ordering a parent to comply with services necessary to ameliorate the abuse or neglect. Orders can also contain provisions regarding visitation between the parent and the child, agency obligations to provide the parent with services, and services needed by the child.

In 2006, approximately 905,000 children were found to be victims of child abuse or neglect (HHS, 2008).

### What happens in substantiated (founded) cases?

If a child has been abused or neglected, the course of action depends on state policy, the severity of the maltreatment, an assessment of the child's immediate safety, the risk of continued or future maltreatment, the services available to address the family's needs, and whether the child was removed from the home and a court action to protect the child was initiated. The following general options are available:

- **No or low risk:** The family's case may be closed with no services if the maltreatment was a one-time incident, the child is considered to be safe, there is no or low risk of future incidents, and any services the family needs will not be provided through the child welfare agency but through other community-based resources and service systems.

- **Low to moderate risk:** Referrals may be made to community-based or voluntary in-home CPS services if the CPS worker believes the family would benefit from these services and the child's present and future safety would be enhanced. This may happen even when no abuse or neglect is found, if the family needs and is willing to participate in services.

- **Moderate to high risk:** The family may again be offered voluntary in-home CPS services to address safety concerns and help ameliorate the risks. If these are refused, the agency may seek intervention by the juvenile dependency court. Once there is a judicial determination that abuse or neglect occurred, juvenile dependency court may require the family to cooperate with in-home CPS services if it is believed that the child can remain safely at home while the family addresses the issues contributing to the risk of future maltreatment. If the child has been seriously harmed, is considered to be at high risk of serious harm, or the child's safety is threatened, the court may order the child's removal from the home or affirm the agency's prior removal of the child. The child may be placed with a relative or in foster care.

In 2006, an estimated 312,000 children were removed from their homes as a result of a child abuse investigation or assessment. Nearly two-thirds (63.6 percent) of the victims who were removed from their homes suffered from neglect; 8.6 percent from physical abuse; 3.2 percent from sexual abuse; and 16.8 percent from multiple types of maltreatment (HHS, 2008).

## What happens to people who abuse children?

People who are found to have abused or neglected a child are generally offered support and treatment services or are required by a juvenile dependency court to participate in services that will help keep their children safe. In more severe cases or fatalities, police are called upon to investigate and may file charges in criminal court against the perpetrators of child maltreatment. In many states certain types of abuse, such as sexual abuse and serious physical abuse, are routinely referred to law enforcement.

Whether or not criminal charges are filed, the perpetrator's name may be placed on a state child maltreatment registry if abuse or neglect is confirmed. A registry is a central database that collects information about maltreated children and individuals who are found to have abused or neglected those children. These registries are usually confidential and used for internal child protective purposes only. However, they may be used in background checks for certain professions, such as those working with children, so children will be protected from contact with individuals who may mistreat them.

### What happens to children who enter foster care?

Most children in foster care are placed with relatives or foster families, but some may be placed in group homes. While a child is in foster care, he or she attends school and should receive medical care and other services as needed. The child's family also receives services to support their efforts to reduce the risk of future maltreatment and to help them, in most cases, be reunited with their child. Parents may visit their children on a predetermined basis. Visits also are arranged between siblings, if they cannot be placed together.

Every child in foster care should have a permanency plan that describes where the child will live after he or she leaves foster care. Families typically participate in developing a permanency plan for the child and a service plan for the family. These plans guide the agency's work. Except in unusual and extreme circumstances, every child's plan is first focused on reunification with parents. If the efforts toward reunification are not successful, the plan may be changed to another permanent arrangement, such as adoption or transfer of custody to a relative. Whether or not they are adopted, older youth in foster care should receive support in developing some form of permanent family connection, in addition to transitional or independent living services to assist them in being self-sufficient when they leave foster care between the ages of 18 and 21.

Federal law requires the court to hold a permanency hearing, which determines the permanent plan for the child, within 12 months after the child enters foster care and every 12 months thereafter. Many courts review each case more frequently to ensure that the agency is actively pursuing permanency for the child.

In fiscal year 2003, 55 percent of children leaving foster care were returned to their parents. The median length of stay in foster care was 12 months. The average age of a child exiting foster care was ten years old (HHS, 2006).

## Summary

The goal of the child welfare system is to promote the safety, permanency, and well-being of children and families. Even among children who enter foster care, most children will leave the child welfare system safely to the care of their birth family, a relative, or an adoptive home.

## References

Badeau, S. and Gesiriech, S. (2003). *A child's journey through the child welfare system*. Washington, DC: The Pew Commission on Children in Foster Care. Retrieved April 20, 2006, from http://pewfostercare.org/docs/index.php?DocID=24.

Goldman, J. and Salus, M. (2003). *A coordinated response to child abuse and neglect: The foundation for practice* (The User Manual Series). Washington, DC: U.S. Department of Health and Human Services. Retrieved April 20, 2006, from www.childwelfare.gov/pubs/usermanuals/foundation/index.cfm.

McCarthy, J., Marshall, A., Collins, J., Milon, J., Arganza, G., Deserly, K. (2003). *A family's guide to the child welfare system*. Washington, DC: National Technical Assistance Center for Children's Mental Health at Georgetown University Center for Child and Human Development. Retrieved May 1, 2007, from www.tapartnership.org/advisors/ChildWelfare/resources/AFamilysGuideFINAL%20WEB%20VERSION.pdf.

U.S. Department of Health and Human Services. (2008). *Child maltreatment 2006*. Washington, DC: U.S. Government Printing Office. Retrieved April 1, 2008, from www.acf.hhs.gov/programs/cb/pubs/cm06/index.htm.

U.S. Department of Health and Human Services. (2006). *Child welfare outcomes 2003: Annual report*. Washington, DC: U.S. Government Printing Office. Retrieved May 1, 2007, from www.acf.hhs.gov/programs/cb/pubs/cwo03/index.htm.

Chapter 36

# Kinship Caregivers and the Child Welfare System

## Different Types of Kinship Care

Children may come to live with their grandparents or other relatives in a number of ways, and only some of these ways involve the child welfare system. Kinship care arrangements fall roughly into three categories: 1) private kinship care, 2) voluntary kinship care, and 3) kinship foster care.

### Private Kinship Care

Private kinship care, sometimes called informal kinship care, refers to arrangements made by the parents and other family members, without any involvement from either the child welfare system or the juvenile court system. A parent may leave children with a grandparent while he or she is sent overseas, or an aunt may care for nephews whose parents are ill or otherwise unable to care for them. In this type of arrangement, the legal custody of the children remains with the parents, and the parents can legally take back the children at any time. The kin caregivers in these circumstances may have difficulty enrolling the children in school, obtaining health insurance, authorizing medical care, and obtaining some other benefits, because they do not have legal custody of the children. Generally, the only type of

Text in this chapter is excerpted from "Kinship Caregivers and the Child Welfare System," Child Welfare Information Gateway, U.S. Department of Health and Human Services (HHS), updated September 18, 2008.

financial assistance available to kin caregivers in this type of arrangement is the child-only temporary assistance for needy families (TANF) benefit.

**Physical custody** refers to where the child lives. If your grandchildren or niece and nephew live with you, you have physical custody of them. You may feed and clothe them, help them with their homework, and take care of them when they are sick.

**Legal custody** refers to the legal right to make decisions about the children, such as where they live. Parents have legal custody of their children unless they voluntarily give custody to someone else (the parent is sent overseas) or a court takes this right away and gives it to someone else. For instance, a court may give legal custody to a relative or to a child welfare agency. Whoever has legal custody can enroll the children in school, give permission for medical care, and give other legal consents.

The same person does not necessarily have both physical and legal custody. For instance, as a grandparent, you may have physical custody of your grandchildren because they live with you, but their mother may still have legal custody or the state agency may have legal custody.

### Voluntary Kinship Care

Voluntary kinship care refers to situations in which the children live with relatives and the child welfare system is involved, but the state does not take legal custody. In some cases, children have been placed with relatives by a court, and in other cases an arrangement is made by the child welfare agency with no court involvement. This type of kinship care covers a wide variety of circumstances and varies greatly from state to state. Some situations that might result in voluntary kinship care include the following:

- Child welfare workers find signs of abuse or neglect by the parents, but the evidence is not serious enough to take the children into state legal custody; instead, the caseworkers, parents, and kin work out a voluntary kinship care arrangement where the children move in with the kin.

- Under the guidance of child welfare workers, parents voluntarily place their children with relatives while they (the parents) receive treatment for substance abuse or mental illness.

Some jurisdictions will require the parents to sign a voluntary placement agreement with the child welfare agency when the children are placed with relatives. In many situations, the kinship care arrangement comes about because the parents understand that if they refuse to voluntarily place the children with kin, the child welfare agency will go to court and ask the judge to remove the children from the parents' care and award legal custody to the state.

In voluntary kinship care, the children are in the physical custody of the relatives, but they may remain in the legal custody of the parents, or the parents may sign over temporary legal custody to the kin. Some states have consent forms that parents can sign to allow kin caregivers to have some temporary decision-making power regarding the children (for instance, to seek medical treatment or enroll the children in school).

### Kinship Foster Care

Kinship foster care, also known as formal kinship care or public kinship care, refers to cases in which the children are placed in the legal custody of the state by a judge, and the child welfare system then places the children with grandparents or other kin. In these situations, the child welfare agency, acting on behalf of the state, has legal custody and must answer to the court, but the kin have physical custody. The child welfare agency, in collaboration with the family, makes the legal decisions about the children, including deciding where they live. The child welfare agency is also responsible for ensuring that the children receive medical care and attend school. If the court has approved visitation with parents, the child welfare system is responsible for making sure that the visits occur between parents and children. In kinship foster care, the child's relative caregivers have rights and responsibilities similar to those of non-relative foster parents.

## How the Child Welfare System Becomes Involved in Kinship Care

The involvement of the child welfare system in kinship care situations varies from state to state, since each state has its own laws and practices that govern these situations; it also varies from case to case, depending on the children's age, safety needs, the legal custody, and other differences. If American Indian or Alaska Native children are involved, the Federal Indian Child Welfare Act must be followed.

The child welfare caseworker may be the person who initially approaches a grandparent or other relative and asks that person to take care of the children. In other situations, the family may contact the child welfare system for help. Some examples follow of these two types of contact.

### The Child Welfare System Makes the Contact

- **A report of child abuse or neglect is made:** Child protective services screen reports of child abuse and neglect, according to state policies and practices. If investigators believe that children are in danger in their own home, they may be removed immediately. The caseworkers often look for a relative to keep the children until the case goes to court. If the case goes to court and the charges are proven, the court and the child welfare system may select relatives to care for the children until a parent can safely care for them, or an alternative placement may be made.

- **Parents are arrested:** Police may arrest a parent or parents but be willing to leave the children with a relative. The police then notify the child welfare agency of this temporary placement. Depending on the state laws and practice, the agency may leave the children with the relatives, take them into the state's legal custody and place them into non-relative foster care, or take them into state custody but place them with the relatives.

- **Parents die:** In the event that both parents die or the parent with custody dies, the child welfare system may be responsible for locating relatives with whom the children can live. If no relatives can be located who are willing to take the children, they come into the legal custody of the state and may be placed into non-relative foster care.

### Parents or Other Family Members Make the Contact

- **A parent leaves the children with grandparents or other relatives and does not return:** This abandonment by a parent, even if it is temporary, may prompt the kin caregivers to call child welfare services and ask for help. In these situations, caseworkers may be able to offer services or they may help the kin to seek temporary legal custody through the court. However, if the parent remains missing and the kin cannot continue to care for the children, the children may be taken into the state's legal custody and placed in another home.

- **Grandparents or other kin are no longer able to care for children under a private arrangement:** In these situations, the kin caregiver may have planned to care for the children for a long time without agency help, but an unexpected circumstance forces them to seek help from the child welfare agency. For instance, the caregiver may become ill, a child may suddenly need special services, or the caregiver may lose a job and no longer be in a position to financially support the children. The child welfare worker may be able to help arrange services for the kin caregiver or arrange other placements for the children.

- **Parents voluntarily give up custody due to their own illness:** Parents suffering from mental illness or from a debilitating illness such as human immunodeficiency virus (HIV)/acquired immune deficiency syndrome (AIDS) may contact the child welfare agency themselves and ask the agency to take their children into legal custody. In such situations, caseworkers may seek out relatives with whom the children can be placed (physical custody), rather than placing them with unrelated foster parents.

- **Parents no longer want a child or children to live with them:** In such situations, the parents may turn over custody to the child welfare agency. This is more common when the children are teenagers. Most child welfare agencies are reluctant to take custody in these situations. However, if they do, the child welfare workers may look for relatives with whom the children can live.

## What to Expect from the Child Welfare System

After the children are placed in their home, kin caregivers may wonder what they can expect in their future dealings with the child welfare system. Much of the ongoing relationship with child welfare will depend on whether the legal custody of the children remains with the parents or kin caregiver (voluntary kinship care) or with the state or child welfare agency (kinship foster care).

### *Voluntary Kinship*

Voluntary kinship caregivers may expect a range of assistance from child welfare caseworkers. In states where this type of arrangement is accepted and promoted by child welfare, kinship caregivers may find that caseworkers are involved in the following ways:

- **Ensuring safety:** Caseworkers may need to ensure that the kin caregivers and their homes meet minimal requirements for the safety of the children.

- **Visiting:** In some states, the caseworker may make periodic visits to ensure that the children remain in a safe environment.

- **Offering services:** Some states have services available for children and families in voluntary kinship care. For instance, these might include referrals to therapy for the children.

- **Changing the custody status:** If the children's parent is not meeting the requirements set out in the service plan or if the children are placed in dangerous situations by the parent who has legal custody, the caseworker may help the kin caregiver to petition the court for temporary legal custody of the children. Or, the caseworker may go to court and petition to have the children placed in the legal custody of the state.

In some voluntary kinship cases, there may be very limited contact with the child welfare agency. Once the caseworker has completed background checks on the kin, the caseworker may be satisfied that the children are in a safe environment and may not contact kin again. In such situations, kinship caregivers who need help or services may need to contact the caseworker or locate community services themselves.

### Kinship Foster Care

Kinship foster care includes much more involvement with the child welfare system, because the state has legal custody of the children. All states have requirements that non-kin foster parents must meet before they can care for children in their home through the foster care system. For kin caregivers in the foster care system, some states currently offer different requirements or will waive some of the standard foster care requirements. Also, kin caregivers are usually given some flexibility in the amount of time needed to meet the state's requirements, because the placement of the children is often unexpected.

Compared to voluntary kinship placement, caregivers in kinship foster care will find that they have more structured involvement with the child welfare system, as well as access to more services. Caregivers may find that some of this structure is helpful in dealing with the children's parents, schools, or medical care arrangements; on the other hand, caregivers have less freedom to make decisions on their own about the children. The following are some of the ways that the child welfare system may be involved in kinship foster care:

- Ensuring safety or licensing standards
- Supervision and support
- Arranging visitation with parents
- Service planning including: 1) a permanency goal for each child, and 2) actions toward reunification or other permanency goals

Service plans should be reviewed at least every six months to see if everyone is meeting their goals. Kinship foster caregivers should be involved in or consulted about the creation of the plan and should receive copies of the plan.

Questions for the new kin caregiver to ask the child welfare caseworker about taking responsibility for the children:

- Who has legal custody of the children?
- What rights and responsibilities does legal custody give in this state? Physical custody?
- May I receive a copy of the signed voluntary placement agreement?
- May I be involved in developing the service plan and receive a copy of the plan?
- Will I or the children have to go to court?
- Who is responsible for enrolling the children in school, obtaining health insurance, granting permission for medical care and obtaining it, signing school permission forms, and so forth?
- Will someone from child welfare services visit my home on a regular basis?
- What are the requirements for me and my home if I want the children to live with me?
- Are the requirements different if the children are with me just temporarily?
- What services are available for me and for the children, and how do I apply?
- Are there restrictions on the discipline I can use (such as spanking) with the children?

- What subsidies or financial assistance is available? What do I need to do to apply?

- Am I eligible to become a licensed foster parent and receive a foster care subsidy?

## *Services*

The child welfare agency is often involved in providing services to children and families or making referrals to other groups that provide services. Services and referrals are more likely to be available to children in kinship foster care than to those in voluntary kinship care. Early on in their involvement with the child welfare system, kin caregivers should ask about available services.

Some of the different types of services include the following.

**Therapy and counseling:** Children who have experienced abuse or neglect should be assessed to see what services they may need. Such services may include therapy or counseling. These may be available through child welfare agency referrals or through the schools.

**Financial support:** Many grandparents and other relative caregivers struggle to provide for the children under their care. Depending on a number of factors, including the caregiver's age, caregiver's income, child's income, child's disability status, number of siblings, and the legal status of the caregiving arrangement (voluntary or foster care), there may be financial support available. Some of the programs include the following:

- **The Temporary Assistance to Needy Families (TANF)** program is designed to provide financial assistance while helping low-income families become self-sufficient. Caregivers do not need to have legal custody in order to apply for TANF benefits, but they do need to meet their state's TANF definition of a kin caregiver. A caseworker can provide information or refer a caregiver to the correct place to find information on eligibility for TANF. In these situations, only the children's income is considered for eligibility. If the children have little or no income, it is likely that they will be eligible to receive TANF benefits, and these benefits will be available until their 18th birthday.

- **Food stamps** are available to families with incomes below a certain level. In this case, the entire household's income is considered, and the relative children can be included in family size for determining benefit amount.

- **Supplemental Security Income (SSI)** may be available to children or caregivers who are disabled. This is also available to anyone over age 65.

- **Foster care payments or kinship care payments** may be available to relative caregivers. The requirements for receiving these payments vary from state to state. Relative caregivers who are licensed foster parents taking care of children placed with them by their local child welfare agency or court may be eligible for such payments. Foster care payments are generally higher than other forms of reimbursement, such as TANF.

**Health insurance:** Many children being raised by relatives are eligible for medical insurance through either Medicaid or the Children's Health Insurance Program (CHIP). Every state permits grandparents or other kin caregivers to apply for Medicaid or a CHIP on behalf of the children for whom they are caring. Most states do not require the caregiver to have legal custody in order for the children to be eligible.

**Respite care:** Grandparents and other relative caregivers seeking a break from full-time childcare may find some relief in respite care. Availability of respite care may be limited, and such availability may depend on the needs of the caregiver and/or the child. The child welfare agency should have more information about the availability of such programs, and caregivers should ask about these programs.

## Involvement of the Courts

Kin caregivers who are part of the foster care system are likely to have some involvement with the court—in most states, this occurs in a family or juvenile court. Whenever possible, grandparents or other relative caregivers should make arrangements to attend court hearings; they may even be asked to testify at them. It is important for kin caregivers to give their view of the situation and to get a full understanding of the court's decisions. It is also important for the caregiver to be there to support the children if they appear before the judge.

Questions to ask the child welfare caseworker about court hearings:

- When and where is the hearing?

- Is this a permanency hearing or a review hearing?

- What will be decided at the hearing?
- Who will be present?
- Who will have a lawyer?
- Do I need a lawyer? If so, who can help me find one?
- Who will represent the child or children? May I speak to that person?
- May I speak at the hearing?
- What is the schedule of future hearings?

## Permanent Living Arrangements for the Children

Permanency is a term used by child welfare workers to mean a permanent living arrangement for a child. A permanency plan is a plan for determining where a child will grow up. Some of the options that might be considered by the court for permanency for children in kinship foster care include the following:

**Reunification:** Returning the children home and reuniting them with a parent or parents is the first choice of child welfare agencies when this option will ensure the safety and well-being of the children and provide a permanent situation for them.

**Guardianship:** Guardianship is a legal option for permanency, and it may be especially appropriate in kinship care. Federal law encourages states to consider a relative rather than an unrelated person when seeking a guardian for a child who cannot return home.

**Adoption:** Some kin caregivers choose to adopt their grandchildren, nieces, nephews, or other relative children in order to give them a permanent home. As with foster care and guardianship, the child welfare agency will have to ensure that the home and prospective adoptive parents meet certain state standards for the safety and well-being of the children. Children can be adopted only after the court has terminated all the legal rights of the parents or the parents have voluntarily surrendered all of their rights permanently. A court must finalize the adoption. Once the adoption is finalized, the grandparent or other relative becomes the legal parent of the child; there is generally no further involvement by the child welfare agency after that finalization, except in circumstances involving adoption assistance.

Questions to ask the child welfare caseworker regarding long-term arrangements:

1.  What is the current permanency goal for each child? (Siblings may not have the same goal.)

2.  What are options for the children if they can never return to their parents?

3.  What are my options if the children cannot return to their parents?

4.  Under what circumstances can I receive a subsidy to help pay for the children's care?

5.  Will the legal arrangement be affected when the children turn 18?

6.  How will the child welfare agency continue to be involved with my family?

## Conclusion

Dealing with the child welfare agency can be confusing and, sometimes, even frustrating for grandparents and other relatives who are trying to provide the best care they can for children whose parents cannot care for them. It may be helpful to keep in mind that child welfare caseworkers are following federal and state requirements to ensure the safety and well-being of all children. Using the information in this chapter may help kin caregivers work with the child welfare system to provide the best outcome and permanent living arrangements for their relative children.

# Chapter 37

# *Child Protective Services (CPS)*

## *Chapter Contents*

Section 37.1

## *Services Provided by CPS*

Excerpted from "Child Maltreatment 2006: Chapter 6,"
Administration for Children and Families, 2008.

Child protective services (CPS) agencies provide services to prevent future instances of child abuse and neglect and to remedy conditions that have come to the attention of child welfare agencies. There are two categories of CPS services:

- Preventive services are provided to parents whose children are at risk of abuse or neglect. These services are designed to increase parent's and other caregiver's understanding of the developmental stages of childhood and to improve their child-rearing competencies. Examples of preventive services include respite care, parenting education, housing assistance, substance abuse treatment, daycare, home visits, individual and family counseling, and homemaker help.

- Post-investigation services are offered on a voluntary basis by child welfare agencies or ordered by the courts to ensure the safety of children. These services address the safety of the child and are usually based on an assessment of the family's strengths, weaknesses, and needs. Examples of post-investigation services include individual counseling, case management, family-based services (services provided to the entire family, such as counseling or family support), in-home services, foster care services, and court services.

During federal fiscal year (FFY) 2006:

- an estimated 3.8 million children received preventive services;

- nearly 60 percent of victims received post-investigation services; and

- an estimated 312,000 children received foster care services as a result of an investigation.

## Preventive Services

For FFY 2006, 50.7 children per 1,000 children in the population received preventive services. This results in a national estimate of approximately 3.8 million children. During 2005, it was estimated that 25.7 children per 1,000 children or approximately two million children received preventive services.

This significant increase from 2005 to 2006 of the number of children who received preventive services is due, in part, to improved data collection and estimation. During 2006, state counts of both families and children who received preventive services were used for the national estimate; in prior years only the counts of children were used. Some states are able to report the number of families who received services funded by a specific funding source, but are not able to report the number of children.

States and local communities determine who will receive preventive services, what services will be offered, and how the services will be provided. Preventive services were funded by the following federal programs, as well as by state-funded programs.

- Section 106 of Title I of the Child Abuse Prevention and Treatment Act (CAPTA), as amended [42 U.S.C. 5106 et seq.]: The Child Abuse and Neglect State Grant (Basic State Grant) provides funds to states to improve CPS systems. The grant serves as a catalyst to assist states in screening and investigating child abuse and neglect reports, creating and improving the use of multidisciplinary teams to enhance investigations, improving risk and safety assessment protocols, training CPS workers and mandated reporters, and improving services to infants disabled with life-threatening conditions.

- Title II of CAPTA, as amended [42 U.S.C. 5116 et seq.]: The Community-Based Grants for the Prevention of Child Abuse and Neglect assist each state to support community-based efforts to develop, operate, expand, enhance, and network initiatives aimed at preventing child abuse and neglect; support networks of coordinated resources and activities to strengthen and support families; and foster appreciation of diverse populations.

- Title IV-B, Subpart 2, Section 430, of the Social Security Act, as amended Promoting Safe and Stable Families [42.U.S.C. 629 et seq.]: This legislation has the goal of keeping families together by funding such services as preventive intervention so that children do not have to be removed from their homes, services to develop alternative placements if children cannot remain safely in the home, and reunification services to enable children to return to their homes, if appropriate.

- Title XX of the Social Security Act, Social Services Block Grant (SSBG), [42 U.S.C. 1397 et seq.]: Under this grant, states may use funds for such preventive services as child daycare, child protective services, information and referral, counseling, and foster care, as well as other services that meet the goal of preventing or remedying neglect, abuse, or exploitation of children.

## Post-Investigation Services

More than three-quarters of states have policies requiring workers to provide short-term services, if needed, during an investigation. A similar percentage of states require workers to assist with the planning of ongoing services. Nearly 60 percent (58.9%) of child victims received post-investigation services. Of the children who were not found to be victims of maltreatment, 30.3 percent of children received such services. These data result in national estimates of 533,000 victims and 808,000 non-victims who received services. With a few exceptions, the state data on the average number of days to the provision of services fall within the timeframe allowed for an investigation or shortly thereafter. The average time from the start of investigation to provision of service was 43 days.

Children may be removed from their homes during or after an investigation. Some children who are removed on an emergency basis spend a short time in foster care, while others spend a longer time. Approximately one-fifth of victims (21.5%) were placed in foster care as a result of an investigation compared to 21.7 percent for FFY 2005. Although the national percentage of victims who were removed from home or received foster care services at the time of the investigation is 21.5 percent, several states reported more than 40 percent of victims received foster care services.

In addition, 4.4 percent of non-victims experienced removal. Nationally, it is estimated that 312,000 children were removed from their homes as a result of a child maltreatment investigation. Nearly two-thirds (63.6%) of the victims who were removed from their homes suffered from neglect, 8.6 percent from physical abuse, 3.2 percent from sexual abuse, and 16.8 percent from multiple types of maltreatment.

Court-appointed representatives were assigned to 12.9 percent of child victims. This number is understood within the context of two other statistics—states report that 15.2 percent of victims were the subject of court proceedings and 21.5 percent were placed in foster care as a result of an investigation. Given the statutory requirement in CAPTA that "in every case involving an abused or neglected child which results in a judicial proceeding, a guardian ad litem...who may be an attorney or a court appointed special advocate...shall be appointed to represent the child in such proceedings," many states are working to improve their reporting of the court appointed representative data element. Nearly one-third of child victims (31.0%) had received family preservation services and 8.1 percent had received family reunification services within the previous five years.

## Factors Influencing the Receipt of Services

A multivariate analysis was used to examine which factors influenced the receipt of services, and among children who received services, which factors influenced the removal of victims from their homes. Three analyses were conducted. The first analysis focused on all victims and examined factors associated with receipt of any post-investigation service, either in-home, foster care, or both. The second and third analyses focused on only victims who received any post-investigation services; one examined factors associated with receipt of in-home services only and the other examined factors associated with any placement in foster care. The results of these analyses are the inverse of each other, but they provide two different perspectives on the factors contributing to the type of services provided.

### Receipt of Post-Investigation Services

Only some children and families with reports of maltreatment receive post-investigation services or family reunification services, due to a variety of factors. Including that services are not usually available for all families, and the waiting lists may be very long. The characteristics of a child's case may also influence the receipt of services. Case-level data submissions were analyzed to examine which factors influenced whether or not a victim or the victim's family received post-investigation services. Highlights of the findings are listed:

- Child victims who were reported with a disability were two times more likely to receive post-investigation services than children without a disability.

- When compared with physical abuse victims, victims of multiple maltreatments were 65 percent more likely and victims of neglect were 20 percent more likely to receive services. Victims of sexual abuse were 24 percent less likely to receive services.

- African-American child victims were 22 percent more likely and Hispanic child victims were 16 percent more likely to receive services when compared with White victims.

- Child victims who were abused or maltreated by nonparental perpetrators were 60 percent less likely to receive post-investigation services than child victims who were abused or maltreated by their mothers alone. Child victims who were abused by both parents, or by their mothers along with another person, were significantly more likely to receive services than child victims who were maltreated by their mothers alone.

### Receipt of In-Home Services

For this analysis, only victims who received any post-investigation service were included. Findings related to these child victims who received or whose families received only services provided in the home or the community, and not foster care placement, include the following.

- Child victims with reported disabilities were 39 percent as likely to receive only in-home services as child victims without reported disabilities.

- Children who were sexually abused or had "other abuse" types were more likely to receive exclusively in-home services than children who were physically abused. Children who were neglected or who were maltreated in more than one way were significantly less likely to receive only in-home services.

- When compared with infants, older children were significantly more likely to receive exclusively in-home services. Children age 8–11 were twice as likely to receive in-home services.

- Child victims who were abused or maltreated by their fathers were twice as likely to receive only in-home services as child victims who were abused or maltreated by their mothers.

- Victims referred by mental health and educational personnel were more than twice as likely to receive only in-home services as victims who were referred by the social services personnel.

### *Receipt of Foster Care Services*

For this analysis, only victims who received any post-investigation service were included. Findings related to these child victims who received services include the following.

- Among children who received any services, prior child victims were 63 percent more likely to be placed in foster care than children with no prior victimization.

- Child victims reported with a disability were two and a half times more likely to be placed in foster care than child victims with no reported disability.

- When compared with victims of physical abuse, victims of multiple maltreatments were 79 percent more likely to be placed in foster care, and victims of neglect were 22 percent more likely to be placed in foster care.

- When compared with White child victims, African-American child victims were 27 percent more likely and victims of "other" or multiple races were 52 percent more likely to be placed in foster care.

- Children who were victimized by their fathers were 50 percent less likely to be placed in foster care than children who were victimized by their mothers.

- Victims referred by mental health personnel were 53 percent less likely and victims referred by educational personnel were 50 percent less likely to be placed in foster care than victims referred by social services personnel.

## Section 37.2

# Differential Response by CPS to Reports of Child Abuse and Neglect

Excerpted from "Differential Response to Reports of Child Abuse
and Neglect," Child Welfare Information Gateway, U.S. Department
of Health and Human Services (HHS), 2008.

## Defining Differential Response

Differential response is a child protective services (CPS) practice that allows for more than one method of initial response to reports of child abuse and neglect. Also called dual track, multiple track, or alternative response, this approach recognizes variation in the nature of reports and the value of responding differently to different types of cases (Schene, 2001).

While definitions and approaches vary from state to state, differential response generally uses two or more tracks or paths of response to reports of child abuse and neglect. Typically, these responses fall into two major categories:

- **Investigation:** These responses involve gathering forensic evidence and require a formal determination regarding whether child maltreatment has occurred or the child is at risk of abuse or neglect. In a differential response system, investigation responses are generally used for reports of the most severe types of maltreatment or those that are potentially criminal.

- **Assessment (alternative response):** These responses—usually applied in low- and moderate-risk cases—generally involve assessing the family's strengths and needs and offering services to meet the family's needs and support positive parenting. Although a formal determination or substantiation of child abuse or neglect may be made in some cases, it is typically not required.

However, not all jurisdictions that employ differential response focus simply on choosing an assessment or investigation track. In some areas, there is more variation in types of response. Additional tracks may include a resource referral/prevention track for reports that do not meet screening criteria for CPS but suggest a need for community services, or a law enforcement track for cases that may require criminal charges.

## Similarities between Differential Response and Traditional CPS

While introducing a more flexible way of responding to reports, differential response systems still share many underlying principles with the traditional child protection approach. Both:

- focus on the safety and well-being of the child;

- promote permanency within the family whenever possible;

- recognize the authority of CPS to make decisions about removal, out-of-home placement, and court involvement, when necessary; and

- acknowledge that other community services may be more appropriate than CPS in some cases.

Differential response systems acknowledge that investigations are necessary in some cases. They typically allow for changes in the response track if circumstances change or information emerges that indicates a different type of response is needed to ensure child safety or better respond to the family.

The National Study of Child Protective Services Systems and Reform Efforts (U.S. Department of Health and Human Services, 2003a), which included a survey of a nationally representative sample of local CPS agencies, found that despite the differences in focus, many of the approaches and practices used in conducting investigations and alternative responses were similar. During investigations, almost all agencies reviewed CPS records, interviewed or formally observed the child, and interviewed the caregiver. A slightly lower proportion of agencies conducted the same activities during alternative responses. Under both responses, a majority of agencies sometimes discussed the case with other CPS workers or with a multidisciplinary team, visited the family, and interviewed professionals.

## Differences between Assessment and Investigation Approaches

In traditional child protection practice, all accepted reports receive an investigation response. Investigations are conducted to determine if children have been harmed or are at risk of being harmed and to provide protection if needed. In differential response systems, investigations are no longer the singular focus of CPS response to reports of child maltreatment. While investigations are conducted for some reports (typically the more serious and severe), assessment is used for most other screened-in reports.

In comparison to investigations, assessment responses tend to:

- be less adversarial;

- focus more on understanding the conditions that could jeopardize the child's safety and the factors that need to be addressed to strengthen the family;

- tailor approaches and services to fit families' strengths, needs, and resources;

- place importance on engaging parents to recognize concerns that affect their ability to parent and to participate in services and supports;

- tap into community services and the family's natural support network; and

- offer voluntary services.

Unlike investigations, assessment responses typically do not require caseworkers to make a formal finding regarding whether child abuse or neglect occurred, identify victims and perpetrators, or enter perpetrator names into central registries.

## Why the Growing Interest in Differential Response?

A number of factors explain the growing national interest in differential response. Some of the most significant include limitations of traditional CPS practice, recognition of the importance of family engagement, and an increased focus on accountability and outcomes.

### Limitations of Traditional CPS Practice

In the two decades following the passage of the Child Abuse Prevention and Treatment Act (CAPTA) of 1974, reports of abuse and neglect rose sharply, reaching three million per year in the mid-1990s without a corresponding increase in available staff. In response, CPS practice became more bureaucratic, standardized, and legalistic. A

**Table 37.1.** Comparison between Investigation and Assessment Approaches[1]

| | Investigation | Assessment |
|---|---|---|
| **Focus** | • Did an incident of child abuse or neglect occur?<br>• Who was responsible?<br>• What steps need to be taken to ensure the child's safety? | • What underlying conditions and factors may jeopardize the child's safety?<br>• What strengths and resources exist within the family and community?<br>• What areas of family functioning need to be strengthened? |
| **Goal** | To determine the findings related to allegations in the report and identify perpetrators and victims. | To engage parents, extended family, and community partners in identifying problems and participating in services and supports that address family needs. |
| **Disposition** | A decision must be made whether to substantiate the allegation of maltreatment. | Caseworkers are not typically required to make a formal finding regarding whether child maltreatment occurred. |
| **Central Registry** | Perpetrators' names are entered into a central registry, in accordance with State statutes and policies. | Alleged perpetrators' names are not entered into a central registry. |
| **Services** | If a case is opened for services, a case plan is generally written and services are provided. Families can be ordered by the court to participate in services if CPS involves the court in the case. | Voluntary services are offered. If parents do not participate, the case is either closed or switched to another type of response. |

[1] Adapted from Schene, 2005, p.5.

growing dissatisfaction with traditional CPS practices contributed to the emergence of differential response systems.

### Recognition of the Importance of Family Engagement

Family-centered practices, such as family team meetings, are generally understood to improve the level of cooperation with services compared to investigations that lack more comprehensive assessments and

**Table 37.2.** States with Policies, Practices, and Statutes Reflecting Differential/Alternative Response (*continued on next page*)

| State | Identified in Policy/ Practice Protocols | Author- ized by Statute | Statewide Implemen- tation | Local/ County/ Regional Implemen- tation | Other Experi- ence* |
|---|---|---|---|---|---|
| Alaska | X | | | X | |
| Arizona | | | | | X |
| California | | | | X | X |
| Delaware | | X | | | |
| Florida | | | | X | X |
| Georgia | X | | X | | |
| Hawaii | X | | X | | |
| Idaho | X | | | | |
| Iowa | | | | | X |
| Kansas | X | | X | | |
| Kentucky | X | X | X | | |
| Louisiana | X | X | | X | |
| Maine | X | | X | | |
| Massachusetts | | | | | X |
| Michigan | | | X | | X |
| Minnesota | X | X | X | | |
| Missouri | X | X | X | | |
| Nevada | X | | | | |
| New Jersey | | X | | X | |
| New Mexico | | | | | X |

individualized service planning. Family involvement in the assessment and service planning process fosters a shared understanding about how the family got to the point of a maltreatment report, what needs to change, what services might help, and who is expected to do what, by when. Differential response systems leverage opportunities to engage families, identify motivations to change, build on family strengths, and involve extended family networks and community supports in protecting children.

**Table 37.2.** States with Policies, Practices, and Statutes Reflecting Differential/Alternative Response (*continued from previous page*)

| State | Identified in Policy/ Practice Protocols | Author- ized by Statute | Statewide Implemen- tation | Local/ County/ Regional Implemen- tation | Other Experi- ence* |
|---|---|---|---|---|---|
| North Carolina | X | X | X | | X |
| North Dakota | | | | | X |
| Oklahoma | X | X | X | | |
| Pennsylvania | X | X | X | | |
| South Carolina | | | | | X |
| South Dakota | X | | X | | |
| Tennessee | X | X | | X | |
| Texas | | | | | X |
| Utah | X | | | | |
| Vermont | X | | X | | |
| Virginia | X | X | X | | |
| Washington | X | | X | | |
| West Virginia | X | | | X | |
| Wisconsin | | | | | X |
| Wyoming | X | X | X | | |
| Total | 22 | 12 | 16 | 7 | 12 |

* Other experience includes states that previously had a differential response system but are not currently operating under the system. It also includes states that have incorporated some elements of differential response into their system or that are operating a pilot project but do not have a formal differential response system.

## *Increased Focus on Accountability and Outcomes*

The introduction of the Child and Family Services Reviews (CFSR) has heightened awareness within the child welfare community that the work of child protection should be measured against the outcomes of safety, permanency, and child well-being. Many jurisdictions are paying attention to the value of responding more individually to reports and learning more about what has to change in each family to achieve and sustain a better end result.

## Conclusion

Differential response has been a positive development in child protection. Evaluations demonstrate that:

- children are at least as safe as in traditional practice;
- parents are engaging in services; and
- families, caseworkers, and administrators are supportive of the approach.

Jurisdictions implementing differential response still face hurdles. For example, collaboration and coordination with other agencies and broader community stakeholders is an area likely to receive more attention as CPS shares more of the responsibility for the protection of children with local communities. In addition, limited resources—including services, supports, and time for caseworkers to facilitate connections to these resources—will be a continuing challenge.

Nonetheless, building from lessons learned, states and agencies continue to move forward, refining existing differential response systems and expanding into new jurisdictions. And, as they do, they draw upon flexible, family-centered practices and community resources to more effectively strengthen our nation's families and promote the safety and well-being of children.

# Chapter 38

# *Child Neglect Assessment and Interventions*

## Chapter Contents

# Section 38.1

# *CPS Assessments*

Text in this section is from "Child Neglect: A Guide for Prevention, Assessment, and Intervention: Chapter 5," Child Welfare Information Gateway, U.S. Department of Health and Human Services (HHS), updated September 18, 2008. The complete document is available at http://www .childwelfare.gov/pubs/usermanuals/neglect/chapterfive.cfm.

## *Assessment of Child Neglect*

Child protective services (CPS) is responsible for receiving and evaluating reports of suspected child abuse and neglect, determining if the reported information meets statutory and agency guidelines for child maltreatment, and judging the urgency with which the agency must respond to the report. In addition, CPS provides the public, as well as individuals who report allegations of child abuse or neglect (frequently referred to as reporters), with information about state statutes, agency guidelines, and the roles and responsibilities of CPS.

After receiving a report, CPS conducts an initial assessment or investigation, which may include the following:

- A determination of whether the report of child maltreatment is substantiated.

- A safety assessment to determine if the child's immediate safety is a concern. If it is, CPS develops a safety plan with interventions to ensure the child's protection while keeping the child within the family or with family members (for example, kinship care or subsidized guardianship), if at all possible and appropriate.

- A risk assessment to determine if there is a risk of future maltreatment and the level of that risk.

- A service or case plan, if continuing agency services, is needed to address any effects of child maltreatment and to reduce the risk of future maltreatment.

During the initial assessment or investigation, CPS must determine whether child abuse or neglect occurred and can be substantiated and whether to conduct an evaluation to determine the risk of maltreatment occurring in the future. The initial assessment identifies the risk and safety factors of concern in the family. The family assessment:

- considers the relationship between the strengths and the risks; and

- identifies what must change in order to:

  - keep children safe,

  - reduce the risk of (future) neglect,

  - increase permanency, and

  - enhance child and family well-being.

Consequently, while the initial assessment identifies problems, the family assessment promotes an understanding of the problems and becomes the basis for the prevention and intervention, or the case plan.

## Intake

When a referral is made to CPS, a decision is made whether it should be "screened in" or "screened out" for investigation or assessment. For a case to be screened in, there usually has to be a specific allegation of maltreatment or an imminent threat or danger to the child. Cases that are screened in then receive an initial assessment or investigation. Families may be referred to CPS multiple times without having a referral screened in because each incident in question may not meet the state or local standards for neglect that are used by the particular CPS agency. In cases of neglect where no actual injury occurred, it often is difficult for a CPS caseworker to determine if a child is at risk of being harmed or how great the risk is; therefore, these cases may be screened out.

Many CPS agencies only screen in the most serious cases. Consequently, cases in which it is reported that a child may be at risk for neglect (for example, a child living in a dirty house with used drug needles on the floor), but actually has not been harmed, may not be investigated. Unfortunately, some children and families who could benefit from services are not receiving them either due to being screened out or to having an unsubstantiated case. In addition, families who have unsubstantiated incidences of neglect and do not receive services are likely to be referred later for incidences that are more serious. Receiving even one form of service may reduce the likelihood that a neglectful family would be re-referred. For the safety and well-being of the child, it would be more beneficial for these families to receive services to prevent neglect from occurring.

## Initial Assessment or Investigation

Determining whether child neglect has occurred is based on the answers to two primary questions: "Do the conditions or circumstances indicate that a child's basic needs are unmet?" and "What harm or threat of harm may have resulted?" Answering these questions requires sufficient information to assess the degree to which omissions in care have resulted in significant harm or significant risk of harm. CPS caseworkers also must make their determination of whether neglect has occurred based on state or local statutes. Unlike the other forms of maltreatment, this determination may not be reached by examining one incident; the decision often requires considering patterns of care over time. The analysis should focus on examining how the child's basic needs are met and on identifying situations that may indicate specific omissions in care that have resulted in harm or the risk of harm to the child.

### Home Accidents

Home accidents pose a significant risk to young children and often occur because of a lack of supervision. More than 90 percent of all fatalities and injuries to children younger than five years of age can be attributed to accidents within the home. Since almost all accidents are preventable, an evaluation of hazardous home conditions is essential to ensure a safe environment for children.

### Lack of Supervision

While state statutes vary, most CPS professionals agree that children under the age of eight years who are left alone for any substantial amount of time are being neglected. In determining whether neglect has occurred, the following issues should be considered:

- The child's age, physical condition, mental abilities, coping capacity, maturity, competence, knowledge regarding how to respond to an emergency, and feelings about being alone.

- The type and degree of indirect adult supervision. For example, is there an adult who is regularly checking in on the child?

- The length of time and frequency with which the child is left alone. Is the child being left alone all day, every day? Is he or she left alone all night?

- The safety of the child's environment, neighborhood, and home.

## Distinguishing Risk and Safety Assessments

Assessing risk differs from assessing safety. A risk assessment is the collection of information to determine the degree to which a child is likely to be abused or neglected in the future. A safety assessment involves the identification and evaluation of the imminent risk of harm regarding the specific vulnerability of a child. Depending on where they fall on a continuum of severity and chronicity, factors are typically relevant to both risk and safety assessments. Caseworkers should work with families to develop an effective and accomplishable safety plan. This is usually an in-home or out-of-home service strategy created after the initial assessment or investigation that specifically addresses and manages risk of harm. In addition, risk and safety assessments should be ongoing throughout the life of the case, not just during the initial assessment.

## Family Assessment Process

The family assessment is a comprehensive process for identifying, considering, and weighing factors that affect the child's safety, permanency, and well-being. It is designed to gain a greater understanding about the strengths, needs, and resources of the family. The assessment should be conducted in partnership with the family to help parents or caregivers recognize and remedy conditions so that children can be safe and the risk of neglect can be reduced. Family assessments must be individualized and tailored to the unique strengths and needs of each family. When possible and appropriate, this assessment also should be undertaken through family decision-making meetings and other means designed to involve the extended family and support network.

Based on the information obtained in the initial assessment or investigation, the caseworker should develop a list of issues to address during the family assessment process.

While the CPS caseworker has primary responsibility for conducting the family assessment, other community providers frequently may be called upon to assist when there is a specific client condition or behavior that may require additional professional assessment.

## Analyze Information and Make Decisions

To individualize the response to a particular child and family, the caseworker identifies the critical risk factors by examining the information in terms of cause, nature, extent, effects, strengths, and the family's perception of the neglect. The caseworker and family then should identify the necessary changes, translate them into desired outcomes, and match the outcomes with the correct intervention to increase safety, well-being, and permanency for the children.

# Section 38.2

# *CPS Interventions*

Text in this section is from "Child Neglect: A Guide for Prevention, Assessment, and Intervention: Chapter 6," Child Welfare Information Gateway, U.S. Department of Health and Human Services (HHS), updated September 18, 2008. The complete document is available at http://www .childwelfare.gov/pubs/usermanuals/neglect/chaptersix.cfm.

## Child Neglect Prevention and Intervention

The goal of the initial prevention or intervention should be to address safety and other emergency needs and to increase the caregiver's readiness for change-oriented practices or behaviors. By the time families experiencing neglect come to the attention of CPS agencies, they often have acute and chronic needs that require long-term intervention. These families are significantly more likely to experience recurrence of child neglect than abusive families. In some CPS agencies, families experiencing neglect are given less priority than those dealing with physical or sexual abuse, even though their risk of recurrence may be particularly high.

Effective ways must be found to target and serve these at-risk families as soon as they are identified to minimize risks that could lead to child neglect and abuse.

## Principles for Effective Prevention and Intervention

Efforts targeting single risk factors may be as effective in preventing neglect and its recurrence as programs that are individualized and offer multiple services. Either way, services must be based on principles that empower families, build upon strengths, and respect cultural diversity. The following are some basic principles for practitioners who intervene with families when children's basic needs are unmet:

- Have an ecological-developmental framework
- Carry out a comprehensive family assessment
- Establish a helping alliance and partnership with the family
- Utilize an empowerment-based practice
- Emphasize family strengths
- Develop cultural competence
- Ensure developmental appropriateness

## Interventions for Neglect Cases

### Concrete Support

- Housing assistance
- Emergency financial, food, or other assistance
- Transportation
- Clothing, household items
- Availability or accessibility to community resources
- Hands-on assistance to increase safety and sanitation of home (home management aids)
- Free or low-cost medical care
- Available and affordable quality child care

### Social Support

- Individual social support (parent aide, volunteer)
- Connections to faith-based activities
- Mentor involvement
- Social support groups

- Development of neighborhood child care and respite care services
- Neighborhood-centered activities
- Social networking
- Recreation programs
- Cultural festivals and other activities

## Developmental

- Therapeutic child care
- Individual assistance with developmental skills (parenting)
- Home visits with focus on developmental needs of family members
- Peer groups (often at schools) geared to developmental tasks
- Mentors to provide nurturing, cultural enrichment, recreation, and role modeling

## Cognitive and Behavioral

- Social skills training
- Communication skills building

**Table 38.1.** Possible Responses to Families

| Types of Cases | Responses Suggested | Organizations Responsible |
|---|---|---|
| Mild Risk | Early intervention, family support, formal or informal services, parent education, housing assistance, community neighborhood advocacy | Community programs |
| Moderate Risk | Appropriate formal services, coordinated family support, safety plans, community support services | CPS and community programs |
| Severe Risk | Intensive family preservation or reunification services, child removal, court-ordered services, foster care, adoption, criminal prosecution | CPS and law enforcement |

- Teaching of home management, parent-child interaction, meal preparation, and other life skills
- Individual or group therapeutic counseling (regarding childhood history)
- Parenting education
- Employment counseling and training
- Financial management counseling
- Problem-solving skills training

## *Individual*

- In- and out-patient counseling and detoxification for substance abuse
- 12-step programs
- Mental health in-patient and out-patient counseling
- Crisis intervention
- Stress management
- Play therapy

## *Family System*

- Home-based, family-centered counseling regarding family functioning, communication skills, home management, and roles and responsibilities
- Center-based family therapy
- Enhancing family strengths
- Building nurturing behaviors
- Refining family dynamics and patterns

## Key Steps in the Intervention Process

Regardless of which intervention approaches and models are implemented, certain steps are necessary to make them appropriate for the needs of the child and family, including the following:

- Building a relationship with the family
- Developing case and safety plans

- Establishing clear, concrete goals
- Targeting outcomes
- Tracking family progress
- Analyzing and evaluating family progress

## Conclusion

Although child neglect is the most common type of maltreatment, its causes, effects, prevention, and treatment often are not as prominently discussed and explored as are those for physical or sexual

**Table 38.2.** Matching Risks to Outcomes

| Risk or Problem | Desired Client Outcomes |
|---|---|
| Condemned housing (no heat or running water, children diagnosed with lead poisoning, safety hazards for young children) | • Household safety<br>• Financial management skills<br>• Problem-solving skills |
| Acting out behavior (refusing to listen, throwing temper tantrums, fights with peers) | • Behavioral control<br>• Social skills<br>• Impulse control |
| Communication problems or conflicts (domestic violence, parent-child conflict) | • Conflict management skills<br>• Decision-making skills<br>• Impulse control<br>• Family functioning |
| Frequent moves (in and out of placement, numerous schools, numerous caregivers) | • Financial management<br>• Problem-solving skills |
| Parental addiction | • Recovery from addiction |
| Inappropriately harsh parenting, inappropriate expectations of children | • Parenting knowledge<br>• Emotional control |
| Fear of expressing feelings, verbally abusive, not recognizing feelings of others | • Communication skills<br>• Empathy |
| Lack of social supports | • Supportive linkages with sources of formal and informal support |

abuse. Neglect, like other types of maltreatment, has many contributing factors at the individual, familial, and community levels. The complexities of neglect present difficulties not only for an overburdened child welfare system, but also for community- and faith-based programs, researchers, legislators, and other service providers. It is key, therefore, that these groups work collaboratively to develop promising and effective practices for preventing neglect and for mitigating its effects on children and society. Part of this process is providing individuals, families, and communities with the knowledge, resources, and services to deal with the challenges associated with neglect. Child welfare agencies can only provide a part of the solution. Neglect must be viewed not only as an individual or a family problem, but also as a community issue requiring a community response.

# Chapter 39

# *Children's Advocacy Centers*

Children's advocacy centers (CACs) play an increasingly significant role in the response to child sexual abuse and other child maltreatment in the United States. First developed in the 1980s, CACs were designed to reduce the stress on child abuse victims and families created by traditional child abuse investigation and prosecution procedures and to improve the effectiveness of the response. According to several experts, child victims were subjected to multiple, redundant interviews about their abuse by different agencies, and were questioned by professionals who had no knowledge of children's developmental limitations or experience working with children. Child interviews would take place in settings like police stations that would further stress already frightened children. Moreover, the response was hampered because the multiple agencies involved did not coordinate their investigations, and children's need for services could be neglected.

CACs aimed to correct these problems by coordinating multidisciplinary investigation teams in a centralized, child-friendly setting; employing forensic interviewers specially trained to work with children; and assisting children and families in obtaining medical, therapeutic, and advocacy services. The CAC movement is based on the

This chapter includes text from "Evaluating Children's Advocacy Centers' Response to Child Sexual Abuse," *Juvenile Justice Bulletin*, Office of Juvenile Justice and Delinquency Prevention, August 2008. The complete document is available online at http://www.ncjrs.gov/pdffiles1/ojjdp/218530.pdf.

341

belief that the response system should focus on the needs of the child and family and is most effective when the skills of multiple agencies are coordinated.

The number of children's advocacy centers in the United States has grown dramatically in the last 20 years. The first CAC was created in 1986 and by 1994, there were 50 CACs established nationwide. As of 2006, the National Children's Alliance (NCA), the accrediting organization for CACs, reported more than 600 CACs.

Accrediting standards that NCA established require that CACs provide evidence of the following:

- **A child-appropriate, child-friendly facility:** CACs must provide a welcoming environment that is private and physically and psychologically safe. Typically this is geographically separate from police stations, child protective services (CPS), and courthouses. Facilities are designed to provide a child- and family-friendly environment for interviews and family meetings.

- **A multidisciplinary investigation team and coordinated forensic interviews:** A multidisciplinary team typically consists of law enforcement officers, CPS investigators, prosecutors, and mental health and medical professionals. The team members coordinate their response to increase the investigation's effectiveness and reduce stress for children. Methods may include interviews in which one trained forensic interviewer collects information from the child while multiple team members watch through a one-way mirror or closed-circuit television. The single interview informs multiple agencies, reducing the need for children to be interviewed more than once.

- **Case reviews:** In the weeks after the initial interview, the team reviews the case to give professionals further opportunities to refine planning, share new information, engage in team problem solving, and refer a child for additional services.

- **Medical evaluation, therapeutic intervention, and victim advocacy services:** CACs have formal links with medical professionals and arrange for medical examinations, as needed. Many have medical staff and facilities onsite. NCA membership standards require that CACs work with a victim's family to secure needed services, such as child psychotherapy and victims' advocacy services.

## CAC Evaluation Findings

Researchers collected information on an extensive number of variables to examine the many potential effects of CACs on investigation processes and outcomes. This section presents an overview of the effects that CACs have had on child abuse investigations.

### CAC Characteristics

While all the CACs met NCA standards and shared the same philosophy and essential capabilities, they varied considerably in many structures and processes. They differed in their organizational base (large children's hospital versus small, independent family services center), their stage or organizational development, their referral process (referrals based on a professional's judgement versus a standard protocol) and their specific emphasis (criminal justice versus human services).

### Investigations and Child Interviewing

Improving investigation methods and child forensic interviews following allegations of child abuse is a central aim of CACs. Overall, communities with CACs showed more evidence of coordinated investigations than comparison communities. CAC cases more often used multidisciplinary team interviews (28 percent of CAC cases versus six percent of comparison cases), videotaping of interviews (52 percent versus 17 percent), joint CPS-police investigations (81 percent versus 52 percent), and multidisciplinary case reviews (56 percent versus seven percent). CACs were more likely to have police involvement in interviewing the child in CPS child sexual abuse investigations than comparison communities (55 percent versus 43 percent).

All CACs in the study provided separate, private, and comfortable facilities specially designed for interviewing children, and 81 percent of child interviews in the CAC sample were conducted in these facilities. Contrary to researchers' hypotheses, children interviewed in CACs and comparison communities underwent about the same number of interviews.

### Disclosure

The steps that CACs take to reduce stress on children who have been abused may make it easier for the victims to disclose the abuse in the forensic interview. Disclosure during a forensic interview is

343

often not the child's first statement about the abuse. The majority of the allegations in CAC and comparison communities arose because children first told a parent, counselor, or other person. Disclosure in the forensic interview is important for several reasons. Disclosure allows investigators to make an accurate decision about allegations, to prepare legal and child protection interventions if needed, and to explore the impact of the abuse on the child.

### Medical Exams

CACs strive to improve access to forensic medical exams. Medical examinations can be an important part of the response to suspected child sexual abuse. They increase the likelihood of timely medical care for the child and provide information to support legal decision making. Many professionals recommend that all reported child sexual abuse victims have a medical evaluation.

The percentage of children who had medical examinations was significantly greater in CACs (48 percent) than in comparison communities (21 percent). The difference in medical examinations between the CAC and comparison communities was particularly pronounced in cases where the sexual abuse did not involve penetration. CAC cases not thought to involve penetration were four times more likely to receive exams than similar cases in comparison communities.

### Mental Health Services

Sexual abuse victims are at high risk for emotional and behavioral problems. The CAC model strives to improve victim access to mental health services. CACs referred a higher proportion of victims to mental health services (72 percent) than comparison communities (31 percent). CACs directly provided mental health services for 30 percent of their cases. In the remaining cases, the CAC referred the child to community and private mental health practitioners. However, interviews with caregivers in the CAC study found no difference in rates of access to child mental health services in CAC and comparison sites.

### Child Protection

Investigations of child sexual abuse occasionally lead to the CPS agency removing a child from the home, if the agency finds that the child is in danger of further maltreatment. An investigation through a CAC could increase removal rates because of more thorough investigation procedures and more aggressive protection strategies, or it could decrease removal rates if work with families and non-offending caregivers increased safety levels in the home.

### Criminal Justice Outcomes

Improving criminal justice outcomes for child sexual abuse cases helps protect children and is a critical goal for many CACs. However, effecting change in criminal charges and convictions could be difficult for CACs. Many factors can influence these outcomes, including state law and a variety of processes among police, prosecutors, and the courts. Moreover, it is difficult to measure the effect CACs may have on the criminal justice system because of the relatively small percentage of sexual abuse cases that make their way through the entire criminal justice process. This evaluation found few indications that CAC communities prosecuted sexual abuse cases more effectively than comparison communities, except in two sites where the CACs had strong involvement with police and prosecutors.

### Families' Experiences with the Investigation

Almost all CAC programs are intended to improve the experience for children and families. This outcome might be considered one of the primary tests of the agencies' success. Overall, caregiver satisfaction with the investigation was moderately high across samples, but satisfaction was greater in the CAC samples than in the comparison communities. When asked about satisfaction with the investigation process, 70 percent of caregivers in CAC communities reported high levels of satisfaction versus 54 percent of the caregivers from comparison communities. Additionally, 83 percent of caregivers who worked with CACs reported high satisfaction with the interview procedures compared with 54 percent of the comparison sample. These positive findings for CACs held even when accounting for other variables (caregiver support for the child, agency involvement in the case, and case outcomes).

### Community-Level Outcomes

CACs intervene at the level of individual children and families, but they also help their communities as a whole. The CACs in the study provided a number of services to their communities: training to other professionals, consultation to other agencies and departments with which they worked, child abuse prevention activities, and community education on child maltreatment. The CACs are regarded as community leaders and experts in the area of child abuse.

## The Impact of CACs

In this study, CAC cases demonstrated several apparent advantages over comparison communities. Multi-agency investigations of child sexual abuse were more likely to be coordinated and more likely to involve police. Children were more likely to receive referrals for forensic medical evaluations and mental health services, although analyses could not identify referrals that were not recorded in agency records. Non-abusive caregivers reported a higher average level of satisfaction, both with child interviewing and with the investigation as a whole. Children tended to report feeling less scared during CAC interviews. However, no evidence suggested that children were subjected to multiple forensic interviews in either CACs or comparison communities.

Other similarities between CAC and comparison communities are harder to explain. CACs did not affect whether children thought to have been sexually abused disclosed the abuse in a forensic interview. This finding may stem from factors like prior disclosure in the community and child age. The fact that parents reported that their children received mental health services at the same rate in CAC and comparison communities could indicate that a mental health referral does not translate into follow-through on services. Another possibility is that the caregivers who participated in interviews were more likely to seek mental health services than other caregivers in both the CAC and comparison communities.

Most CACs did not differ from comparison communities on criminal justice variables (filing charges, offender confessions, and convictions). Establishing a CAC in a community does not guarantee effective prosecution for child abuse cases. Police and prosecutors must be substantially involved in and committed to the mission of prosecuting child abuse and the CAC method for CACs to help bring about the successful prosecutions of offenders. CAC communities with better criminal justice outcomes than comparison communities generally had involved and committed police and prosecutors.

Many different factors contribute to successful prosecution of child abuse. These include effective methods of gathering corroborative evidence and special training of prosecutors. Criminal justice professionals need to improve these investigation and prosecution methods to impact child abuse prosecution.

Chapter 40

# Working with the Courts in Child Protection

## Chapter Contents

# Section 40.1

## *Court System and Child Protection*

Excerpted from "Working with the Courts in Child Protection:
Chapter 2," Child Welfare Information Gateway, U.S. Department of
Health and Human Services (HHS), updated September 18, 2008.

State courts, including county and municipal courts, are responsible
for resolving a wide variety of issues and do so increasingly in diverse
ways. In addition to going to court for child abuse and neglect cases, child
protective services (CPS) caseworkers often also must be involved in court
proceedings for child support, domestic violence, criminal conduct, juvenile delinquency, child custody, mental health, and directly related proceedings such as termination of parental rights (TPR) and adoption. How
courts are organized and how they divide their caseloads vary widely by
state and even within a state. Thus, it is important for CPS caseworkers
to know which courts hear which kinds of cases in their communities.

### *Jurisdiction*

To hear and to decide a case, a court must have jurisdiction or "authority" over that type of case, as specified by state law. The allegations
of the petition initiating the case must satisfy the statutory criteria for
cases of that type. The court must have jurisdiction over the parties
against whom the case is brought, such as the parents of a child removed from the home. It is the judge's responsibility to decide at the
outset whether the court has jurisdiction over the subject matter of the
case and over the parties. Objections to jurisdiction, although infrequent
in child abuse and neglect cases, can be complex and require CPS to
have legal representation.

### *Juvenile Court*

The juvenile court decides whether children have been victimized
by maltreatment, as defined by state law. It then assumes responsibility for ordering services and monitors cases to ensure that its interventions are as beneficial and effective as possible.

The juvenile court operates according to the legal power of *parens patriae*. The *parens patriae* doctrine stipulates that the state has the legal authority to act as the guardian of children whose parents are unable to provide adequate protection or meet their needs sufficiently.

Today, juvenile court judges hear cases alleging child abuse and neglect, delinquency, and status offenses. Most also hear TPR cases and adoption matters. Some juvenile courts have responsibility for mental health commitment and admission hearings, abortion consent waivers for minors, and petitions for emancipation.

## How Juvenile Courts Are Different from Other Courts

Juvenile courts operate like other courts when deciding whether a child was abused or neglected, or committed a delinquent act or a status offense. What is unique about juvenile courts is that they also make extensive use of experts, including CPS caseworkers, juvenile probation officers, psychologists, mental health professionals, physicians, domestic violence specialists, educators, child development specialists, foster parents, relative caretakers, and others. The court utilizes the expertise of these individuals to understand children and their families better, why events occurred that necessitated court intervention, and how to prevent recurrence. Juvenile courts attempt to look beyond individual and family deficits to understand the family and child as a whole. They aim to make well-informed decisions to address needs for housing, childcare, in-home services, domestic violence advocacy, mental health or substance abuse treatment, paternity establishment, child support, educational services, or employment. Also unique to the juvenile court, particularly in CPS cases, are the frequent review of parents and the assessment of agency performance.

## Powers of the Court

Courts and judges often are viewed as possessing enormous power and influence. The power of the courts is ever changing, and the authority of judges varies considerably from state to state. Some courts exercise the authority to dictate to CPS where children should be placed, sometimes including specific foster homes. Other states are more prescriptive in their statutory laws about placement options for children in state custody and give less discretion and authority to the courts. CPS caseworkers who recognize and know how to access the powers of the court will find them advantageous to the resolution of their cases. Seven different powers held by the court include the following:

- **Power to subpoena witnesses:** A subpoena is a court order that directs a person to appear in court.

- **Power to subpoena documents and records:** This subpoena commands a person to produce in court certain designated documents or records.

- **Power to assist CPS investigations:** Some states have granted courts the authority to order parents to allow CPS to examine and to interview their children and to compel others who have information relevant to a child maltreatment investigation to make that information available for CPS examination.

- **Power to make negative "reasonable efforts" determinations:** A court can find that CPS has failed to make "reasonable efforts" to:
  - avoid a child's removal from the home;
  - reunite a child with the family from which the child was removed; or
  - secure an adoptive home or other permanent placement for a child.

- **Power to hold individuals in contempt:** Civil contempt is the willful failure to do something that a court has ordered. Indirect criminal contempt is a willful violation of a court's order. Direct criminal contempt occurs in the presence of the judge and usually involves some disruptive or disrespectful behavior.

- **Power to order treatment:** Some states specifically authorize courts to order parents to participate in mental health or substance abuse treatment.

- **Inherent power of the position:** Most of the professionals involved with child maltreatment respect the position and authority of the court and are responsive to judicial requests or inquiries. When a judge calls a meeting to address a particular issue or invites stakeholders in a child abuse or neglect case to a meeting, they usually attend.

## The Rights of Parents and Children in Child Maltreatment Cases

The court system accords both parents and children certain legal rights and entitlements, depending on the type of proceeding in which they are involved, including the following:

- The right to family integrity
- The right to notice of the proceedings
- The right to a hearing
- The right to counsel
- The right to a jury trial
- The CAPTA requirement of a guardian ad litem or court-appointed special advocate
- The entitlement to reasonable efforts

Parents and children must not only be informed of their rights, but they also must understand the protections those rights afford them. Court representatives and CPS caseworkers can educate families about their rights and help them feel empowered in an otherwise intimidating process.

Except in certain aggravated circumstances, parents and children are entitled under the Adoption Assistance and Child Welfare Act (P.L. 96-272) and the Adoption and Safe Families Act (ASFA) (P.L. 105-89) to have state agencies make reasonable efforts to keep them together, or if a child has been removed from the family, to make reasonable efforts to reunify the family. ASFA also states that children who are not going to be reunited with their families are entitled to reasonable efforts by state agencies or departments to secure a permanent placement for them.

Federal law further requires that judges decide at each critical stage of an abuse or neglect case whether the agency has complied with the reasonable efforts requirement. The obligation to make reasonable efforts applies to CPS alone, not to the parents, any other individuals, or service providers.

## Section 40.2

# *Juvenile Court Process*

Excerpted from "Working with the Courts in Child Protection: Chapter 4,"
Child Welfare Information Gateway, U.S. Department of Health and
Human Services (HHS), updated September 18, 2008.

Other than judges or attorneys, most people find court proceedings
intimidating and confusing. Child protective services (CPS) caseworkers and families involved in juvenile court face the daunting task of
understanding the court process, the roles of court personnel, the complex legal jargon, and the court's expectation of them. CPS caseworkers need to be competent in navigating the juvenile court process to
achieve positive outcomes for children and families.

### *The Petition for Removal*

Cases of any type begin with the filing of an initial pleading with
a court. A child protection proceeding is initiated by filing a petition.
The petition usually will be captioned "In re Jane Doe," meaning it is
brought regarding her. The state or county is the petitioner and the
parents, caretakers, or child may be referred to as respondents. They
are not defendants and the petition does not charge them with child
abuse or neglect. The petition contains the essential elements of the
conduct that is alleged to be child maltreatment. It does not need to
contain all the facts known to the petitioner, but should include
enough to establish the court's jurisdiction.

The decision to file a child maltreatment petition is made by the
CPS caseworker and supervisor, often in consultation with the
agency's lawyer. Most states allow only CPS to initiate child protection proceedings, but some also permit other public officials or even
private citizens to do so.

The requirements for reasonable efforts have resulted in more
attempts to "remove the harm and not the child" by effectively addressing maltreatment without going to court. These attempts include
diverting families to community-based programs and services, such
as residential mental health treatment, substance abuse treatment

combined with the placement of the child with a relative, housing subsidies, childcare, or financial support; in-home services ranging from
intensive family preservation to periodic monitoring; and ordering violent or sexually abusive adults out of the child's home.

### Petitions and Removals

State and local practices regarding the filing of petitions, emergency removals, and prior authorization of removals by judicial officers are not governed by federal law and vary widely between and
within states. Ideally, no child should be removed from a family until
after a petition is filed and the court has conducted a hearing at which
the parents were present and had an opportunity to be heard. In reality, most removals are authorized by *ex parte* orders and the first
hearing is conducted after the removal has occurred.

Petitions alleging maltreatment do not have to include a request
that the child be removed. It sometimes may be useful to file a petition without asking for removal. An example would be a case in which
maltreatment is substantiated and removal does not appear necessary, but the parents are resistant to CPS intervention. The court may
be convinced to exercise its powers of persuasion, or even coercion, to
promote parental cooperation.

### Continuances, Adjournments, Postponements, and Delays

Continuances (postponements of a date of a trial, hearing, or other
court appearance to a later date) or adjournments (temporary postponements of the proceedings of a case until a specified future time)
should be avoided, if at all possible. They waste court time and in-
convenience the parties, CPS caseworkers, attorneys, guardian ad
litem (GAL) or court-appointed special advocate (CASA), volunteers,
and witnesses. Typically, the impact of these delays is felt most acutely
by the children and families involved. Most importantly, they delay
resolution of the case and permanency for the child.

### The Initial Hearing

The first event in court after the filing of a petition is the initial
hearing, known also as the preliminary protective hearing, shelter
care hearing, detention hearing, emergency removal hearing, or temporary custody hearing. It occurs soon after the filing of the petition
or the removal of the child from the home. The precise deadline for
this hearing depends on state law. Ideally, it should occur on the first

day following the filing of the petition, upon removal of the child, or as soon as possible thereafter.

The initial hearing is the most critical stage in the child abuse and neglect court process. Many important decisions are made and actions taken that chart the course for the remainder of the proceeding. At this hearing, the relationships between those involved in the process also are established, and the tone is set for their ongoing interactions.

The main purpose of the initial hearing is to determine whether the child should be placed in substitute care or remain with or be returned to the parents pending further proceedings. The critical issue is whether in-home services or other measures can be put in place to ensure the child's safety.

## Pretrial Conferences

Some courts use pretrial conferences, also known as settlement conferences, in child maltreatment cases. These conferences are opportunities for the parents, their attorneys, and the child's advocates to discuss a settlement in the form of stipulated, or agreed to, facts that would make a trial unnecessary. In courts where there are no formal pretrial conferences, these settlement negotiations often occur among attorneys by phone or at the courtroom and as late as right before the scheduled adjudication. The judge may or may not participate, depending on the jurisdiction and the nature of the case, and some judges will initiate such negotiations themselves.

### *Mediation*

An increasing number of juvenile courts across the country are using mediation and other non-adversarial dispute resolution methods, such as family group conferencing, to settle child maltreatment and termination of parental rights (TPR) cases. The mediation process usually is called "dependency mediation" and is similar in many ways to settlement conferences, except that there is a skilled and trained mediator facilitating the discussion. Family group conferencing also utilizes a facilitator, but tries to involve the child's extended family more fully and encourages family members to craft their own plans for the support of the child and parent. When settlement conferences and mediation fail to produce agreement on the entire case, they nevertheless may produce agreement on some issues and at least shorten the time necessary for the adjudication.

## Discovery

Discovery is a pretrial process that allows each party to obtain information relevant to the case from the other parties. It is intended to avoid "trial by ambush," to narrow the contested issues, and to expedite settlement. Discovery in child maltreatment cases usually involves the parents' and child's attorneys asking CPS for its records. In most states, they are entitled to those records. While details of the initial and investigative reports are revealed, the name of the reporter is not.

## The Adjudication Hearing

If the case is not settled by agreement of the parties, it will go to adjudication. Once the petition is filed, the court schedules an adjudication hearing (also known as the fact-finding hearing or jurisdictional hearing). At the adjudication hearing, the court decides whether CPS can prove the allegations in its petition. The CPS attorney will present evidence through the testimony of the CPS caseworker, law enforcement officers, or other witnesses, including any experts. Documents such as medical records or photographs also may be entered into evidence. The attorneys for the parents and the child will have the right to question or to cross-examine the witnesses and to present evidence. The parents may testify, as may other family members or neighbors who have knowledge of the facts alleged in the petition or of the care the parents provided their children.

### Parent Testimony

Because child maltreatment cases in juvenile court are civil as opposed to criminal, the parents do not enjoy the right against self-incrimination contained in the Fifth Amendment to the U.S. Constitution. Therefore, they can be called to testify by CPS, the other parent, or the GAL. They still can "take the Fifth," however, and refuse to testify on the grounds that their answers may incriminate them.

### Burden of Proof

CPS holds the burden of proof, and its attorney needs to present enough evidence to convince the judge that the maltreatment of the child alleged in the petition occurred. The burden of proof is either the greater weight (or preponderance) of the evidence or clear and convincing evidence, depending on the state. In determining whether the burden of proof has been met, the judge will take into account the quantity, quality, credibility, and convincing force of the evidence.

### Order

At the conclusion of an adjudication in favor of CPS (whether it is by agreement or after a contested hearing), the judge needs to enter an order finding specific facts regarding the child's maltreatment and the problems that must be resolved before the child can return home safely. Other issues to be addressed include whether CPS has made reasonable efforts to avoid placement or to achieve reunification, the child's placement, all incomplete or unresolved issues from the initial hearing, and the disposition hearing date.

## The Disposition Hearing

At the disposition hearing, the court decides whether the child needs help from the court and, if so, what services will be ordered. For example, the court may enter an order that mandates counseling and rehabilitative services. The court also may enter orders providing for out-of-home placements, or visitation schedules, or for controlling the conduct of the parent. It also can order CPS to conduct follow-up visits with the family to ensure the child's protection. Essentially, the disposition hearing determines what will be required to resolve the problems that led to CPS intervention.

The rules of evidence are relaxed in disposition hearings, and they are generally less formal than adjudications, although witnesses sometimes testify and are cross-examined. While the disposition hearing is sometimes held on the same day as the adjudication hearing, the National Council of Juvenile and Family Court Judges recommends that the disposition hearing be separate and follow the adjudication within 30 days.

## Court Report

CPS must prepare a disposition court report and present it to the court, the counsel for all parties, and any GAL or CASA at least seven calendar days prior to the hearing or by the time specified in any local court rules.

## The Case Plan

Before the disposition hearing, CPS should confer with the parents and develop with them a case plan that identifies the problems that led to CPS involvement with the family and are specified in the adjudication order. The case plan will state the goal for the child's permanent placement.

## The Placement Decision

Placement is the key issue at the disposition hearing. The child can be:

- left with or returned to the parents, usually under CPS supervision;
- kept in an existing placement;
- moved to a new placement; or
- placed in substitute care for the first time if removal was not ordered previously.

The option that the court chooses will depend on the circumstances of the case, principally the risk of harm to the child in the home and the possibilities for reducing that risk to a safe level. The options for placement will depend on the needs of the child and include:

- either or both parents;
- the extended family or kinship care;
- foster care; or
- a group home or institutional care.

As a part of its reasonable efforts inquiry, the court needs to scrutinize carefully any CPS recommendation that the child be placed outside the home.

## Review Hearings

Review hearings are the next stage of a continuing process that begins with the initial hearing and continues through adjudication and disposition. The review hearing is an opportunity to evaluate the progress that has been made toward completing the case plan and any court orders and to revise the plan as needed.

### Timing of Review Hearings

Federal law, through Title IV-E of the Social Security Act (42 U.S.C. 675(5)(B)), requires that states make provision for cases to be reviewed at least every six months after the child is placed in substitute care.

## The Permanency Hearing

Review hearings are intended primarily to monitor compliance with the case plan, adjust the plan as necessary, and ensure that the case is progressing toward resolution. The permanency hearing is fundamentally different as it is the point at which a definitive decision is made about the child's permanent placement. The Adoption and Safe Families Act (ASFA) requires that the permanency hearing occur no later than 12 months from the date the child is considered to have entered foster care.

In making the determination about the permanent placement of the child, the court must weigh which option is in the child's best interest. In some cases, concurrent planning may be pursued. Under concurrent planning, an alternative, permanent placement is developed at the same time as family reunification is attempted. With this approach, the child can be moved quickly to a stable home if reunification with the birth family cannot take place.

### Timing of Permanency Hearings

In some cases, the permanency hearing is the last stage of child maltreatment litigation. It determines whether the final plan will be to reunite the child and parent or to pursue an alternative, permanent home. It is a more formal hearing than reviews. The permanency hearing usually is held after one year. However, if it becomes readily apparent earlier that a reunification plan will not be successful, the permanency hearing should be scheduled as soon as possible.

## Appeals

Parents and CPS have the right to appeal some decisions of the juvenile court in child abuse and neglect and TPR cases. At the very least, the right to appeal attaches at the conclusion of any adjudication, disposition, or TPR trial. Some states may allow appeal from other trial court orders or decisions, but generally, only final decisions are appealed or accepted for appellate review.

Appellate courts decide cases based on the written record, or a videotape in some locations, from the trial court. They examine the record and determine whether:

- the trial judge abused his or her discretion in finding the facts;
- the facts support the judge's conclusions of the law; and if

- the judge correctly applied the law to the facts.

Although the child is the subject of the litigation, the child is not a party and, depending on the laws of that state, may not have an independent right to appeal. In states that have intermediate appellate courts, appeals most likely will be addressed to these courts. In other states, the appeal will be made directly to the state supreme court.

It is not uncommon for this process to take more than a year from the time of the trial court's decision until an appellate opinion is published. Meanwhile, the child, parents, and foster or adoptive parents are in limbo. Some state appellate courts have attempted to correct this problem by prioritizing the completion of cases.

## Section 40.3

# *Grounds for Involuntary Termination of Parental Rights*

Excerpted from "Grounds for Involuntary Termination of Parental Rights," Child Welfare Information Gateway, U.S. Department of Health and Human Services (HHS), updated April 3, 2009.

Every state, the District of Columbia, American Samoa, Guam, the Northern Mariana Islands, Puerto Rico, and the U.S. Virgin Islands have statutes providing for the termination of parental rights by a court. Termination of parental rights ends the legal parent-child relationship. Once the relationship has been terminated, the child is legally free to be placed for adoption, with the objective of securing a more stable, permanent, family environment that can meet the child's long-term parenting needs.

Termination may be voluntary or involuntary. Birth parents who wish to place their children for adoption may voluntarily relinquish their rights. When addressing whether parental rights should be terminated involuntarily, most states require that a court:

- determine, by clear and convincing evidence, that the parent is unfit; and

- determine whether severing the parent-child relationship is in the child's best interest.

## Grounds for Termination of Parental Rights

The grounds for involuntary termination of parental rights are specific circumstances under which the child cannot safely be returned home because of risk of harm by the parent, or the inability of the parent to provide for the child's basic needs. Each state is responsible for establishing its own statutory grounds, and these vary by state.

The most common statutory grounds for determining parental unfitness include the following:

- Severe or chronic abuse or neglect

- Abuse or neglect of other children in the household

- Abandonment

- Long-term mental illness or deficiency of the parent(s)

- Long-term alcohol- or drug-induced incapacity of the parent(s)

- Failure to support or maintain contact with the child

- Involuntary termination of the rights of the parent to another child

Another common ground for termination is a felony conviction of the parent(s) for a crime of violence against the child or another family member, or a conviction for any felony when the term of incarceration is so long as to have a negative impact on the child, and the only available provision of care for the child is foster care.

The Adoption and Safe Families Act (ASFA) requires state agencies to file a petition to terminate parental rights, with certain exceptions, when:

- a child has been in foster care for 15 of the most recent 22 months; and

- a court has determined:

    - a child to be an abandoned infant; or

    - that the parent has committed murder or voluntary manslaughter of another child of the parent; aided, abetted, attempted, conspired, or solicited to commit such a murder or voluntary manslaughter; or committed a felony assault that has resulted in serious bodily injury to the child or another child of the parent.

In response to ASFA, many states have adopted limits to the maximum amount of time a child can spend in foster care before termination proceedings can be initiated. Typically, states have adopted the ASFA standard of 15 out of the most recent 22 months in care. Some states, however, specify shorter time limits, particularly for very young children. The laws in most states are consistent with the other termination grounds required under ASFA.

## Exceptions

ASFA requires that proceedings to terminate parental rights be initiated when the child has been in foster care for 15 of the most recent 22 months. An exception may be made under some circumstances, including:

- the child has been placed under the care of a relative;

- the state agency has documented in the case plan a compelling reason to believe that terminating the parent's rights is not in the best interests of the child; or

- the parent has not been provided with the services required by the service plan for reunification of the parent with the child.

## Effects of Termination

A termination action can sever the rights of one parent without affecting the rights of the other parent. If the rights of both parents are terminated, the state assumes legal custody of the child along with the responsibility for finalizing a permanent placement for the child, either through adoption or guardianship, within a reasonable amount of time.

In a few states, if a permanent placement has not been achieved within a specific timeframe, a petition may be filed with the court requesting reinstatement of the parent's rights. If the court determines that the parent is now able to provide a safe home for the child, the request may be granted.

# Chapter 41

# *Foster Care and Adoption*

## *Chapter Contents*

# Section 41.1

# *Numbers and Trends in Foster Care*

This section includes excerpts from "Foster Care Statistics," Child Welfare Information Gateway, U.S. Department of Health and Human Services (HHS), 2007; and excerpts from "The AFCARS Report–Preliminary FY Estimates as of January 2008 (14)," Administration for Children and Families, HHS, 2008.

## *Foster Care Statistics*

The Adoption and Foster Care Analysis and Reporting System (AFCARS) uses the definition of foster care found in the Code of Federal Regulations (CFR), where it is defined as "24-hour substitute care for children outside their own homes." Foster care settings include, but are not limited to, non-relative foster family homes, relative foster homes (whether payments are being made or not), group homes, emergency shelters, residential facilities, and pre-adoptive homes.

### *Permanency Goals*

The ultimate goal for children in care is permanency with caring parents. Permanency goals refer to the goals for permanent placement that are reported to AFCARS.

**Point in time:** Of the estimated 513,000 children in foster care as of September 30, 2005:

- 51 percent had a goal of reunification with parent(s) or primary caregiver(s);
- 20 percent had a goal of adoption;
- 7 percent had a goal of living with a relative or guardian;
- 7 percent had a goal of long-term foster care;
- 6 percent had a goal of emancipation; and
- 8 percent had not yet had a permanency goal established.

**Trends:** The most dramatic change between fiscal year (FY) 2000 and FY 2005 occurred in the proportion of children with a goal of reunification, which posted an increase of ten percentage points.

## *Length of Stay*

Length of stay in foster care refers to the amount of time between entering and exiting foster care. It may be days, months, or years, depending on a number of factors.

**Exits:** Of the estimated 287,000 children who exited foster care during FY 2005:

- 17 percent had been in care less than one month;
- 33 percent had been in care for 1–11 months;
- 22 percent had been in care for 12–23 months;
- 11 percent had been in care for 24–35 months;
- 9 percent had been in care for 36–59 months; and
- 8 percent had been in care for five or more years.

**Trends:** The median amount of time children spent in foster care remained stable between FY 2000 and FY 2005 at 12.0 months. However, when the time periods are broken down, it becomes apparent that fewer children were in foster care less than one month or longer than three years and more children were in foster care from 1–23 months in FY 2005, compared to FY 2000.

## *Race and Ethnicity*

AFCARS tracks children's race or ethnicity. Using U.S. Bureau of Census standards, children of Hispanic origin may be of any race. Beginning in FY 2000, children could be identified with more than one race designation.

**Point in time:** Of the estimated 513,000 children in foster care as of September 30, 2005:

- 41 percent were White/non-Hispanic;
- 32 percent were Black/non-Hispanic;
- 18 percent were Hispanic; and
- 8 percent were other races or ethnic origins.

**Trends:** The percentage of Black/non-Hispanic children in care as of September 30 dropped seven percentage points (from 39 to 32 percent) between FY 2000 and FY 2005, while the percentage of White/non-Hispanic children and the percentage of Hispanic children each rose three points. Percentages for other race and ethnicity categories remained the same.

## The Adoption and Foster Care Analysis and Reporting System (AFCARS) Report

**Note:** Data from both the regular and revised submissions received by January 16, 2008 are included in the following information. Missing

**Table 41.1.** Ages of Children in Foster Care

Mean Years        9.8
Median Years      10.2

| Age of child | Percent | Number of children |
|---|---|---|
| Less than one year | 6% | 30,418 |
| 1 year | 7% | 34,344 |
| 2 years | 6% | 30,367 |
| 3 years | 5% | 26,966 |
| 4 years | 5% | 24,384 |
| 5 years | 5% | 23,021 |
| 6 years | 4% | 21,574 |
| 7 years | 4% | 20,760 |
| 8 years | 4% | 20,025 |
| 9 years | 4% | 19,263 |
| 10 years | 4% | 18,958 |
| 11 years | 4% | 19,475 |
| 12 years | 4% | 21,532 |
| 13 years | 5% | 25,706 |
| 14 years | 6% | 30,949 |
| 15 years | 8% | 38,259 |
| 16 years | 8% | 42,272 |
| 17 years | 8% | 39,624 |
| 18 years | 3% | 13,303 |
| 19 years | 1% | 5,488 |
| 20 years | 1% | 3,316 |

data are not used in the calculation of percentages. Due to rounding, percentages in some tables may not total 100% and numbers in some tables may not equal the total number of children in the population described.

There were 510,000 children in foster care on September 30, 2006. Tables 41.1, 41.2, and 41.3 give specific information about the ages, placement settings, and gender of the children.

During fiscal year 2006, 303,000 children entered foster care; and 289,000 children exited foster care.

**Table 41.2.** Placement Settings of Children in Foster Care

| Setting | Percent of children | Number of children |
|---|---|---|
| Pre-adoptive home | 3% | 17,351 |
| Foster family home (relative) | 24% | 124,571 |
| Foster family home (non-relative) | 46% | 236,911 |
| Group home | 7% | 33,433 |
| Institution | 10% | 53,042 |
| Supervised independent living | 1% | 5,872 |
| Runaway | 2% | 12,213 |
| Trial home visit | 5% | 26,606 |

**Table 41.3.** Gender of Children in Foster Care

| Gender | Percent of children | Number of children |
|---|---|---|
| Male | 52% | 267,027 |
| Female | 48% | 242,973 |

## Children Waiting for Adoption

As of September 30, 2006, 129,000 children were waiting to be adopted. Waiting children are identified as children who have a goal of adoption or whose parental rights have been terminated. Children 16 years old and older whose parental rights have been terminated and who have a goal of emancipation have been excluded from the estimate. Tables 41.4 and 41.5 provide specific information about waiting children.

**Table 41.4.** Number of Months Waiting Children Have Been in Continuous Foster Care

| Months | Percent of children | Number of children |
|---|---|---|
| Mean months | 39.4 | |
| Median months | 28.9 | |
| Less than one month | 1% | 656 |
| 1–5 months | 4% | 4,843 |
| 6–11 months | 9% | 11,079 |
| 12–17 months | 14% | 17,463 |
| 18–23 months | 14% | 17,557 |
| 24–29 months | 12% | 15,536 |
| 30–35 months | 9% | 11,767 |
| 36–59 months | 20% | 25,792 |
| 60 or more months | 19% | 24,307 |

**Table 41.5.** Racial/Ethnic Distribution of the Waiting Children

| Race/ethnicity | Percent of children | Number of children |
|---|---|---|
| American Indian/Alaskan Native/non-Hispanic | 2% | 2,223 |
| Asian/non-Hispanic | 1% | 651 |
| Black/non-Hispanic | 32% | 41,591 |
| Hawaiian/Pacific Islander/non-Hispanic | 0% | 301 |
| Hispanic | 20% | 25,481 |
| White/non-Hispanic | 38% | 49,637 |
| Unknown/unable to determine | 3% | 3,362 |
| Two or more, non-Hispanic | 4% | 5,754 |

Note: Using U.S. Bureau of the Census standards, children of Hispanic origin may be of any race. Beginning in FY 2000, children could be identified with more than one race designation.

As of September 30, 2006, 79.000 children in foster care had their parental rights terminated for all living parents. Public agencies were involved with 51,000 adoptions of children. Tables 41.6, 41.7, and 41.8 provide specific information about children who were adopted from the public foster care system.

**Table 41.6.** Age of Children When They Were Adopted from the Public Foster Care System

| Child's age | Percent of children | Number of children |
|---|---|---|
| Less than one year | 2% | 1,099 |
| 1 year | 11% | 5,567 |
| 2 years | 13% | 6,735 |
| 3 years | 11% | 5,647 |
| 4 years | 9% | 4,666 |
| 5 years | 8% | 3,914 |
| 6 years | 7% | 3,562 |
| 7 years | 6% | 3,063 |
| 8 years | 5% | 2,686 |
| 9 years | 5% | 2,422 |
| 10 years | 4% | 2,138 |
| 11 years | 4% | 2,012 |
| 12 years | 4% | 1,785 |
| 13 years | 3% | 1,618 |
| 14 years | 3% | 1,378 |
| 15 years | 2% | 1,070 |
| 16 years | 2% | 830 |
| 17 years | 1% | 636 |
| 18 years | 0% | 148 |
| 19 years | 0% | 17 |
| 20 years | 0% | 6 |

**Table 41.7.** Racial/Ethnic Distribution of Children Adopted from the Public Foster Care System

| Race/ethnicity | Percent of children | Number of children |
|---|---|---|
| American Indian/Alaskan Native-non Hispanic | 1% | 693 |
| Asian-non Hispanic | 1% | 289 |
| Black-non Hispanic | 27% | 13,783 |
| Hawaiian/Pacific Islander-non Hispanic | 0% | 125 |
| Hispanic | 19% | 9,569 |
| White-non Hispanic | 45% | 22,979 |
| Unknown/unable to determine | 2% | 1,049 |
| Two or more-non Hispanic | 5% | 2,512 |

Note: Using U.S. Bureau of the Census standards, children of Hispanic origin may be of any race. Beginning in FY 2000, children could be identified with more than one race designation.

**Table 41.8.** Relationship of Adoptive Parents to the Child Prior to the Adoption

| Relationship | Percent | Number |
|---|---|---|
| Non-relative | 15% | 7,646 |
| Foster parent | 59% | 29,997 |
| Step-parent | 0% | 36 |
| Other relative | 26% | 13,321 |

# Section 41.2

# *Criminal Background Checks for Prospective Foster and Adoptive Parents*

Excerpted from "Criminal Background Checks for Prospective
Foster and Adoptive Parents," Child Welfare Information Gateway,
U.S. Department of Health and Human Services (HHS), 2008.

All states, the District of Columbia, Guam, and Puerto Rico have
statutes or regulations requiring background investigations of prospective foster and adoptive parents and all adults residing in their
households. In most states, the background investigation includes a
check of federal and state criminal records. Many states also require
checks of child abuse and neglect registries. States may deny approval
of a foster care license or adoption application if any adult in the
household has been convicted of certain crimes, such as sexual abuse
of a minor.

## *Federal Requirements*

State statutes requiring criminal background checks are supported
by federal legislation, in Title IV-E of the Social Security Act. The Adoption and Safe Families Act (ASFA) of 1997 amended Title IV-E (42 U.S.C.
671(a)(20)) to require criminal record checks for any prospective foster or adoptive parent when foster care maintenance payments or adoption assistance payments are to be made under Title IV-E. The Adam
Walsh Child Protection and Safety Act of 2006 (P.L. 109-248) further
amended Title IV-E to require a fingerprint-based check of a national
crime information database before any prospective foster or adoptive
parent may be approved for placement of a child, regardless of whether
foster care maintenance payments or adoption assistance payments are
to be made on behalf of the child.

Under Title IV-E, approval of the foster or adoptive home may not
be granted if either of the following is found:

- The applicant has ever been convicted of felony child abuse or
  neglect; spousal abuse; a crime against children (including child

371

pornography); or a crime involving violence, including rape, sexual assault, or homicide, but not including other physical assault or battery.

- The applicant has been convicted of a felony for physical assault, battery, or a drug-related offense within the past five years.

The Child Abuse Prevention and Treatment Act (CAPTA), as amended in June 2003, extends the requirement for criminal background checks to all adults residing in prospective foster or adoptive family households. The Adam Walsh Act (P.L. 109-248) also requires a check of the state child abuse and neglect registry(s) for all adults living in prospective foster and adoptive homes. These checks must be conducted in every state where each individual lived during the previous five years.

## State Requirements for Prospective Foster Parents

All states require a criminal record check as part of the background investigation that is conducted when an individual has applied for licensure as a foster parent. Requirements for the types of background checks and the individuals who must be included in the checks may be found in statute or regulation. As of April 2008:

- state or local criminal record checks of the foster parent applicant are required in all states, the District of Columbia, and Puerto Rico;

- federal criminal record checks also are required in approximately 38 states;

- fingerprinting, in addition to name-based checks, is required as part of the criminal record check in 38 states;

- child abuse and neglect record checks are required in 40 states, the District of Columbia, Guam, and Puerto Rico;

- checks of the state sex offender registries are required in Illinois, Iowa, Nebraska, Oklahoma, South Carolina, and Puerto Rico;

- criminal record checks are required for all adult members of the prospective foster parents' household in 42 states and the District of Columbia;

- criminal record checks are required for all adults and older children in the prospective foster parents' household in ten states; and

- criminal records checks are required for all members of the prospective foster parents' household, regardless of age, in five states.

An application for foster parent licensure may be rejected when a check reveals that the prospective foster parent or other household member has been convicted of a crime that would raise concerns about the family's ability to provide a safe and stable home environment for the child.

## State Requirements for Prospective Adoptive Parents

Nearly all states require a criminal record check as part of the background investigation for approving an adoptive placement. In most states, the requirements for adoptive parents are similar to those for foster parents, although the specifics may vary. An example of this is the requirement to check the state's sex offender registry: Alaska requires checks for adoptive parents, but not foster parents, while Iowa and Nebraska require checks for foster parents but not adoptive parents. All three states examine conviction records for sex offenses for both foster and adoptive parents.

Requirements for the types of background checks and the individuals who must be included in the checks may be found in statute or regulation. These include:

- state or local criminal record checks of the adoptive parent applicant are required in approximately 48 states, the District of Columbia, Guam, and Puerto Rico;

- federal criminal record checks also are required in 31 states;

- fingerprinting and name-based checks are required as part of the criminal record check in 31 states;

- child abuse and neglect record checks are required in 37 states, the District of Columbia, Guam, and Puerto Rico;

- checks of the state sex offender registries are required in Alaska, Illinois, Oklahoma, South Carolina, and Puerto Rico;

- criminal record checks are required for all adult members of the prospective adoptive parents' household in approximately 31 states and the District of Columbia;

- criminal record checks are required for all adults and older children in the prospective adoptive parents' household in seven states; and

- criminal record checks are required for all household members, regardless of age, in Idaho and Montana.

The information contained in criminal background histories and child abuse reports is incorporated into the adoption home study that is used to help determine whether the adoptive parents' home will be safe and appropriate for placement of a child. An unfavorable home study may be issued, and the adoption petition may be denied, when a check reveals that the prospective adoptive parent or other household member has been convicted of a crime that would raise concerns about that family's ability to provide a safe home for a child.

## Disqualifying Crimes

Approximately 15 states and the District of Columbia will disqualify an applicant if he or she or any household member has ever been convicted of felony child abuse or neglect, spousal abuse, a crime against children (including child pornography); or a crime of violence, including rape, sexual assault, or homicide; or has been convicted of physical assault or battery or a drug-related offense within the last five years. In most states, other crimes, including any crime of violence, arson, kidnapping, illegal use of weapons or explosives, fraud, forgery, or property crimes such as burglary and robbery may lead to disqualification. In 22 states, an applicant may be disqualified if he or she has a registry record of substantiated or founded child abuse or neglect.

# Section 41.3

# *Supporting the Social-Emotional Development of Infants and Toddlers in Foster Care*

This article is reprinted with permission from the Centre of Excellence for Child Welfare (CECW) in Canada. CECW fosters research, develops policy, and disseminates knowledge about the prevention and treatment of child abuse and neglect. For more information, visit http://www.cecw-cepb.ca. The research for this information sheet was funded by the Centre of Excellence for Child & Youth Mental Health at CHEO, the Alberta Centre for Child Family and Community Research, Infant Mental Health Promotion at the Hospital for Sick Children (Sick Kids), and Alberta Health Services. The CECW is one of the Centres of Excellence for Children's Well-Being funded by Public Health Agency of Canada (PHAC). Production of this information sheet has been made possible through a financial contribution from PHAC. However the views expressed in this article do not necessarily represent the official policy of the CECW's funders.

The social-emotional development of infants and toddlers in foster care who have been neglected, abused, or traumatized can differ from other children. This section offers practical strategies to caseworkers and foster parents for supporting the social-emotional development of foster children under the age of five.

## *What do young children need for healthy social-emotional development?*

All infants and young children need the opportunity to form a close emotional tie with a consistent adult. They need someone who will act as a safe haven in times of stress and who will take delight in their exploration and accomplishments. Forming a consistent relationship with at least one caring adult in the first few years of life lays the foundation for healthy development in virtually all aspects of life—intellectual, social, physical, emotional, behavioral, and moral.[2] The crucial importance of an infant's need to develop an early connection with an adult cannot be overstressed.

The development of these early parent-child relationships occurs simultaneously with all aspects of children's social-emotional development.

One important component of social-emotional development is the acquisition of self-regulation skills which is a key milestone in learning to relate to others.[3] Self-regulation refers to the ability to achieve some level of control over one's emotions, behaviors, and attention. Self-regulation also refers to the ability to manage positive and negative emotional states such as excitement or distress when needed. Children learn how to self-regulate early in life through their interactions with supportive caregivers.[4]

***Why does the social-emotional development of foster children differ from other children?***

When young children have been frightened, abused, or neglected by their primary caregiver, or when they have repeated changes in caregivers, several things may happen that can interfere with these children's social-emotional development and their relationships with new caregivers:

- Maltreated infants and toddlers frequently develop problems giving accurate cues about their emotional needs, often because these cues were not responded to consistently in the past.[5] This can cause them to miscue their new caregiver about their feelings. They can, for example, appear to neither want nor need nurturing or they might whine, pester, or tantrum to enlist reassurance and support from a caregiver.

- In some situations, these children can behave in ways that made sense in their previous environment but are confusing or misleading to a new caregiver. For example, an infant who has witnessed violence between his or her parents from a crib might become unexpectedly agitated when placed in a crib. If foster parents are not aware of the child's history, they can be confused about the child's real need.

- Well-meaning foster parents may view some of these children's behaviors as purposeful when in fact they are not. For example, under normal circumstances a child who tantrums at mealtimes might be seen as manipulative; for many foster children however, mealtimes are especially difficult to manage because of past deprivation.

- Foster parents may unwittingly set expectations that are reasonable for other children the same age, but that the foster child cannot meet due to his or her lack of self-regulation skills. For example, it is not unreasonable to expect a five-year-old child to sit still and wait his or her turn or to share a toy. A child with self-regulation difficulties may not be able to handle this expectation. If the foster parent sets up a consequence for behavior the child is incapable of producing, this can set off an escalating negative cycle between the child and the foster parent in which worsening behavior is met with increasing dismay.

### What kinds of problems do young children in foster care display?

Along with disturbed parent-child relationships and abusive early experiences, other biological or environmental factors (such as congenital problems or prenatal exposure to drugs and alcohol) can add to a foster child's emotional problems and further interfere with his or her ability to communicate feelings and needs effectively. Researchers estimate that the majority of children in foster care have some type of emotional, behavioral, or developmental delay such as impairments in language, learning ability, or physical development, that are frequently undiagnosed.[6] Some of these children have not learned how to handle strong emotions, focus their attention, or cooperate with others.[7] Other children might display inappropriate sexual behaviors, or they might display odd self-soothing behavior such as head-banging or masturbating.[8] Foster parents should be well prepared for having foster children with this combination of emotional, developmental, and parent-child relationship problems. This will reduce the likelihood of foster parents either misunderstanding the reasons why some foster children have difficulties behaving in expected ways, or becoming discouraged if children with these behaviors do not respond to strategies foster parents have used successfully with other children.

### How can caseworkers help foster parents understand their foster child's problem behaviors?

- Along with an initial medical assessment, all young children in foster care should be screened for physical, developmental, and emotional problems once the child has had a stable placement for at least two months. When concerns are identified, a developmental specialist or multi-disciplinary team should be consulted. A prenatal history, birth record, and previous health information are crucial to maximize the contributions of specialists.

- Foster parents need detailed information about what life was like for the foster child before coming to their home and how the child's history might affect his or her behavior and development.

- Foster parents might need special help to understand their foster child's behavioral cues and develop effective responses.[9] Offering an empathetic response to some behavioral cues without encouraging attention-seeking behavior can be challenging. Foster parents may require help developing strategies to address the child's underlying needs without encouraging problem behaviors.

- Foster parents can differ in their ability to tolerate various kinds of challenging behavior in foster children.[10] For example, foster parents who value independence might be less understanding of a needy or clingy foster child. Foster parents may find that their tolerance increases once they become more aware of their own behavioral "triggers."

### *How can foster parents build a relationship with a young foster child?*

1. **Child-led play:** Child-led play is an excellent strategy for building a relationship[11] and teaching play skills to children of all ages, even very young infants. Find a 15–20 minute period several times a week to play one-to-one with the foster child. Foster parents can babble with the baby, imitate his or her sounds, make facial expressions, and so on. Older foster children can be offered a limited selection of toys with the rules of "no breaking anything" and "no hurting anybody." The child is in charge of the play and the foster parent follows his or her lead. The goal of child-led play is to help the child enjoy a relationship with an adult rather than to teach academic skills.

2. **"Time-ins":** Isolating children when they misbehave as a discipline tool (which is called "giving a time-out") can be effective when used properly; however, some traumatized children can become distressed or panic when placed in a time-out. Instead of using time-outs with these children, try employing a "time-in" strategy: view the misbehavior as a mistake and increase supervision of the child by maintaining close physical proximity and engaging the child in a positive interaction.

Use a verbal cue such as, "I see you are having trouble sharing your truck, I'm going to help you with that. Why don't the three of us play together for a little while?"

3.  **Learn when to take charge and always use empathy:** Try to anticipate when meltdowns are likely to occur and intervene before problems escalate. The use of a kind, calming voice, empathic statements, and gentle touch can be effective in curtailing emotional outbursts and can encourage a child to view the foster parent as someone who will help him or her feel better. Make sure the child is capable of producing the desired behavior before attaching rewards or consequences to it.

4.  **Be persistent with withdrawn children:** Sometimes withdrawn children can be easy to overlook. They need to be engaged by their caregiver even though it may take some effort and persistence.[12] The use of quiet activities and a soft tone of voice can entice the withdrawn child into a social interaction. Gentle games like "this little piggy" allow the foster parent to playfully introduce soothing touches that can be pleasing for withdrawn children.

### How can foster parents promote self-regulation in young foster children?

-   **Think younger (sometimes much younger):** Young foster children who are struggling might not have the ability to do certain things independently such as use the bathroom or feed themselves. They may find it difficult to control their impulsive behavior or to handle the sharing and turn-taking required to play well with other children. Expectations in all of these areas can become more realistic by thinking of children at their emotional age, rather than their chronological age.

-   **Modify the environment:** Foster children can become overstimulated or distracted by noisy, busy environments or clutter. Even exciting activities such as local fairs or trips to the mall might be difficult for some foster children. If the foster child is overly active, distractible, or quick to tantrum, try turning off the television or radio, removing clutter, and storing toys and other play activities until needed. Try as much as possible to create an environment that is quiet, consistent, and highly predictable.

- **Moderate the activity level:** As children grow, they establish a daily activity pattern; they will sleep through the night, be alert in the morning, and have periods of quiet followed by more boisterous activity throughout the day. Foster children often do not have established patterns.[13] They may become overstimulated and have difficulty regaining equilibrium. Recognize signs of overstimulation, such as the child becoming too lively or loud, and signal the child with a consistent verbal cue such as, "let's take a rest" so he or she can anticipate the next step. Guide the child to a calmer activity that includes nurturing, such as sitting together with a book or hand puppet. Some foster children will start to recognize when they need help regaining self-control and will signal their foster parent on their own.

Whenever possible, follow the foster child's lead and take delight in his or her accomplishments. Whenever necessary, take charge, use a calm tone of voice, and support the expected behavior.[14]

## Tips for Caseworkers

1. Language delays are common in foster children but are often misdiagnosed as learning or behavior problems.[15] Encourage foster parents to consult with community speech-language resources or early intervention programs and ask for strategies that they can use at home to promote the language development of children in their care. Many of these strategies have the added benefit of building positive relationships between children and their caregivers (child-led play is one example).

2. Case workers should listen empathically to the concerns of foster parents and address their priorities promptly. When problems arise, professionals should aim to instill patience and confidence rather than impart advice or give directions.

3. High-quality preschool programs can provide foster children with enriched and supportive environments in which to thrive. These programs can be a source of continuity through placement changes and can offer needed respite for foster parents. A preschool program that includes psychology and speech-language pathology services is ideal because these support services raise the overall quality of the program offered, and they help to ensure that foster children with delays are identified and linked to the necessary services.

# References

1. This information sheet is based on the peer-reviewed article, Wotherspoon, E., O'Neill Laberge, M., and Pirie, J. (2008). Meeting the emotional needs of infants and toddlers in foster care: The collaborative mental health care experience. *Infant Mental Health Journal*, 29(4), 377–397.

2. National Scientific Council on the Developing Child (2004). *Young children develop in an environment of relationships* (Working Paper No.1). Retrieved August 8, 2008 from: www .developingchild.net/pubs/wp/environment_of_ relationships .pdf

3. Schore, A. (2001a). Effects of a secure attachment relationship on right brain development, affect regulation, and infant mental health. *Infant Mental Health Journal*, 22(1–2), 7–66.

4. Ibid.

5. Dozier, M., Higley, E., Albus, K.E., & Nutter, A. (2002). Intervening with foster infants' caregivers: Targeting three critical needs. *Infant Mental Health Journal*, 25, 541–554.

6. Community Paediatrics Committee, Canadian Paediatric Society (2008). Special considerations for the health supervision of children and youth in foster care. *Paediatrics & Child Health*, 13(2), 129–32.

7. Silver, J., Amster, B., and Haecker, T. (1999). *Young children and foster care*. Baltimore, MD: Brookes Publishing.

8. Perry, B. (2001). Bonding and attachment in maltreated children: Consequences of emotional neglect in childhood. Caregiver Education Series, Child Trauma Academy. Retrieved August 16, 2008 from www.childtrauma.org/ ctamaterials/AttCar4_03 _v2.pdf.

9. Dozier, M., Higley, E., Albus, K.E., & Nutter, A. (2002). Intervening with foster infants' caregivers: Targeting three critical needs. *Infant Mental Health Journal*, 25, 541–554.

10. Ibid.

11. Dozier, M., Lindhiem, O., & Ackerman, J. (2005). Attachment and biobehavioral catch-up: An intervention targeting empirically identified needs of foster infants. In L. Berlin, Y. Ziv, L.

Amaya-Jackson, & M. T. Greenberg (Eds.), *Enhancing early attachments: Theory, research, intervention, and policy* (pp. 178–194). New York: Guilford Press.

12. Dozier, M., Higley, E., Albus, K.E., & Nutter, A. (2002). Intervening with foster infants' caregivers: Targeting three critical needs. *Infant Mental Health Journal*, 25, 541–554.

13. Dozier, M., Manni, M., Gordon, M. K., Peloso, E., Gunnar, M. R., Stovall-McClough, K., et al. (2006). Foster children's diurnal production of cortisol: An exploratory study. *Child Maltreatment*, 11, 189–197.

14. Circle of Security (1998). *Twenty-five words*. Retrieved August 8, 2008 from: http://www.circleofsecurity.org/ downloads.html.

15. Canadian Association of Speech Language Pathologists and Audiologists (2006). General Speech and Hearing Fact Sheet. Retrieved July 21, 2008 from: http://www.caslpa.ca/english/ resources/factsheets.asp.

# Section 41.4

# *Foster Parents Considering Adoption*

Text in this section is from "Foster Parents Considering Adoption: Factsheet for Families," Child Welfare Information Gateway, U.S. Department of Health and Human Services (HHS), updated September 18, 2008.

This section is written for foster parents who are considering adopting one or more of the children in their care. It provides information on the differences between foster care and adoption, and it explores some of the things for foster parents to consider when making the decision about whether to adopt a child in their care.

## *Differences between Foster Parenting and Adopting*

There are a number of significant differences between foster care and adoption for the foster/adoptive family involved, even when a child remains in the same household. Compared to foster care, adoption brings the following changes for the parents:

- Full legal responsibility for a child: Legal responsibility was held by the agency during the time the child was in foster care.

- Full financial responsibility for the child: Even if the family receives adoption assistance or a subsidy on behalf of the child, families are still responsible for financial obligations such as childcare and extracurricular activities.

- Full decision-making responsibility: While the child was in foster care, decision-making was shared with the agency and birth parent. When the child is adopted, adoptive parents take on this full responsibility.

- Attachment differences: The family is no longer working with the agency to help the child reunify with his/her parents; rather, they are now working to incorporate the child as a permanent member of their own family.

## Trends in Foster Parent Adoption

National adoption and foster care statistics show that foster parent adoptions accounted for over half of the adoptions of children adopted from foster care each year from fiscal year (FY) 1998 through the end of fiscal year (FY) 2002. According to the Adoption and Foster Care Analysis and Reporting System (AFCARS), in FY 2002, 27,567 (or 52 percent) of the 53,000 children adopted from foster care that year were adopted by their foster parents (U.S. Department of Health and Human Services, 2005).

## Benefits of Foster Parent Adoption

Adoption by the foster family has the potential to benefit not only the child being adopted, but also the foster family and the child welfare agency. There are a number of reasons that a child's foster parents may be the best adoptive parents for that child:

- Foster parents have a greater knowledge of a child's experiences prior to placement and know what behaviors to expect from the child. If they have sufficient background information about what happened to a child before this placement, some knowledge of how children generally respond to such experiences, and extensive information about this child's specific behavior patterns, the foster family is better able to understand and respond to the child's needs in a positive and appropriate way.

- Foster parents usually have fewer fantasies and fears about the child's birth family, because they often have met and know them as real people with real problems.

- Foster parents have a better understanding of their role and relationship with the agency—and perhaps a relationship with their worker (if the same worker stays throughout the duration of the child's placement).

### Benefits for the Child

The biggest benefit of foster parent adoption for a child is the fact that the child does not have to move to a new family. Even very young infants may grieve the loss of the familiar sights, sounds, smells, and touch of a family when they must move. Staying in the same placement means the child will not leave familiar people and things, such as:

- familiar foster parents and family;
- school, classroom, classmates, and teachers;
- pets;
- friends;
- sports teams and other extracurricular activities; or
- bedroom, house, or apartment.

Since the foster family may have met or cared for a child during the child's visits with the birth family, the foster family is better able to help the child remember important people from the past and maintain important connections.

### Benefits for Others

Foster parent adoption also benefits the birth parents in many cases by allowing them to know who is permanently caring for their children. For foster parents, receiving the agency's approval to adopt affirms the family's love and commitment to the child. Agencies benefit from this practice as it enables them to move children into permanency more quickly (since finalization of adoption requires that a child be in a placement at least six months, and this requirement has already been fulfilled in foster parent adoptions).

## *Characteristics of Foster Families Who Adopt Successfully*

Child welfare experts have identified characteristics of foster families who adopt the children in their care. The National Resource Center for Family-Centered Practice and Permanency Planning provides characteristics of successful "permanency planning resource families."

- These families like to give and help.
- They are satisfied with their lives.
- They are resourceful.
- They are tolerant of loss, anxiety, and ambiguity.
- They have a sense of humor.
- They are involved with the child in the community.

Researchers who studied foster/adoptive families in the early 1980s found that the families who successfully adopted the children in their care had the following characteristics:

- They expected the children would be placed long-term and had the children in their home for a longer period of time than foster parents who did not choose to adopt.

- They enjoyed the children and were able to be actively involved with them.

- The foster parents had some acceptance of the birth family's positive attributes and were able to talk about them with their children. However, these foster families also perceived the children to be similar to the foster family in some way.

- The children who were adopted by their foster families had successfully resolved their ties to their birth families and were younger than children not adopted by their foster families.

This same study also found the following:

- Visits with birth parents were beneficial to the adoption process. Visits with the birth families did not inhibit the adoption process—in fact, just the opposite was true. The families who adopted their foster children were more likely to have met their child's birth parents in the year they were considering adopting the child. The benefits of birth parent visiting for the child include the fact that, through visits with their birth parents, children gain a more realistic view of their birth parents and a sense of their own identity. Of course, the family circumstances for each child are unique, and visits with birth family members may not be indicated for some children.

- A positive interaction cycle was established between the parents and child. Foster parents had the sense that things were "getting better" as the placement progressed. This positive cycle in which everyone's needs were met was found to a greater extent in the families who chose to adopt versus those families who chose not to adopt, and it was noticeably absent at the point of adoption disruption in the adoptions that failed. Families may remain responsive to their children only if they think their efforts are justified and their children are responsive. Children will respond to parents only under similar conditions.

## Foster Families Whose Adoptions Fail

Child welfare experts identified the following characteristics of resource families who did not adopt successfully:

- Unresolved losses in the past and present, resulting in a need to revisit past relationships and an inability to meet the child's needs
- Possessiveness of the child and an unwillingness to acknowledge and work with important people from the child's past
- Desperation for a child, resulting in unrealistic expectations of foster care and adoption
- High stress and anxiety levels
- Aggressiveness
- Power and control issues

A study of foster families in the early 1980s found that the foster families in the adoptions that failed were rigid and did not allow for changes easily. They might have had difficulty sharing parenting with the agency or the birth families. These families were poorly prepared for adoption and did not have open communication or an open relationship with their social worker. Some families felt coerced by their worker into agreeing to adopt the child. These families also experienced more worker turnovers than the families who were successful in their adoptions.

## Conclusion

The decision by a foster family to adopt a child in their care will be based on the unique factors associated with the child, family, and circumstances. To help with such decision-making, many states use mutual, informed decision-making in their training for foster/adoptive parents.

Foster families who decide to pursue adoption should inform themselves as much as possible and work with their agency to ensure a smooth transition for the child and themselves. Successful foster parent adoptions are the result of a mutual decision by the foster parents and the agency about what is best for a specific child.

## Section 41.5

# *Helping Your Foster Child Transition to Being Your Adopted Child*

Excerpted from "Helping Your Foster Child Transition to Your Adopted Child: Factsheet for Families," Child Welfare Information Gateway, U.S. Department of Health and Human Services (HHS), updated September 18, 2008.

For foster families who choose to adopt the child or children in their care, there are a number of ways to help these children make the emotional transition from being a ward of the state or the court to being a son or daughter of specific parents. While parents may appreciate the difference in the child's role within their family, children may not clearly comprehend the difference between being a foster child versus being an adopted child when they continue to live in the same family. There are specific things families can say and do to help children understand these differences.

## *Talking with Children about the Changes*

In preparing to talk to children about the changes that occur with adoption, parents and other caring adults in children's lives should remember to engage the child in the process and listen carefully to the words the child uses and to the questions the child asks. Questions about the birth family and their status may need to be addressed. It is important to always tell the truth—even if it is painful—and to validate the child's experience and feelings. While these talks may bring up painful feelings for children, and for parents who love them, helping children to grieve can also help them to move on to a feeling of permanency in their foster or adoptive family.

Talks between parents and children about the differences in status within the foster family and the adoptive family will probably need to be repeated several times and in a variety of ways, so children can fully understand at their own level. It is best if these conversations take place when the parent and child are engaged in activities together. Adoption professional H. Craig-Oldsen (1988) offers the following suggestions for making these talks beneficial for the child:

- **Plan the discussion:** In collaboration with the social worker, the parents should decide if they want to talk with the child first and have the social worker reinforce what was said in a later conversation, or if they would like to talk to the child together about the change from being in foster care to being adopted. Parents should be prepared to answer the child's questions that may be raised by the discussion.

- **Help the child talk about the perceived difference in his or her own words:** The parents should ask open-ended questions of the child such as, "How do you think being adopted will be different from being in foster care?" or "What do you think the biggest difference will be, when you're adopted?"

- **Use analogies:** Help the child draw analogies to something in the child's own life. For instance, a parent might say, "This is like the time when . . . ."

There are a number of changes in status that will affect the child, and these should be discussed, depending on the child's developmental level.

1. To help the child understand the legal differences between foster care and adoption, foster parents might talk about how the adoption court hearing is different from other court hearings

the child might have remembered from foster care. Some parents may explain adoption by using marriage as an analogy. The court hearing is like the marriage ceremony, and the adoption certificate is like the marriage certificate that makes the relationship legal and permanent. (Parents who use this analogy should be prepared for questions about divorce, depending on the child's experience.)

2. Older children who are aware of the foster care board payment or adoption assistance their parents receive might be helped to understand the financial differences inherent in foster care and adoption. These payments might be compared to a child's allowance; older children may be able to understand the payments as costs to meet the child's needs. Experienced adoptive parents note the importance of honesty, compassion, and developmental appropriateness in conversations with children regarding these issues.

3. To help children understand the parenting differences between foster care and adoption, parents might remind the child that when in foster care, the parents had to get a permission slip signed by an agency social worker to go on a field trip, spend the night at a friend's house, or travel across state lines; now that their foster parents are their legal parents, the parents can sign permissions for these types of things without needing to go through an agency or court.

## Helping Children Understand Their Own History

Parents can help children review and understand their previous life experiences to clarify what happened to them in the past and help them integrate those experiences so they will have greater self-understanding. Foster or adoptive parents and children's therapists and social workers can help children in answering important questions about their lives—both to assess their readiness for and to prepare them for staying permanently in their family.

There are many ways families can help children in answering these important questions and in understanding their unique history. Life books, eco-maps, life maps, and life paths are all tools used by foster or adoptive parents and children's therapists to help children of various ages understand and find ways to visually represent the answers to questions of how they came to be separated from their birth family and where they will ultimately belong.

389

- A life book, is essentially an account of the child's life in words, pictures, photographs, and documents. While life books can take many forms, each child's life book will be unique to that child. Foster parents can assist in creating a life book for a child by gathering information about a child and taking pictures of people and places that are—or were—important to the child.

- An eco-map is a visual representation of a person and the important people and activities in his or her life. A child's eco-map may have a circle in the middle of the page with a stick figure of a child, along with the question "Why am I here?" Lines are drawn out from the circle like spokes to other circles representing the court, other foster families, siblings, school, or to other topics such as "things I like to do" to visually represent what and who is important to a child and to help the child understand how he or she came to live with the adoptive family.

- Life maps or life paths are visual representations to help children understand the paths their lives have taken and the decision points along the way. They may have stepping stones to represent a child's age and a statement about where and with whom they lived at that age. They may have lines that go to a drawing of a house representing any foster homes a child lived in, the years the child lived there, and a mention of who lived with the child at that house, if known.

Possible items to collect or include in a child's life book include the following:

- Developmental milestones (when a child first smiled, crawled, walked, talked)

- Common childhood diseases and immunizations, injuries, illnesses, or hospitalizations

- Pictures of a child's birth parents and/or birth relatives and information about visits

- Members of the foster family's extended family who were/are important to the child

- Pictures of previous foster families, their homes, and their pets

- Names of teachers and schools attended, report cards, and school activities

- Any special activities such as scouting, clubs, or camping experiences
- Faith-based activities
- What a child did when he or she was happy or excited and ways a child showed affection
- Cute things the child did, nicknames, favorite friends, activities, and toys
- Birthdays or religious celebrations or any trips taken with the foster family

The most important information to include in any of these tools to help children understand their past history is information about the child's birth and an explanation of why and how the child entered foster care and how decisions about moves and new placements were made. A baby picture and pictures of birth parents should be included, if possible. If no information is available, children can draw a picture of what they might have looked like. Statements such as, "there is no information about Johnny's birth father in his file," at least acknowledge the father's existence. The importance of honesty, developmental appropriateness, and compassion in any explanation of difficult and painful circumstances that bring children into care is important for children.

Working with these tools provides an opportunity for the child to experience and work through the feelings of loss; therefore, they are beneficial therapeutic methods to help children with the grieving process.

## Helping Children Adjust to Losses

Adoption experts acknowledge the importance of helping children integrate their previous attachments to important people in their lives in order to be able to transition that emotional attachment to a new family. Integration is a way of helping children cope with the painful realities of the separation from their birth families that often impact their future behaviors and can create extraordinary stress between them and their foster or adoptive parents. The five-step integration process, first described by adoption pioneer K. Donley (1988), is an effort to clarify the child's permission to be in foster care, to live with new parents, to be loved by them, and to love them back.

### Steps in the Integration Process

- Create an accurate reconstruction of the child's entire placement history. Creating a life book, life map, or eco-map with a child helps a child to see and understand his or her own history.

- Identify the important attachment figures in the child's life. Foster parents might be able to learn who these important people in a child's life are by listening to the child talk about people from previous placements. These attachment figures might be parents, but they could be siblings, former foster parents, or other family members.

- Gain the cooperation of the most significant of the attachment figures available. If possible, parents should cooperate with the birth mother during a child's visits or gain the cooperation of a birth grandparent or relative to whom the child was attached. Even if the birth family is not happy about a child's permanency goal of adoption, there is likely to be one important person (a teacher, a former neighbor) who will be willing to work with foster or adoptive parents or the agency to make a child's transition to adoption easier.

- Clarify the permission message. It is important for children to hear and feel from people who are important to them that it is all right to love another family. The important person in a child's life who is available to give the child that message should be sought out to do so.

- Communicating it to the child. Whether the "permission to love your family" comes in the form of a letter or phone call from grandma or from the birth parent during family visits, it is important that children hear from that person that it is not their fault they are in foster care and that it is all right to love another family. This permission will go a long way to helping a child relax and transfer his or her attachment to the new family.

In working with children during this transition phase it will be important for parents and others working with the child to use the following skills:

- Engaging the child
- Listening to the child

- Telling the truth
- Validating the child's life story
- Creating a safe space for the child
- Realizing that it is never too late to go back in time
- Embracing pain as part of the process

## *Helping Children Transfer Attachments*

Once it is clear that a child will be adopted by the foster family, there are many things parents can do to signal to a child that his or her status within the family has changed. Some of these include:

- encouraging the child to start calling the adoptive parents mom and dad;
- adding a middle name to incorporate a name of family significance;
- hanging pictures of the child on the wall;
- involving the child in family reunions and similar extended family activities;
- including the child in family rituals;
- holding religious or other ceremonies to incorporate the child into the family;
- making statements such as, "In our family, we do it this way" in a supportive way; and
- sending out announcements of the adoption.

## *Conclusion*

While on the surface it may seem easy for a child to stay in the family in which he or she was living as a foster child, in reality, the internal process for a child and family is much more complicated. Allowing children to just drift into adoption without acknowledging the very significant changes for the family may lead to later difficulties. Foster or adoptive parents need to help children consider and understand their own history and reasons why they cannot live with their birth family, help them adjust to this loss, and help them transfer their attachments to the foster or adoptive family. In helping children, families will need to consider each child's needs as they are related to the child's age, health, personality, temperament, and cultural and racial experiences.

## For More Information

### *National Foster Care and Adoption Directory*
Website: http://www.childwelfare.gov/nfcad/index.cfm

The National Foster Care and Adoption Directory has a list of foster and adoptive support groups in each state.

Chapter 42

# Family Reunification: What the Evidence Shows

## Research on Family Reunification

It is clear from a review of the state child and family services review (CFSR) final reports that numerous factors interact and play important roles in a state's ability to reunify children in foster care with their birth families. Family engagement, assessment, case planning, and service delivery are key factors. Systemic supports related to funding for services; support from the courts; and stable, competent staff also appear to impact, directly and indirectly, the achievement of reunification goals. A review of the relevant literature sheds additional light upon state CFSR findings regarding the factors in achieving timely, stable reunifications.

## Family Engagement Is Fundamental to Successful Reunification

Much of the literature addresses three dimensions of family engagement:

- the relationship between the caseworker and the family;
- parent-child visitation; and
- the involvement of foster parents.

Excerpted from "Family Reunification: What the Evidence Shows," Child Welfare Information Gateway, U.S. Department of Health and Human Services (HHS), updated September 18, 2008.

The relationship between the caseworker and the family. Both the frequency and the nature of the caseworker's contact with the family are important. Family reunification appears to be facilitated by more frequent caseworker contact. However, parents are sometimes mistrustful of child welfare professionals and thus unwilling to share information or establish a relationship with agency representatives. In a study examining engagement in a sample of 63 families receiving child protective services, the interpersonal relationship with the caseworker was determined to be the strongest predictor of the family's self-report of engagement.

These studies, as well as engagement research in related fields, suggest that the following caseworker behaviors are important in mitigating families' fears and building the rapport necessary for effective helping:

- Establishing open, honest communication with parents
- Requesting family participation and feedback in the planning process
- Providing instruction and reinforcement in the performance and completion of mutually agreed upon activities

**Parent-child visitation:** Research supports the significance of parent-child visitation as a predictor of family reunification. A study of reunification in a sample of 922 children aged 12 and younger found that children who were visited by their mothers were ten times more likely to be reunited.

Effective visitation practice goes far beyond attention to the logistics of scheduling and transportation; it provides an opportunity to build parental skills and improve parent-child interaction. Studies suggest that visitation should have a therapeutic focus. Thus, it is important that anyone supervising visits has clinical knowledge and skills.

**The involvement of foster parents:** Foster parents may facilitate family reunification through both the mentoring of the birth parents and the support of their visitation. The development of a positive relationship between the foster and birth parents may allow children to avoid the stress of divided loyalties and position foster parents to play a supportive role after reunification. However, when selecting foster parents to work with birth parents, agencies should consider their experience, maturity, communication skills, their ability to handle these multiple roles, and the possible need for additional training.

## *Accurate, Individual Assessment and Case Planning Are Crucial for Successful Reunifications*

Child maltreatment is a complex phenomenon with a number of underlying causes. Accurate differential assessment is therefore essential. Differential assessment involves developing an individualized, family-centered understanding of a child and family's circumstances, environment, and potential in order to identify each family's unique needs, determine the extent of the risk to the child, and to construct an appropriate intervention plan.

Research has demonstrated that adequate assessment often does not occur in child welfare, and this failing may be linked to the instability of reunification. In a review of 62 failed reunifications, Peg McCartt Hess and her colleagues found that "poor assessment or decision-making by the caseworker or service provider" was a factor in 42 cases.

The use of standardized tools to aid assessment is an emerging area of child welfare research that offers some promise of improving practice in this area. The North Carolina Family Assessment Scales for Reunification (NCFAS-R), developed by Ray Kirk, Ph.D., at the University of North Carolina at Chapel Hill, is the only validated instrument designed specifically for use in reunification. The NCFAS-R, an adaptation of the original North Carolina Family Assessment Scale used in family preservation, has proven to be an effective tool in assessing readiness for reunification and parent and child ambivalence.

## *Services Should Be Practical and Comprehensive, Addressing All Aspects of Family Life*

Services should be designed to promote an environment in which a child can be safely returned, and to help maintain that environment after reunification. A number of studies have supported the use of interventions that have a behavioral, skill-building focus and that address family functioning in multiple domains, including home, school, and community. Cognitive-behavioral models have been demonstrated to reduce physical punishment and parental aggression in less time than alternative approaches. The most effective treatment involves all members of the family and addresses not only parenting skills, but also parent-child interaction and a range of parental life competencies such as communication, problem solving, and anger control.

## *Literature Reports on the Effectiveness of Several Types of Services*

**Concrete services:** The provision of concrete services such as food, transportation, and assistance with housing and utilities has been demonstrated to be an important aspect of family reunification services. A study reviewing effective family-centered service models identified concrete services as critical elements of practice. The most effective programs studied not only provided services to meet concrete needs, but offered families instruction in accessing community resources so that they could do so independently in the future. In a study of 1,014 families participating in a family reunification program in Illinois, the 50 percent of families who experienced reunification demonstrated high utilization of concrete services such as financial assistance and transportation.

**Substance abuse treatment:** The well-documented incidence of parental substance abuse as a factor in the placement of children into foster care supports the critical importance of readily available resources for the assessment and treatment of addiction. A few agencies have established alliances with drug treatment centers or brought addiction professionals into the agency to ensure more effective assessment of drug-related needs, treatment planning, and monitoring of progress. Others have undertaken more intensive training of staff in addictions and the process of recovery. Research has shown promising results with three types of service delivery:

- **Intensive case management:** Significant results were reported when substance-involved families received intensive case management that included "recovery coaches" to facilitate assessments, conduct service planning, and eliminate barriers to accessing substance abuse treatment.

- **Tailoring programs for women with children:** The provision of treatment services specifically developed to meet the needs of women with children appears to hold promise for retaining women in treatment and decreasing subsequent drug use.

- **Strong social support:** Because social support appears to be an important factor in the successful treatment of addiction, assessment and intervention should involve the entire family, especially spouses or partners, and include consistent, ongoing support from caseworkers and treatment providers.

**Home-based services:** Many home-based service models originally developed to prevent out-of-home placement have shown some success in effecting family reunification. In one experimental study, families in the treatment group received intensive casework services, parenting and life skills education, family-focused treatment, and help in accessing community resources. The treatment group had a reunification rate three times that of the control group and remained intact at a far higher rate seven years later. It is important to note, however, that while some short-term intensive models have demonstrated success in achieving family reunification, not all such programs appear to reduce the risk of re-entry into foster care substantially. Many families who have experienced placement of one or more children in foster care require longer-term intervention and support.

**Post-reunification services:** Data from the Multistate Foster Care Data Archive indicate that about 25 percent of all children who go home will return to care at some point, often within one year. Reunification, although a positive milestone for the family, is also a time of readjustment, and a family already under stress can have difficulty maintaining safety and stability. The difficulty is compounded when children or parents have numerous or more complex personal needs, or when environmental factors, such as extreme poverty and a lack of social supports, are present. Research suggests that follow-up services that enhance parenting skills, provide social support, connect families to basic resources, and address children's behavioral and emotional needs must be provided if re-entry into foster care is to be prevented. Post-reunification services are especially important when parental drug or alcohol use is a concern.

Chapter 43

# Going to a Therapist: Information for Children and Teens

Eric went to therapy a couple of years ago when his parents were getting divorced. Although he no longer goes, he feels the two months he spent in therapy helped him get through the tough times as his parents worked out their differences.

Melody began seeing her therapist a year ago when she was being bullied at school. She still goes every two weeks because she feels therapy is really helping to build her self-esteem.

Britt just joined a therapy group for eating disorders led by her school's psychologist, and her friend Dana said she'd go with her.

When our parents were in school, very few kids went to therapy. Now it's much more common and also more accepted. Lots of teens wonder if therapy could help them.

## What Are Some Reasons That Teens Go to Therapists?

When teens are going through a rough time, such as family troubles or problems in school, they might feel more supported if they talk to a therapist. They may be feeling sad, angry, or overwhelmed by what's been happening—and need help sorting out their feelings, finding

---

solutions to their problems, or just feeling better. That's when therapy can help.

Just a few examples of situations in which therapy can help are when someone:

- feels sad, depressed, worried, shy, or just stressed out;

- is dieting or overeating for too long or it becomes a problem (eating disorders);

- cuts, burns, or self-injures;

- is dealing with an attention problem (attention deficit/hyperactivity disorder [ADHD]) or a learning problem;

- is coping with a chronic illness (such as diabetes or asthma) or a new diagnosis of a serious problem such as human immunodeficiency virus (HIV), cancer, or a sexually transmitted disease (STD);

- is dealing with family changes such as separation and divorce, or family problems such as alcoholism or addiction;

- is trying to cope with a traumatic event, death of a loved one, or worry over world events;

- has a habit he or she would like to get rid of, such as nail biting, hair pulling, smoking, or spending too much money, or getting hooked on medications, drugs, or pills;

- wants to sort out problems like managing anger or coping with peer pressure;

- wants to build self-confidence or figure out ways to make more friends.

In short, therapy offers people support when they are going through difficult times.

Deciding to seek help for something you're going through can be really hard. It may be your idea to go to therapy or it might not. Sometimes parents or teachers bring up the idea first because they notice that someone they care about is dealing with a difficult situation, is losing weight, or seems unusually sad, worried, angry, or upset. Some people in this situation might welcome the idea or even feel relieved. Others might feel criticized or embarrassed and unsure if they'll benefit from talking to someone.

Sometimes people are told by teachers, parents, or the courts that they have to go see a therapist because they have been behaving in ways that are unacceptable, illegal, self-destructive, or dangerous. When therapy is someone else's idea, a person may at first feel like resisting the whole idea. But learning a bit more about what therapy involves and what to expect can help make it seem okay.

## What Is Therapy?

Therapy isn't just for mental health. You've probably heard people discussing other types of medical therapy, such as physical therapy or chemotherapy. But the word "therapy" is most often used to mean psychotherapy (sometimes called "talk therapy")—in other words, psychological help to deal with stress or problems.

Psychotherapy is a process that's a lot like learning. Through therapy, people learn about themselves. They discover ways to overcome difficulties, develop inner strengths or skills, or make changes in themselves or their situations. Often, it feels good just to have a person to vent to, and other times it's useful to learn different techniques to help deal with stress.

A psychotherapist (therapist, for short) is a person who has been professionally trained to help people deal with stress or other problems. Psychiatrists, psychologists, social workers, counselors, and school psychologists are the titles of some of the licensed professionals who work as therapists. The letters following a therapist's name (for example: medical doctor [MD], doctor of philosophy [PhD], doctor of psychology [PsyD], doctor of education [EdD], masters degree [MA], licensed clinical social worker [LCSW], licensed professional counselor [LPC]) refer to the particular education and degree that therapist has received.

Some therapists specialize in working with a certain age group or on a particular type of problem. Other therapists treat a mix of ages and issues. Some work in hospitals, clinics, or counseling centers. Others work in schools or in psychotherapy offices, often called a "private practice" or "group practice."

## What Do Therapists Do?

Most types of therapy include talking and listening, building trust, and receiving support and guidance. Sometimes therapists may recommend books for people to read or work through. They may also suggest keeping a journal. Some people prefer to express themselves using art or drawing. Others feel more comfortable just talking.

When a person talks to a therapist about which situations might be difficult for them or what stresses them out, this helps the therapist assess what is going on. The therapist and client then usually work together to set therapy goals and figure out what will help the person feel better or get back on track.

It might take a few meetings with a therapist before people really feel like they can share personal stuff. It's natural to feel that way. Trust is an essential ingredient in therapy—after all, therapy involves being open and honest about sensitive topics like feelings, ideas, relationships, problems, disappointments, and hopes. A therapist understands that people sometimes take a while to feel comfortable sharing personal information.

Most of the time, a person meets with a therapist one on one, which is known as individual therapy. Sometimes, though, a therapist might work with a family (called family therapy) or a group of people who all are dealing with similar issues (called group therapy or a support group). Family therapy gives family members a chance to talk together with a therapist about problems that involve them all. Group therapy and support groups help people give and receive support and learn from each other and their therapist by discussing the issues they have in common.

## What Happens during Therapy?

If you see a therapist, he or she will talk with you about your feelings, thoughts, relationships, and important values. At the beginning, therapy sessions are focused on discussing what you'd like to work on and setting goals. Some of the goals people in therapy may set include things like:

- improving self-esteem and gaining confidence;
- figuring out how to make more friends;
- feeling less depressed or less anxious;
- improving grades at school;
- learning to manage anger and frustration;
- making healthier choices (for example, about relationships or eating) and ending self-defeating behaviors.

During the first visit, your therapist will probably ask you to talk a bit about yourself. Depending on your age, the therapist will also likely meet with a parent or caregiver and ask you to review information regarding confidentiality.

The first meeting can last longer than the usual "therapy hour" and is often called an "intake interview." This helps the therapist understand you better, and gives you a chance to see if you feel comfortable with the therapist. The therapist will probably ask about problems, concerns, and symptoms that you may be having, or the problems that parents or teachers are concerned about.

After one or two sessions, the therapist may talk to you about his or her understanding of what is going on with you, how therapy could help, and what the process will involve. Together, you and your therapist will decide on the goals for therapy and how frequently to meet. This may be once a week, every other week, or once a month.

With a better understanding of your situation, the therapist might teach you new skills or help you to think about a situation in a new way. For example, therapists can help people develop better relationship skills or coping skills, including ways to build confidence, express feelings, or manage anger.

Sticking to the schedule you agree on with your therapist and going to your appointments will ensure you have enough time with your therapist to work out your concerns. If your therapist suggests a schedule that you don't think you'll be able to keep, be up front about it so you can work out an alternative.

## How Private Is It?

Therapists respect the privacy of their clients and they keep things they're told confidential. A therapist won't tell anyone else—including parents—about what a person discusses in his or her sessions unless that person gives permission. The only exception is if therapists believe their clients may harm themselves or others.

If the issue of privacy and confidentiality worries you, be sure to ask your therapist about it during your first meeting. It's important to feel comfortable with your therapist so you can talk openly about your situation.

## Does It Mean I'm Crazy?

No. In fact, many people in your class have probably seen a therapist at some point—just like students often see tutors or coaches for extra help with schoolwork or sports. Getting help in dealing with emotions and stressful situations is as important to your overall health as getting help with a medical problem like asthma or diabetes.

There's nothing wrong with getting help with problems that are hard to solve alone. In fact, it's just the opposite. It takes a lot of courage and maturity to look for solutions to problems instead of ignoring or hiding them and allowing them to become worse. If you think that therapy could help you with a problem, ask an adult you trust—like a parent, school counselor, or doctor—to help you find a therapist.

A few adults still resist the idea of therapy because they don't fully understand it or have outdated ideas about it. A couple of generations ago, people didn't know as much about the mind or the mind-body connection as they do today, and people were left to struggle with their problems on their own. It used to be that therapy was only available to those with the most serious mental health problems, but that's no longer the case.

Therapy is helpful to people of all ages and with problems that range from mild to much more serious. Some people still hold on to old beliefs about therapy, such as thinking that teens "will grow out of" their problems. If the adults in your family don't seem open to talking about therapy, mention your concerns to a school counselor, coach, or doctor.

You don't have to hide the fact that you're going to a therapist, but you also don't have to tell anyone if you'd prefer not to. Some people find that talking to a few close friends about their therapy helps them to work out their problems and feel like they're not alone. Other people choose not to tell anyone, especially if they feel that others won't understand. Either way, it's a personal decision.

## What Can a Person Get Out of Therapy?

What someone gets out of therapy depends on why that person is there. For example, some people go to therapy to solve a specific problem, others want to begin making better choices, and others want to start to heal from a loss or a difficult life situation.

Therapy can help people feel better, be stronger, and make good choices as well as discover more about themselves. Those who work with therapists might learn about motivations that lead them to behave in certain ways or about inner strengths they have. Maybe you'll learn new coping skills, develop more patience, or learn to like yourself better. Maybe you'll find new ways to handle problems that come up or new ways to handle yourself in tough situations.

People who work with therapists often find that they learn a lot about themselves and that therapy can help them grow and mature. Lots of people discover that the tools they learn in therapy when they're young make them feel stronger and better able to deal with whatever life throws at them even as adults. If you are curious about the therapy process, talk to a counselor or therapist to see if you could benefit.

Chapter 44

# Therapy Models for Families Impacted by Child Abuse

## Chapter Contents

# Section 44.1

# *Parent-Child Interaction Therapy*

"Guide to Effective Programs for Children and Youth:
Parent-Child Interaction Therapy (PCIT)," © 2007 Child Trends
(www.childtrends.org). Reprinted with permission.

## *Overview*

Parent-child interaction therapy (PCIT) is a program designed to prevent physical child abuse among families with a history of previous physical abuse or child neglect. In the program, parents and children are treated together in therapy sessions. Sessions focus on enhancing parent-child relationships by dealing with negative behaviors appropriately and reinforcing positive parent-child interaction. An evaluation of PCIT found that it was effective in reducing repeat cases of physical abuse. The PCIT program also reduced parental depression and negative parenting behaviors.

## *Description of Program*

**Target population:** Parents with children ages 2–12 with prior abuse reports who are at-risk for engaging in future physical child abuse.

Parent-child interaction therapy (PCIT) was initially developed for young children who were exhibiting externalizing behavior disorders. This therapy style was modified to be used with physically abusive families and for children up to 12 years old. The PCIT program consists of three different modules and focuses directly on parent's behaviors and interactions with their children. The first focuses on increasing the parent's motivation to complete the treatment through testimonials from previous graduates of the program and understanding of the negative effects of abuse. The second module consists of training sessions in which parents are instructed about how to handle specific situations with their children. During this module, parents and children or therapists and children role-play various daily interactions and therapists teach skills and techniques to use in these interactions. The third and final module is a series of four follow-up sessions which are intended to answer any questions that parents may have about the program and help solve any issues that have come up since the previous sessions. In an evaluation of the PCIT program, researchers estimate that the program costs between $2,208–3,638 for each parent/child pair that completes the program.

## Evaluation(s) of Program[1]

**Evaluated population:** 100 parent/child pairs who were referred to the investigators by a county child welfare office in Oklahoma. Parents had a recent confirmed report of physical child abuse. Parents in the study had, on average, two previous reports of abuse, with 39% of parents reportedly engaging in severely abusive behavior. Sixty-five percent of parents in the study were female, and 62% of children were male. The average age of parents in the study was 32, and the average age of children was eight years. Sixty-two percent of households were living below the federal poverty line, and 64% of households were receiving some sort of public assistance. Additionally, 39% of the parents met guidelines for an antisocial personality disorder, 33% met criteria for a substance abuse disorder, and 20% were classified as significantly depressed.

**Approach:** To qualify for the study, the parent/child pairs had to meet five eligibility criteria: 1) both parent and child had to be available for participation throughout the study; 2) parents had to score above a mean intelligence score of 70; 3) children were between the ages of 4–12 years; 4) parents were not identified as sexual abusers; and 5) both parent and child appeared able to participate in the intervention. All of these criteria were assessed at an initial interview. After the interview, parent/child pairs were randomly assigned to one of three conditions. The first condition was a PCIT intervention which followed the design described in the previous section. The second condition (EPCIT) was a modified PCIT treatment in which parents received additional services to specifically address parental depression, current substance abuse, and family problems. The control condition consisted of a community group (CG) in which parents were referred to a long-standing community service center which conducted a parenting program in a series of 40 sessions.

**Results:** Parents in the PCIT treatment condition were less likely to be re-reported for physical abuse (19%) than parents in the CG control condition (49%) over a period of 850 days following the conclusion of the

411

intervention. Parents in the EPCIT treatment condition scored lower than parents in the community group control condition on the Beck Depression Inventory. Likewise, parents in the PCIT condition scored somewhat lower on the Beck Depression Inventory than parents in the community group condition, but this difference only approached significance. Parents in the EPCIT and PCIT treatment conditions scored lower than parents in the CG control condition on a measure of negative parenting behaviors. No differences between groups were found on measures of parenting attitudes, parent-reported child behavior problems, parental distress, parental loneliness, positive parent behaviors, and child neglect. The authors estimate that the incremental cost required to avert one repeat report of physical abuse would be between $371 and $1,326, compared with the control group treatment approach.

### References

1.  Chaffin, M., Silovsky, J. F., Funderburk, B., Valle, L. A., Breston, E. V., Balachova, T., Shultz, S., and Bonner, B. L. (2003). *Physical abuse treatment outcome project: Application of parent-child interaction therapy (PCIT) to physically abusive parents* (Grant No. 90CA1633). Oklahoma City, OK: University of Oklahoma Health Sciences Center, Center on Child Abuse and Neglect.

## Section 44.2

## *Trauma-Focused Cognitive-Behavioral Therapy*

This cognitive-behavior therapy program is targeted at children who are experiencing symptoms of post-traumatic stress disorder (PTSD). Trauma-focused cognitive-behavioral therapy (TF-CBT) involves individualized therapy sessions in which children are given emotional skills training and later, with the help of trained therapists, children begin to confront the experience which initialized the PTSD symptoms. The studies outlined below found that TF-CBT was effective in reducing the symptoms of PTSD.

## Description of Program

**Target population:** Children and adolescents who have been diagnosed with post-traumatic stress disorder (PTSD)

Trauma-focused cognitive-behavioral therapy (TF-CBT) is used for children and adolescents who have developed clinical levels of PTSD. In young children, this disorder is often the result of sexual or physical abuse. The program seeks to teach children skills to cope with the difficulties that this disorder creates. At the same time, therapy sessions are used to help children confront and deal with painful or scary past experiences.

## Evaluation(s) of Program

Cohen, J. A., Deblinger, E., Mannarino, A. P., and Steer, R. A. (2004). A multisite, randomized controlled trial for children with sexual abuse-related PTSD symptoms. *Journal of the American Academy of Child and Adolescent Psychiatry*, 43, 393–403.

**Evaluated population:** 229 children ages 8–14 (median = 10.76 years) who had met at least five of the six *Diagnostic and Statistical Manual of Mental Disorders, Fourth Edition* (DSM-IV) criteria for PTSD. The sample was 60% White, 28% African-American, 4% Hispanic, 7% biracial, and 1% other ethnicity.

**Approach:** Participants were given an initial screening by evaluators and then randomly assigned to either a TF-CBT group or a comparison group which used a child-centered therapy (CCT) program. CCT programs are focused on the development of a trusting relationship between the child and therapist. During therapy sessions, children choose what topics to discuss and largely lead the direction of the sessions. The TF-CBT treatment program focused on expressing feelings, training in coping skills, understanding relationships between thoughts and behaviors, and gradual exposure to the traumatic event. Both treatments were given once a week and involved two consecutive 45 minute sessions, one for the child and one for the child's parent, for a total of 90 minutes of treatment sessions each week. Additionally, TF-CBT treatment included three joint parent-child sessions which lasted 30 minutes instead of consecutive 45 minute sessions. The total session breakdown for these three weeks was: 30 minutes for joint session, 30 minutes for child's individual session, and 30 minutes for child's parent's individual session. Parents and children attended treatment sessions once per week for a total of 12 weeks.

**Results:** Participants in both conditions improved scores on all measures for post-traumatic stress disorder symptoms over the course of the study; however, TF-CBT therapy participants had significantly lower scores on survey measures of post-traumatic stress disorder (Kiddie-Schedule for Affective Disorders and Schizophrenia (K-SADS), Child Behavior Checklist (CBCL), Children's Depressive Inventory (CDI), Children's Attributions and Perceptions Scale (CAPS), Shame Questionnaire, Beck Depression Inventory (BDI), and Perceived Emotional Response Questionnaire (PERQ)) when compared with children and adolescents in CCT treatment groups indicating that they were displaying fewer symptoms of post-traumatic stress disorder. TF-CBT participants likewise were less likely to be diagnosed with *Diagnostic and Statistical Manual of Mental Disorders, Fourth Edition* (DSM-IV) defined post-traumatic stress disorder (21%, 19 out of 89) at the end of the study when compared with participants in CCT groups (46%, 42 out of 91).

Cohen, J. A., Mannarino, A. P., and Knudsen, K. (2005). Treating sexually abused children: 1 year follow-up of a randomized controlled trial. *Child Abuse & Neglect*, 29, 135–145.

**Evaluated Population:** 82 children and adolescents ages 8–15 years who were referred to a traumatic stress program. Sixty percent of participants were Caucasian, 37% African-American, 2% biracial, and 1% Hispanic. To be included in the study these children and adolescents had to have had contact sexual abuse within the past six months, significant symptoms of PTSD (clinical levels), and an available non-offending caretaker.

**Approach:** After an initial interview which assessed eligibility for the study, participants were randomly assigned to TF-CBT or non-directive supportive therapy (NST). NST therapists fostered the development of therapeutic, trusting relationships and encouraged children and parents to choose which topics the therapy sessions would focus on. TF-CBT treatments focused on the topics of feeling identification, stress inoculation techniques, direct discussion and gradual exposure of traumatic events, education about healthy sexuality, and safety skill building. The therapy sessions for both treatments were individual and lasted a total of 90 minutes with 45 minutes devoted to individual child therapy and 45 minutes devoted to individual therapy for the child's parent. Parents and children attended treatment sessions once per week for a total of 12 weeks.

**Results:** Participants in the TF-CBT group had greater improvement in scores over time on the CDI, State-Trait Anxiety Inventory for Children (STAIC), and Trauma Symptom Checklist for Children (TSCC) (Anxiety, Depression, and Sexual Problems subscales) scales compared to participants in the control group. This improvement in scores indicates that TF-CBT participants exhibited fewer and/or less pervasive symptoms of post-traumatic stress disorder. At a six-month follow-up interval, participants in the TF-CBT group had greater improvement in scores on the STAIC-State, STAIC-Trait, and TSCC (Anxiety, Depression, Sexual Problems, and Dissociation subscales) scales compared with participants in the control group. At a twelve-month follow-up interval, participants in the TF-CBT group had greater improvement in scores on the TSCC (PTSD and Dissociation subscales) scale. All of these results indicate that participants in the TF-CBT group were displaying fewer and/or less pervasive symptoms of post-traumatic stress disorder compared with participants in control groups.

## *References*

Cohen, J. A., Deblinger, E., Mannarino, A. P., and Steer, R. A. (2004). A multisite, randomized controlled trial for children with sexual abuse-related PTSD symptoms. *Journal of the American Academy of Child and Adolescent Psychiatry*, 43, 393–403.

Cohen, J. A., Mannarino, A. P., and Knudsen, K. (2005). Treating sexually abused children: 1 year follow-up of a randomized controlled trial. *Child Abuse & Neglect*, 29, 135–145.

Chapter 45

# Child Physical and Sexual Abuse: Guidelines for Treatment

## General Principles for Treatment of Physical and Sexual Abuse

### Principles of Empirically Supported Treatments

Child victims of physical or sexual abuse very often have complicated histories of multiple victimization and trauma, and exhibit a
variety of disorders, problems, and difficulties that may or may not
be the direct result of abuse. Complex histories and multiproblem
presentations are considerable assessment and treatment challenges
for practitioners. How should children with multiple problems be
treated? Should several treatment protocols be employed, one for each
problem? What about child victims of both sexual and physical abuse
who may have histories of other traumas as well? Should treatments
be combined, delivered concurrently, or staged sequentially? It may
be helpful for practitioners confronted with these difficult children to
use approaches that are shared across empirically supported treatments. The shared theoretical perspectives, treatment procedures, and
clinical skills associated with these protocols can be flexibly applied
depending on the history, problem matrix, and circumstances of these
complex cases.

Information in this chapter is excerpted from "Child Physical and Sexual
Abuse: Guidelines for Treatment," Saunders, B.E., Berliner, L., and Hanson, R.F.
(Eds.) (Revised Report: April 26, 2004), reviewed 2009. © 2004 National Crime
Victims Research and Treatment Center. Reprinted with permission.

Many treatments have been developed for the disorders, conditions, and problems commonly seen in child victims of physical and sexual abuse and their families. Generally, the interventions with the most empirical support tend to be based on behavioral or cognitive behavioral theoretical approaches, utilize behavioral and cognitive intervention procedures and techniques, and intervene at both the individual child and parent/family levels. Many of them share specific treatment procedures and techniques (for example: cognitive restructuring, exposure procedures, behavioral management skills) that are simply applied to different problems. When examined with complex case presentations in mind, empirically supported protocols have certain common principles and treatment components that can be applied to many different problems children and families may have. Therefore, it is important to identify the common principles and components shared by empirically supported treatment protocols.

In general, treatments with empirical support are goal directed. They are designed to address specific, measurable problems identified through systematic assessment of children and their families. Problems are defined and identified such that they can be measured using sound and accepted assessment tools. Once the problems are defined and measured, a treatment plan can be developed for reducing them, and the effect of the treatment can be assessed over time.

Empirically supported treatments tend to be structured in their approach. They have specific procedures and techniques that are used in order to reduce the problems assessed. Little time is devoted to non-goal directed activity other than for the purpose of rapport building and engaging the client in the therapeutic procedures. These treatments often have a sequential staging of treatment components that are designed to build upon one another until the therapeutic goals are reached. Because of their structure, therapists using these treatments are more likely to stay focused on the larger goals of treatment and not get sidetracked by the inevitable daily problems and "crises" that often arise with this client population.

Empirically supported treatments usually emphasize skill building to manage emotional distress and behavioral disturbance. Children are taught specific skills for self-regulation of their thinking, affect, and behavior. Parents are taught skills for managing children. Treatment components often are variations of basic cognitive-behavioral techniques, and usually include didactic procedures such as psychoeducation, expressive procedures such as exposure therapy, cognitive procedures such as cognitive restructuring, and child behavior management techniques.

These procedures are designed to teach and build skills to manage the targeted problems.

Empirically supported treatments typically use techniques involving repetitive practice of skills with therapist feedback. Practice occurs both within treatment sessions and between sessions in the home, school, or community. The use of role-plays and homework is common in these therapies. These learning strategies maximize the likelihood that newly acquired skills will generalize to every day life.

For children, there are several key skills that are common among empirically supported treatments within child mental health, and are also components of many of the supported treatments. These elements include: 1) skills for emotion identification, processing, and regulation; 2) anxiety management skills; 3) skills for the identification and alteration of maladaptive cognitions; and 4) problem solving skills. All of these skills are applicable to reducing the most common problems that may be the direct impact of abuse. However, they also are useful in addressing the additional problems and difficulties that many abused children have. These general skills cut across the treatment of a variety of emotional and behavioral disorders and can be considered basic and fundamental treatment components. Therefore, clinicians working with abused children should be knowledgeable and skilled in the use of these procedures.

When dealing with children, especially if they have concerning abuse related behavioral reactions or externalizing behavior problems, it is necessary to include treatment components that address the child's environment. For most children, this means working closely with their parents or caregivers and their larger family system. The general principle of treatment for parent-child relationships is to promote positive interactions between parents and children while reducing negative interactions. This goal is accomplished through several approaches. Parents are taught to use effective behavior management skills based upon reinforcement of positive behavior, rather than relying primarily on punishment of negative behavior. Parents are taught the importance of consistency and follow through as essential ingredients for changing child behavior. They are taught: 1) skills to reward and reinforce all manifestations of positive behavior; 2) how to strategically ignore minor or irritating behavioral problems; 3) how to give effective instructions; and, 4) how to implement nonviolent consequences such as time-out or the removal of privileges. Parents are also taught how to recognize and avoid the development of negative interactions with their children, and techniques for constructing positive experiences and increasing their frequency.

As can be seen for the treatment descriptions presented, nearly all of the empirically supported treatments contain some form of these therapeutic elements. They are goal-directed, structured in their approach, and teach appropriate skills to children and parents. Therefore, even when confronted with complex situations of abuse, practitioners can begin with this core set of approaches and adapt and add to them as necessary.

## General Principles of Treatment

While each case of intrafamilial child abuse presents unique challenges, current scientific knowledge about the effects of child abuse and the efficacy of intervention suggests several general principles of treatment that can be applied to most cases. They are based upon the relevant scientific literature, and findings from the field's years of clinical experience treating abused children. Like any guidelines, these principles are not meant to be followed lockstep in every case. Rather, they offer direction and basic precepts that can be used to guide treatment planning.

1.  Children's abuse experiences should be acknowledged and characterized as wrong, unlawful, and harmful in all abuse-specific interventions with children, families, and parents. Child abuse is never acceptable or warranted. Offending parents often have a rationale for their abusive behavior that is based upon distorted ideas of child welfare. Interventions should guard against being co-opted by these rationales.

2.  Children's physical and emotional safety should be assessed and given significant weight in treatment planning and the interventions undertaken. It is unlikely that any child can be placed in an absolutely safe environment. However, a reasonable and acceptable level of safety should be established in the child's environment prior to treatment for problems related to abuse. It is unlikely that children continuing to live in situations that they consider to be dangerous or threatening can be treated successfully. Safety should be maintained throughout course of treatment, and should be a criterion for discharge from treatment.

3.  Systematic clinical assessments of children and parents for both abuse-related and general mental health and behavioral problems should be conducted prior to initiating therapy. Results

420

of systematic clinical assessments should form the basis for all treatment plans.

4.  Systematic clinical assessment should include a comprehensive examination of the child's lifetime victimization and trauma history. Such an examination is not a forensic evaluation conducted to gather evidence for legal purposes. Rather, it is a clinical examination designed to assess the child's relevant history, and identify problems that will be the targets of treatment.

5.  Systematic clinical reassessment of children and parents should be conducted at periodic intervals to determine treatment progress and provide information on which to base revisions to treatment plans and treatment focus.

6.  Interventions should be selected and matched to the problems, disorders, and conditions identified in the systematic assessments of abused children and their parents.

7.  Treatment protocols with the highest levels of empirical and clinical support for their effectiveness with the specific problems identified in the assessment process should be used as the first choice interventions for abused children and their parents.

8.  Therapy is not a risk-free endeavor. Clinicians should be aware of potential harmful effects of therapy and assess the potential risks of any treatment. The potential benefits of a treatment should be balanced against its risks in the treatment selection process. Treatments with higher than average levels of risk should not be used unless there is convincing evidence that children will benefit greatly.

9.  Interventions with abused children should be abuse-informed. That is, interventions should explicitly and directly address the abuse incidents experienced by the child, and the consequent emotions, cognitions, and behaviors exhibited by the child as a result of the abuse. The child's maladaptive behaviors, thoughts, and feelings related to the abuse they experienced should be the primary targets of intervention.

10. Children should not be in treatment specifically for abuse-related problems unless the treating clinician agrees that the child has a history of abuse.

11.  Treatment of the abuse-related problems of the child should be the central, organizing focus of treatment, regardless of treatment modality (individual, group, parent-child, or family therapy) or the participants in treatment (the abused child, non-abused siblings, parents, or extended family).

12.  In most cases, the term of treatment for the abused child will be short to moderate (for example, 12–24 sessions). However, this presumption depends on the presenting problems assessed. Individual client differences will affect treatment duration, and a minority of abused children will require more extended treatment.

13.  Treatment should be conducted in the least restrictive environment with the least amount of burden on the family.

14.  The ultimate, long-term functioning and welfare of the abused child should be the guiding principle of all treatment, regardless of modality or participants.

15.  Treatment should have as a goal the prevention of future problems often associated with a history of abuse (for example: substance abuse, delinquency, re-victimization), as well as relief of the current problems experienced by the child.

16.  Parental acknowledgment of the abuse, belief of the child, and support of the child should be encouraged as part of treatment.

17.  Whenever possible, supportive, non-offending parents should be included in the treatment of abused children.

18.  When clinically indicated, parents should receive appropriate treatment to enhance their ability to support, care for, and effectively parent the abused child and to provide a safe environment for the child.

19.  When clinically indicated, offending parents should receive appropriate treatment for their abusive behavior.

20.  When possible, treatment interventions should be used to improve the quality of parent/child relationships in abusive families.

21.  When clients have achieved the therapeutic goals, treatment should end.

22.  If it is clear that clients are not benefitting from treatment or that treatment is being harmful, treatment should be changed or discontinued.

## Conclusion

Physical and sexual abuse of children is a difficult social problem affecting the growth and development of a substantial proportion of American youth. Abused children are at significantly increased risk for suffering a variety of medical, emotional, behavioral, relational, and social problems that can affect them throughout life. Mental health intervention with child victims and their families can help ameliorate current problems and reduce the risk of the development of future ones. However, this beneficial effect can occur only if effective interventions are developed, tested, and most important, actually used with child victims of abuse and their families. Therefore, practitioners in the field need ready access to information describing interventions that are likely to help their clients, and they need training in the proper use of these treatments. The goal of these guidelines is to provide practitioners with some tools for judging the utility of treatment protocols, and to provide them with information and direction concerning treatments commonly used with physically and sexually abused children. Practitioners can then use this information in their treatment planning and abused children and their families will benefit. Ultimately, society at large that will benefit from better services being provided to child victims and their families.

# Chapter 46

# Help for Adult Survivors of Childhood Sexual Abuse

## Survivors of Childhood Sexual Abuse

A sexual assault violates one's most intimate and personal boundaries and triggers a wide range of issues that survivors must confront, on some level, for the rest of their lives. One of the most difficult issues facing survivors of sexual assault is the realization of their vulnerability and powerlessness to protect themselves from such an intimate invasion.

This issue of powerlessness is perhaps most profound for the child victim. Sexual abuse, especially during the developmental stages of childhood, can have devastating and long-lasting effects on the child's growth physically, emotionally, and mentally. Issues concerning trust, self-esteem, and forgiveness can run quite deep and present significant challenges into adulthood.

If your perpetrator was someone you knew and trusted as a child, the effects may be particularly painful. The fact that someone who was supposed to love and protect you caused the violation can be quite frightening.

The powerlessness and shame can sometimes be too difficult to bear. Consequently, some children may successfully bury the memory of the assault until something happens to trigger that memory.

---

"Adults Molested as Children," © Texas Association Against Sexual Assault (www.taasa.org). Reprinted with permission.

## As a Survivor of Childhood Sexual Assault You May Experience...

### *Difficulty Setting Limits and Boundaries*

Past experiences may have given you little hope of having control over what happens to you. However, it is important that you understand that you are no longer a child who is powerless to stop the abuse that was perpetrated on you by the adults in your life. You have more power now, but more importantly you have the right to control what happens to you and to choose your sexual partners.

### *Memories and Flashbacks*

You may experience disruptive memories surrounding the assault. A sudden occurrence of a visual memory is called a flashback. If you have a flashback you may not only see what happened but also experience all of the emotions and feelings that you had at the time of the assault. A flashback can be very frightening and even trigger a panic response. Sounds, smells, people, and places associated with the assault can trigger memories and flashbacks. Remind yourself that these are only memories. You are safe now and have the power to choose if and when you wish to review these memories. When you begin to recognize your personal empowerment these memories will lose their power.

### *Grieving and Mourning*

Victims of childhood sexual abuse experience many losses. There is a loss of innocence, loss of a carefree childhood, loss of security and trust to name a few. There may have been the loss of a normal relationship with parental figures, loss of the opportunity to choose your own sexual experiences and partner, and loss of nurturing. All losses need to be mourned in order to bring the grieving to closure. It is time to name your losses, grieve over them, and put them to rest.

### *Anger*

Although this is one of the most common issues for a survivor of sexual assault, it can be one of the most difficult for the adult survivor of childhood sexual abuse to get in touch with. You have probably spent many years covering up your true emotions. You may have felt powerless to acknowledge and act on your anger and therefore learned to suppress it. The healing process necessarily involves getting in touch with your feelings of anger.

It is important to acknowledge the anger you felt and probably still feel toward the perpetrator and the other adults who were supposed to protect you. You have a right to feel angry and there is nothing wrong with expressing anger in constructive ways. Unexpressed anger can lead to depression.

### Guilt, Shame, and Blame

Many survivors experience feelings of guilt and shame. You may feel guilty that you did not stop the abuse. You may have been afraid to disclose what was happening for fear of not being believed. You must remember that a child can never be responsible for being sexually assaulted. What happened was not your fault. The blame must be placed exactly where it belongs, with the perpetrator. An adult abused their position of authority and must be held accountable.

You may feel ashamed because your body responded to sexual stimulations. You must realize that while the body will respond to certain stimulations this is no indication that you liked or wanted the abuse. Further, children often seek affection from adults and accept any demonstration of affection as affirmation that they are loved. It is the responsibility of the adult to practice and teach appropriate boundaries to the child.

### Trust Issues

Adults who were victimized as children may find it difficult to trust others. You may feel that if you trust and let people near, you will be vulnerable to being hurt and victimized again. This fear is understandable, especially if the person who abused you was someone who you knew and trusted.

Trust does not come automatically. It must be earned. Remember that as an adult you have the power to choose your own relationships. You may choose who you allow to be close to you. You may also choose to stop trusting that person if that trust is violated.

### Intimacy Issues

Survivors of childhood sexual abuse may have difficulty establishing intimacy or a close bond with another person. Intimacy requires trust, respect, love, and sharing. These things can be frightening because of your perceived vulnerability. Or you may find that you cling too tightly to a relationship that makes you feel safe for fear of losing that person. These are difficult issues and many survivors find it helpful to talk with a counselor that can help them develop skills and find the confidence needed to engage in a healthy intimate relationship.

### Sexuality Issues

Survivors of childhood sexual abuse must deal with the difficult fact that their first sexual experiences came as a result of rape or incest. As an adult, these painful memories may be triggered by sexual activity with your partner. This can be disappointing and frustrating since it can interfere with your ability to enjoy your sexuality and engage in consensual sexual relationships. Remember that you are now in control of your body and how you choose to experience your sexuality. You can say "no" or "stop" if you begin to feel uncomfortable. Communicate your feelings and your needs with your partner. Be clear about what you are and are not comfortable with. However, it is important to remember that sexuality, itself, is not shameful. It can be a beautiful expression of intimacy and affection when two adults with equal power choose to share this experience.

### Moving Forward

Survivors of childhood sexual abuse often struggle with the question of forgiveness. You may have asked yourself, "Do I have to forgive the perpetrator?" There is certainly no rule that you must forgive in order to heal. However, fixating on the injustice of the violation, the pain that you have endured, and fantasies of revenge can be damaging. These obsessive thoughts, left unchecked, can become very self-destructive. You may feel that you are not ready, and may never be ready, to forgive. This is fine as long as you do not allow yourself to become consumed with bitterness. This is not helpful and serves no purpose. Every victim must arrive at a place where they are able to "let it go." It may be helpful to seek professional counseling for assistance in putting these issues to rest. Most importantly, forgive yourself. What happened was not your fault.

Chapter 47

# Help for Substance-Involved Parents and the Children in Their Care

It is estimated that 11 percent of American youth live with a parent who abuses alcohol or other drugs. Moreover, substance abuse has been found to be a factor in seven out of ten cases of child maltreatment. Unfortunately, although substance abuse treatment has been shown to be helpful, many individuals are reluctant to enter treatment programs. Not surprisingly, women with children are especially apt to resist entering treatment for chemical dependency. In a recent study of mothers being investigated for child maltreatment who had been assessed for substance use problems, participants reported multiple barriers to their entering treatment, including embarrassment at having a substance abuse problem, lack of childcare support, considerations about the length and cost of treatment, and—by far the number one concern—fear of being separated from or losing custody of their children.

This chapter summarizes some promising approaches to helping substance-involved parents and the children in their care, and touches on some ethical dilemmas facing professionals attempting to achieve positive outcomes for children and their families.[1]

Text in this chapter is from "Substance Abuse and Child Welfare: Promising Practices and Ethical Dilemmas," National Resource Center for Family-Centered Practice and Permanency Planning, a service of the Children's Bureau, U.S. Department of Health and Human Services (HHS), Spring 2007.

## Co-Location Programs: Linking Foster Care Agencies and Drug Treatment Providers

In this model, professionals from substance abuse facilities are co-located at child welfare agencies, working in tandem with child welfare staff. When a caseworker investigating maltreatment suspects familial substance abuse, the case is referred to the substance abuse counselor, who conducts an assessment and provides referral and monitoring as needed. In New Jersey, the Department of Youth and Family Services (DYFS) piloted a program that purchased the services of substance abuse counselors to augment the expertise of their child welfare staff. Cross-training of foster care workers and drug treatment staff helped the former learn about chemical dependency and the latter learn about child welfare issues. While outcome data on treatment completion and family reunification have not been reported to date, the program did achieve its goal of increasing the percentage of parents who entered substance abuse treatment.

## Family Drug Courts

These programs target substance-abusing parents whose children have been or are in danger of being removed from the home due to maltreatment. Parents deemed motivated are immediately referred for substance abuse treatment in lieu of punishment. A case manager is assigned to facilitate collaboration between the various agencies involved, monitor treatment, and link the parent with resources. Intermittent drug testing and regular meetings of the team assist professionals in making timely decisions regarding permanency. While most programs have yet to conduct formal evaluations due to budgetary constrictions, preliminary data indicates that family drug courts produce parents who comply with court mandates.

## Family-Oriented Preventive Services

Family-centered programs are sometimes embedded in preventive services such as intensive family preservation or early intervention programs. In this model, rather than being blamed for their substance use and its impact on their children, parents partner with case managers to develop the optimum treatment plan for the entire family. Based on the assumption that parents possess the capacity to nurture their offspring, the focus here is on parental strengths rather than inadequacies. Services attempt to respond to family needs, and one-stop shopping is prioritized. Family-oriented services show promise, in that they enable parents to feel empowered and are valued by clients as helpful. In at least one study, family-centered intensive case management was associated with higher rates of family reunification.

## Mother-Child Residential Drug Treatment Programs

These relatively small programs, usually consisting of fewer than 50 mother-child units, allow a female parent to reside in a treatment facility with her children, and provide parenting education along with substance abuse treatment. Two advantages of this model are that families do not experience separation during treatment, and mothers have an opportunity to develop new parenting patterns while simultaneously working on changing their substance use behavior. A potential disadvantage may be the distraction and added stress of continuing to perform parental duties while maintaining sobriety, a challenging enough goal even for those focusing exclusively on their own needs. In a qualitative study conducted at four mother-child treatment facilities in New York City, common processes reported by mothers in recovery were: overcoming shame and guilt; dealing with having their parental behavior scrutinized; cultivating mother-to-mother support; and developing maternal empathy.

## Concurrent Planning

Concurrent planning involves working to reunify the substance-involved family while simultaneously preparing some back-up permanency solution should reunification efforts fail. The aim of concurrent planning is to allow the parent some leeway to engage in the process of recovery, while reducing the amount of time it takes to achieve permanency for the child. As with co-location programs, family drug courts, and mother-child treatment programs, there is as of yet no data available on long-term outcomes for children whose cases are handled through concurrent planning.

## Ethical Issues and Value Dilemmas

Despite some of the innovations described, challenges to reunifying substance involved families remain. One predicament has been characterized as the "conflicting time clocks" of the treatment and legal systems. Under the law, children have the right to a permanent custody decision within 12–18 months. However, treatment providers tend to view addiction as a chronic biopsychosocial disease and recovery as a lifelong process.

The need for standard criteria to guide determination of when and under what circumstances families should be reunified has been noted, and efforts have been made to delineate and categorize indicators for safe reunification. However, questions remain as to what outcomes are expected on what timelines, and how to best measure readiness for safe return of the child. For example, is a child safe when a parent completes treatment? When a parent remains abstinent for a certain amount of time? If so, how much time? Likewise, what are grounds for termination of parental rights? Initial refusal to enroll or failure to complete a treatment program? Multiple failures to enroll or complete treatment? Any reported use of a substance following treatment? Reported use of a substance combined with parental dysfunction? Deciding which client (the adult or the child) has precedence, which time clock to follow, and which criteria to use to judge success creates value dilemmas for caseworkers, agencies, and court officials. One ethical issue that has yet to be fully resolved has to do with confidentiality. Treatment facilities are required by law to protect the privacy of clients in their care. However, to make timely custody decisions, foster care agencies and courts need information about how parents are progressing in treatment. The resulting conflict of interest hinders mutual cooperation and collaboration between caseworkers and treatment staff. To overcome this obstacle, some child welfare agencies request that parents sign a consent form giving them the right to obtain information about their progress in treatment. Alternatively, federal law stipulates that a substance abuse facility may enter into a qualified service organizational agreement (QSOA) with a foster care agency, allowing both programs access to information regardless of client consent. However, to date, few child welfare and substance abuse agencies have established QSOAs.

## Conclusion

While female substance abusers are less likely than their male counterparts to enter alcohol and drug treatment, recent research suggests that, once in treatment, women have similar rates of success. Thus, helping these mothers realize the need for treatment, removing barriers to treatment, and providing gender-specific interventions are key factors to improving outcomes for substance-involved parents and the children in their care.

# Reference

[1] Adapted from Fenster, J. (2005) Substance abuse issues in the family. In G. Mallon, and P. Hess (Eds), *Child welfare in the 21st century: A handbook of children, youth and family services*. NY: Columbia University Press.

# Part Five


# Preventing Child Maltreatment

Chapter 48

# Preventing Child Abuse and Neglect

The statistics can feel overwhelming. In 2006, an estimated 905,000 children in the United States were found to be victims of child abuse and neglect. However, child abuse and neglect can be prevented. State and local governments, community organizations, and private citizens take action every day to protect children. You can help.

Research has shown that parents and caregivers who have support—from family, friends, neighbors, and their communities—are more likely to provide safe and healthy homes for their children. When parents lack this support or feel isolated, on the other hand, they may be more likely to make poor decisions that can lead to neglect or abuse.

Increasingly, concerned citizens and organizations are realizing that the best way to prevent child abuse is to help parents develop the skills and identify the resources they need to understand and meet their children's emotional, physical, and developmental needs and protect their children from harm.

## Prevention Programs

Prevention activities are conducted by many state, local, and tribal governments, as well as community and faith-based organizations. The services they provide vary widely.

This chapter includes text from "Preventing Child Abuse and Neglect," Child Welfare Information Gateway, U.S. Department of Health and Human Services (HHS), 2008; and "You Have the Power to Prevent Child Abuse and Neglect," Child Welfare Information Gateway, HHS, 2005.

437

Some prevention services are intended for everyone, such as public service announcements (PSA) aimed at raising awareness about child abuse within the general population. Others are specifically targeted for individuals and families who may be at greater risk of child abuse or neglect. An example of this might be a parenting class for single teen mothers. Some services are developed specifically for families where abuse or neglect has already occurred, to reduce the negative effects of the abuse and prevent it from happening again.

Common activities of prevention programs include the following:

- Public awareness, such as public service announcements, posters, and brochures that promote healthy parenting, child safety, and how to report suspected abuse

- Skills-based curricula that teach children safety and protection skills—many of these programs focus on preventing sexual abuse

- Parent education to help parents develop positive parenting skills and decrease behaviors associated with child abuse and neglect

- Parent support groups, where parents work together to strengthen their families and build social networks

- Home visitation, which focuses on enhancing child safety by helping pregnant mothers and families with new babies or young children learn more about positive parenting and child development

- Respite and crisis care programs which offer temporary relief to caregivers in stressful situations by providing short-term care for their children

- Family resource centers that work with community members to develop a variety of services to meet the specific needs of the people who live in surrounding neighborhoods

Two elements have been shown to make prevention programs more effective, regardless of the type of service or intended recipients—involving parents and providing evidence-based prevention services. Involving parents in all aspects of program planning, implementation, and evaluation helps ensure that service providers are working in true partnership with families. Parents are more likely to make lasting changes when they are empowered to identify solutions that make sense for them.

Another key to success is providing prevention services that are evidence based. This means that rather than relying on assumptions or common sense, research has been conducted to demonstrate that a particular service improves outcomes for children and families. This helps service providers feel confident in what they are doing. It can also help justify a program's continued funding when resources are scarce.

## Protective Factors

Prevention programs have long focused on reducing particular risk factors, or conditions that have been found through research to be associated with child abuse and neglect in families. Increasingly, prevention services are also recognizing the importance of promoting protective factors, conditions in families and communities that research has shown to increase the health and well-being of children and families. These factors help parents who might otherwise be at risk of abusing or neglecting their children to find resources, supports, or coping strategies that allow them to parent effectively, even under stress.

The following protective factors have been linked to a lower incidence of child abuse and neglect:

- **Nurturing and attachment:** When parents and children have strong, warm feelings for one another, children develop trust that parents will provide what they need to thrive.

- **Knowledge of parenting and of child and youth development:** Parents who understand how children grow and develop can provide an environment where children can live up to their potential.

- **Parental resilience:** Parents who are emotionally resilient have a positive attitude, creatively problem solve, effectively address challenges, and are less likely to direct anger and frustration at their children.

- **Social connections:** Trusted and caring family friends provide emotional support to parents by offering encouragement and assistance in facing the daily challenges of raising a family.

- **Concrete supports for parents:** Parents need basic resources such as food, clothing, housing, transportation, and access to essential services that address family-specific needs (such as child care, health care, and mental health services) to ensure the health and well-being of their children.

## You Have the Power to Prevent Child Abuse and Neglect

As an individual and as a member of your community, you have the power to prevent child abuse and neglect. Here are some ways to contribute your ounce—or more—of effort to prevention.

- **Understand the problem:** Child abuse and neglect affect children of all ages, races, and incomes. Most experts believe that actual incidents of abuse and neglect are more numerous than statistics indicate.

- **Understand the terms:** Child abuse and neglect take more than one form. Federal and state laws address four main types of child maltreatment: physical abuse, physical or emotional neglect, sexual abuse, and emotional abuse. Often more than one type of abuse or neglect occurs within families. Some types of maltreatment, such as emotional abuse, are much harder to substantiate than others, such as physical abuse.

- **Understand the causes:** Most parents don't hurt or neglect their children intentionally. Many were themselves abused or neglected. Very young or inexperienced parents might not know how to take care of their babies or what they can reasonably expect from children at different stages of development. Circumstances that place families under extraordinary stress—for instance, poverty, divorce, sickness, disability—sometimes take their toll in child maltreatment. Parents who abuse alcohol or other drugs are more likely to abuse or neglect their children.

- **Support programs that support families:** Parent education, community centers, respite care services, and substance abuse treatment programs help to protect children by addressing circumstances that place families at risk for child abuse and neglect. Donate your time or money, if you can.

- **Report suspected abuse and neglect:** Some states require everyone to report suspected abuse or neglect; others specify members of certain professions, such as educators and doctors. But whether or not you are mandated by law to report child abuse and neglect, doing so may save a child—and a family. If you suspect a child is being abused or neglected, call the police or your local child welfare agency.

- **Spread the word:** Help educate others in your community about child abuse and neglect.

- **Strengthen the fabric of your community:** Know your neighbors' names and the names of their children, and make sure they know yours. Give stressed parents a break by offering to watch their children. Volunteer. If you like interacting with children, great, but you do not have to volunteer directly with kids to contribute to prevention. All activities that strengthen communities, such as service to civic clubs and participation on boards and committees, ultimately contribute to the well-being of children.

- **Be ready in an emergency:** We've all witnessed the screaming-child-in-the-supermarket scenario. If we are parents, at least once that screaming child has been ours. Most parents take the typical tantrum in stride. But what if you witness a scene—in the supermarket or anywhere else—where you believe a child is being, or is about to be, physically or verbally abused? Responding in these circumstances technically moves beyond prevention to intervention, and intervention is best handled by professionals. Still, if you find yourself in a situation where you believe a child is being or will be abused at that moment, there are steps you can take. Prevent Child Abuse America suggests the following:

  - Talk to the adult to get their attention away from the child. Be friendly.

  - Say something like, "Children can really wear you out, can't they?" or "My child has done the same thing."

  - Ask if you can help in any way—could you carry some packages? Play with an older child so the baby can be fed or changed? Call someone on your cell phone?

  - If you see a child alone in a public place—for example, unattended in a grocery cart—stay with the child until the parent returns.

Finally—and most important if you are a parent—remember that prevention, like most positive things, begins at home. Take time to re-evaluate your parenting skills. Be honest with yourself—are you yelling at your children a lot or hitting them? Do you enjoy being a parent at least most of the time? If you could benefit from some help with parenting, seek it—getting help when you need it is an essential part of being a good parent. Talk to a professional that you trust; take a parenting class; read a book about child development.

## For More Information

### Parents Anonymous, Inc.
675 W. Foothill Blvd., Suite 220
Claremont, CA 91711
Phone: 909-621-6184
Fax: 909-625-6304
Website: http://www.parentsanonymous.org
E-mail: parentsanonymous@parentsanonymous.org

### Prevent Child Abuse America
500 N. Michigan Ave., Suite 200
Chicago, IL 60611
Toll-Free: 800-244-5373
Phone: 312-663-3520
Fax: 312-939-8962
Website: http://www.preventchildabuse.org
E-mail: mailbox@preventchildabuse.org

Chapter 49

# Four Strategies for Preventing Child Sexual Abuse

## Back-to-School Safety In and Out of the Classroom

The beginning of the school year is a great time for adults to review their understanding of the four R's of preventing child sexual abuse—**R**ules, **R**ead, **R**espect, and **R**esponsibility—and to get back to the basics of nurturing kids. Prevention promotes healthy behaviors rather than waiting to punish violations, before there's any need for a cure.

## Four R's of Prevention

**Rules (noun):** Principles set forth to guide behavior or action. Example: Everyone's safer when everyone knows and is clear about the rules for what's considered acceptable behavior.

**Respect (noun):** To show consideration or thoughtfulness in relation to somebody. Example: Support others with respect to live up to the generally accepted rules and expectations for positive interactions, all the time.

**Read (verb):** To interpret the information conveyed by movements, signs, or signals; an understanding of something by experience or

"The Four R's of Prevention," © 2007 Stop It Now! (www.stopitnow). Reprinted with permission.

intuitive means. Example: Regularly read what's going on around you and trust your instincts to stay aware of concerning behaviors.

**Responsibility (noun):** The state, fact, or position of being accountable to somebody or for something. Example: Responsibility for keeping kids safe belongs to every adult in the community, every day.

With the beginning of the school year, teachers, coaches, other kids' parents, even popular students are assuming new roles of influence or authority over children. Clear, shared guidelines—the rules—about what kids should expect from these relationships let everyone know what's acceptable and what's considered questionable, long before there's a problem.

Respect is the cornerstone of sexual abuse prevention—both as a way to define what makes behavior acceptable and as an essential communication tool when concerns arise. Respectful behavior is the opposite of abusive behavior.

Regularly reading the situations where kids play, learn, and work is an important part of prevention. To create sexually safe environments, learn to read and redirect potentially harmful behavior—like ignoring a child's limits around hugs, kisses, or tickling—before a child is harmed. Remember, the focus is prevention, not cure. Signs or signals that someone is struggling to control his or her impulses are often visible long before any sexually harmful actions.

Kids have the right to count on those with authority or influence to stay within the bounds of their particular roles: to take responsibility to follow and enforce the expected rules. Whether the lesson is math or religion, soccer or swimming, successful learning demands a level of openness and intimacy. Good teachers, coaches, and others inspire kids to overcome challenges with imagination, creativity, and humor. But over time, some may consciously or unconsciously begin to ignore or gradually change the terms of the relationship, using things like secret understandings, suggestive jokes, or belittling other authority figures to engage kids. Even when there is no harmful intention, regularly breaking the expected rules can leave everyone guessing about what's okay and create openings to veer off from healthy behaviors.

And don't forget—older siblings, star athletes, popular students, and other kids may need help managing their influence over other children. As they mature, young people increasingly look to peers for cues about rules, often leading to confusion or misinformation. But the ultimate responsibility to provide guidance about safe relationships lies with the adults. Despite what they may say, kids depend on it.

- **Decide on the rules:** Talk with friends about what are appropriate rules for those in different roles of authority or influence. Then make your expectations clear to anyone influencing kids.

- **Practice "reading" children's relationships:** Stay aware of the signs or patterns of change. Honor your instincts. Then speak up. Ask questions. Talk through your concerns with others.

- **Be a role model of respect:** Insist that others act respectfully toward you. Stay aware of how your actions affect others. Use firm, respectful language to insist that others honor the rules.

- **Embrace responsibility:** Be accountable. Start one conversation everyday with a friend or family member about how to fulfill adults' responsibility to keep children safe.

Kids shouldn't have the responsibility to recognize and challenge unsafe behaviors. A whole community of responsible adults, reading behaviors, respectfully supporting kids and other adults to understand and follow the rules—that's the best way to prevent sexual abuse. Our kids are counting on us. And after all, an ounce of prevention is worth a pound of cure.

Chapter 50

# Preventing Child Sexual Abuse within Youth-Serving Organizations

Youth-serving organizations strive to create a safe environment for youth, employees, and volunteers so that youth can grow, learn, and have fun. Part of creating a safe environment is making sure that youth are not harmed in any way while participating in organization-sponsored activities. One risk in any organization working directly with youth is child sexual abuse. It is vital that organizations create a culture where child sexual abuse is discussed, addressed, and prevented.

## Balancing Caution and Caring

The same dynamics that create a nurturing environment, and may ultimately protect against child sexual abuse, can also open the doors to sexually abusive behaviors. Research has shown that youth who are emotionally insecure, needy, and unsupported may be more vulnerable to the attentions of offenders. By promoting close and caring relationships between youth and adults, organizations can help youth feel supported and loved and thus reduce their risk of child sexual abuse. But that same closeness between a youth and an adult can also provide the opportunity for abuse to occur. When developing policies for child sexual abuse prevention, organizations must balance the need to keep youth safe with the need to nurture and care for them.

Excerpted from "Preventing Child Sexual Abuse within Youth-Serving Organizations: Getting Started on Policies and Procedures," Centers for Disease Control and Prevention (CDC), 2007. The complete document is available at http://www.cdc.gov/ncipc/dvp/PreventingChildSexualAbuse.pdf.

## Screening and Selecting Employees and Volunteers

**Goal:** To select the best possible people for staff and volunteer positions and to screen out individuals who have sexually abused youth or are at risk to abuse.

**General principles:** Screening for child sexual abuse prevention should be integrated into the general screening and selection process that organizations already employ to choose the best possible candidates for positions. Child sexual abuse prevention should be one of the many areas considered when deciding whom to select. While employee and volunteer screening and selection are important, they should not be the only efforts adopted to prevent child sexual abuse.

### Critical Strategies for Screening and Selecting Employees and Volunteers

By letting applicants know your organization is serious about protecting youth, you may deter some people at risk of abusing youth from applying for staff or volunteer positions.

- Inform applicants about your organization's policies and procedures relevant to child sexual abuse prevention.

- Share your code of conduct or ethics.

- Require applicants to sign a document describing the policies and procedures of your organization to demonstrate their understanding and agreement.

- Ask applicants if they have a problem with any of the policies and procedures.

**Written application:** The written application provides the information you need to assess the background and interests of applicants. Questions should help you determine whether applicants have mature, adult relationships as well as clear boundaries and ethical standards for their conduct with youth.

**Personal interview:** The personal interview provides an opportunity to meet applicants, determine if they are a good fit for your organization, and ask additional questions to screen for child sexual abuse risk factors.

**Reference checks:** These provide additional information about applicants and help verify previous work and volunteer history.

- Obtain verbal—not just written—references for applicants.

- Match references with employment and volunteer history. Is anyone important missing from the references, such as the supervisor from the applicant's most recent job? To provide a more complete picture of the applicant, the references should come from a variety of sources and should not be limited to family members or friends.

- Be aware that many employers will only provide basic information, such as dates of employment or rehiring eligibility. If a former employer will only provide limited information, clarify whether the person providing the reference is limiting information because of company policy.

**Criminal background checks:** Criminal background checks are an important tool in screening and selection; however, they have limitations. Criminal background checks will not identify most sexual offenders because most have not been caught. When this report was published, an efficient, effective, and affordable national background screening system was not available.

## Guidelines on Interactions between Individuals

**Goal:** To ensure the safety of youth in their interactions with employees and volunteers and with each other.

**General principles:** Guidelines on interactions between individuals should be determined by an organization's mission and activities. For example, organizations that promote one-on-one activities between adults and youth may need different interaction guidelines than programs built around group activities. Organizations should develop interaction policies before situations arise. The strategies that follow should be tailored to the developmental age and maturity of the youth, employees, and volunteers. Strategies should also match the cultural context of the population served by the organization.

### Critical Strategies for Guidelines on Interactions between Individuals

**Appropriate and inappropriate or harmful behaviors:** Appropriate, positive interactions among youth and between employees, volunteers, and youth are essential in supporting positive youth development, making youth feel valued, and providing the caring connections that serve as protective factors for youth. Conversely, inappropriate or harmful interactions put youth at risk for adverse physical and emotional outcomes. Organizations should identify behaviors that fall into the categories of appropriate, inappropriate, and harmful. These categorizations can be spelled out in the code of conduct or ethics. Carefully balance the benefits of appropriate interactions with the risks associated with inappropriate interactions.

**Ratios of employees and volunteers to youth:** The goal of setting ratios for the numbers of employees and volunteers to youth is to ensure the safety of the youth. There is no standard ratio for all situations. Consider contextual variables such as the age and developmental level of youth and employees or volunteers, risk of the activity, and location of the activity when making decisions about ratios.

Encourage employees and volunteers to actively interact with the youth to maintain adequate supervision and monitoring. Even with a satisfactory ratio of employees and volunteers to youth, the youth are not being monitored if all of the employees and volunteers are immersed in their own conversations in a corner of the room.

## Monitoring Behavior

**Goal:** To prevent, recognize, and respond to inappropriate and harmful behaviors and to reinforce appropriate behaviors.

**General principles:** Monitoring involves observing interactions and reacting appropriately. This includes both, employee or volunteer with youth, and youth with youth interactions. Youth leaders often require more supervision and monitoring because they are young, may lack judgment, and are harder to screen. Define areas for monitoring based on the organization's mission and activities.

### Critical Strategies for Monitoring Behavior

**Responding to what is observed:** Your organization must be prepared to respond to interactions among youth and between employees or volunteers and youth.

**Roles and responsibilities:** All employees and volunteers should be responsible for monitoring behavior and interactions within the organization. Everyone needs to know how and what to monitor. Define roles and responsibilities by including monitoring within a job description, specifying what employees or volunteers need to do from the very beginning, and providing training.

**Clear reporting structure within organization:** Your organization should have a well-defined reporting structure so people know who to contact if they observe potentially inappropriate or harmful behavior.

**Observation and contact with employees or volunteers:** Each organization should use multiple monitoring methods to get a clear picture of how individuals are interacting.

**Documentation that monitoring has occurred:** Although it may be clear when other child sexual abuse prevention strategies, such as screening or environmental policies, have been implemented in an organization, it is harder to be sure that adequate monitoring is occurring. Documenting that monitoring has occurred emphasizes to employees and volunteers that it is an essential, nonnegotiable part of the organization's child sexual abuse prevention efforts.

## Ensuring Safe Environments

**Goal:** To keep youth from situations in which they are at increased risk for sexual abuse.

**General principles:** Environmental strategies will vary depending on the organization. Strategies will be different for organizations with physical sites (a day care, school), organizations with multiple sites for activities (some sports and recreation organizations), and organizations with leased or undefined space (mentoring organizations). The risk of the environment should be considered regardless of an organization's physical space. If an organization does not control its own space, back-up strategies should be used to ensure that youth, employees, and volunteers can be monitored.

### Critical Strategies for Ensuring Safe Environments

**Visibility:** Building or choosing spaces that are open and visible to multiple people can create an environment where individuals at risk for sexually abusive behaviors do not feel comfortable abusing.

**Privacy when toileting, showering, changing clothes:** Each organization should develop policies and procedures for reducing risk during activities such as toileting, showering, and changing clothes that consider not just the risk of employee or volunteer sexual abuse, but also the risk of inappropriate or harmful contact among youth.

**Access control:** The organization should monitor who is present at all times.

**Off-site activity guidelines:** Each organization should define and communicate its on-site and off-site physical boundaries.

**Transportation policies:** Each organization should define who is responsible for transporting youth to and from regular activities and special events (field trips, overnight trips).

## Additional Strategies to Consider

**Territoriality:** The goal of this strategy is to visually send a message that the program is unified, cohesive, and not permeable to threats. Some examples of this strategy include making navigation easy with signs and overstating the appearance of staff with uniforms or similar clothing.

**Monitoring devices (video cameras):** This strategy implies that there is an infrastructure or staff behind the monitoring devices. If you install these devices, be sure to provide the infrastructure to uphold that implicit promise.

## Responding to Inappropriate Behavior, Breaches in Policy, and Allegations and Suspicions of Child Sexual Abuse

**Goal:** To respond quickly and appropriately to: 1) inappropriate or harmful behavior; 2) infractions of child sexual abuse prevention policies; and, 3) evidence or allegations of child sexual abuse.

**General principles:** The ultimate aim of child sexual abuse prevention efforts within youth-serving organizations is to prevent child sexual abuse from ever occurring; however, an organization needs to have communicated clearly what it and its employees and volunteers should do if policies are violated or if child sexual abuse occurs.

## *Critical Strategies for Responding to Inappropriate Behavior, Breaches in Policy, and Allegations and Suspicions of Child Sexual Abuse*

It is often difficult to find the balance between being vigilant and protective of youth and being so hyper-vigilant that the positive parts of programs (for example, relationships between adults and youth) are lost. In responding, the need for this balance involves recognizing the tension between over-reacting and under-reacting. By developing policies before any inappropriate behavior occurs, your organization can set reasonable expectations for responding.

**Reporting process:** If evidence of child sexual abuse has surfaced or an allegation has been made, a formal report needs to be made to an outside agency. Ensure that your organization's reporting policies are consistent with current state law.

**Internal records:** Although your organization should not investigate allegations or suspicions of child sexual abuse in lieu of reporting them to the authorities, it should develop a system to track allegations and suspicions of child sexual abuse cases.

**Confidentiality policy:** Because of the sensitive nature of child sexual abuse cases, your organization should decide in advance what information should remain private and what information can be made public.

- Withhold the names of potential victims, the accused perpetrator, and the people who made the report to the authorities.

- Decide whether to inform the community that an allegation has been made.

- Ensure that your organization's confidentiality policy is consistent with state legal requirements.

**Response to the press and the community:** Each organization should decide on a strategy for responding to the press and the community before an allegation has been made.

**Membership or employment of alleged offenders:** Remember that an allegation of child sexual abuse does not equate to guilt. The person alleged to have engaged in sexually abusive behavior should not be labeled as an offender or sexual abuser. However, once a suspicion or allegation has been communicated, it needs to be reported to the authorities, and your organization must take certain steps to protect the youth under its care. A decision must be made whether to suspend membership or employment.

### *Additional Strategies to Consider*

**Support for victims and families:** Organizations may want to provide support for victims and their families to help them cope with the sexual abuse.

- Provide referrals for victims and their families to child sexual abuse organizations and counselors or therapists.

- Reimburse victims and families for counseling.

- Offer restorative justice approaches. Restorative practices are a way to have a respectful and safe dialogue when a misunderstanding or harm has occurred.

Chapter 51

# Respite and Crisis Care Can Prevent Child Maltreatment

Respite provides a temporary safe haven and meaningful experience for a child that allows short-term relief for parents or primary family caregivers to attend to their own and other family members' health, social, or emotional needs. It is a preventive strategy that strengthens families, protects their health and well-being, and allows them to continue providing care at home. Respite is an important component of a continuum of comprehensive family support and long-term services that are available to caregivers not only on a planned basis, but also in the event of a crisis or emergency situation.

According to Community Based Child Abuse and Neglect Prevention Grants (CBCAP), Title II of the Child Abuse Prevention and Treatment Act (CAPTA), the term "respite care services" specifically means:

"Short-term care services provided in the temporary absence of the regular caregiver (parent, other relative, foster parent, adoptive parent, or guardian) to children who—(A) are in danger of abuse or neglect; (B) have experienced abuse or neglect; or (C) have disabilities, chronic, or terminal illnesses. Such services shall be provided within or outside the home of the child, be short-term care (ranging from a few hours to a few weeks of time, per year), and be intended to enable the family to stay

Text in this chapter is from "Respite and Crisis Care," Fact Sheet 14, FRIENDS National Resource Center for Community Based Child Abuse and Neglect Prevention Grants (CBCAP), U.S. Department of Health and Human Services (HHS), September 2007.

together and to keep the child living in the home and community of the child."

## Respite Models

Many models of planned respite exist, ideally to be able to meet the particular needs and preferences of the family. Various respite models are provided through state or local disability organizations such as Easter Seals, United Cerebral Palsy, or The Arc, or are privately owned and operated by profit or non-profit entities or individuals. Many public entities, such as schools or community mental health centers, may also be used to support or provide respite services. Models include, but are not limited to the following:

• In-home respite with trained professionals or volunteer providers

• Out-of-home (childcare centers or schools, family day care homes, foster care homes, hospital, or specific respite facility), also using trained or volunteer providers

• Periodic respite (churches, community centers or other community-based organizations that support periodic respite events)

• Summer camps, recreational, or after-school programs

Each model has its benefits and each may be utilized by families at different times depending on their needs and circumstances. However, a full array of available respite options in a particular community may frequently be limited by too few state or local resources, including a lack of qualified respite providers, volunteers, or agencies which provide respite services. Often weekend, evening, and overnight options are extremely limited.

Increasingly, through Medicaid waivers, state or federally supported family support, or respite programs, and even CBCAP funded efforts, respite is available through vouchers which encourage and support consumer direction. Families are considered the employers and are provided funds to purchase their own respite, often selecting, hiring, and training their own providers, who may be neighbors, friends, other family members, or church or civic group volunteers. Families may also purchase respite from existing agencies or providers.

Crisis respite is defined as temporary emergency care for children, available any time of the day or night, when families are facing a crisis and no other safe child care options are available. Crisis respite services are often also referred to as crisis nurseries. Crisis nurseries were first developed in the early 1970s, primarily for children ages 0–5, though many crisis respite programs now accept children of any age. Crisis nursery and crisis respite programs were also designed to offer an array of support services to the families and caregivers of these children. In addition to dedicated center-based crisis respite facilities, crisis respite can be offered in conjunction with homeless or domestic violence shelter services, or in foster or family day care homes.

## Who needs respite and are these families being served?

As a primary prevention service, it could be argued that all families with children face stress and hardship that place them in need of respite at some time in their lives. However, planned and emergency respite services are most often requested and utilized by families of children with physical or emotional disabilities or chronic conditions; families at risk of abuse or neglect who are in or out of the child protective services (CPS) system; grandparents and other kinship care providers; foster and adoptive families; and families in domestic violence situations or in temporary crisis resulting from homelessness, illness, job loss, or other emergency situations.

In 2001, 9.4 million children under age 18 were identified with chronic or disabling conditions. Without adequate family supports, children with disabilities are almost four times more likely to be victims of neglect, physical abuse, or emotional abuse, and almost three times more likely to be victims of sexual abuse than children without disabilities. About 30% of children in foster care have severe emotional, behavioral, or developmental problems, requiring foster families to look to respite for support and a necessary break from caregiving. In addition, approximately 150,000 children ages 5–17 with at least one disability are adopted, increasing the pool of families who could benefit from respite, but may not know how or where to find or pay for the supportive service.

Compound this picture with the growing number of grandparent or kinship caregivers. In the United States (U.S.), 6.7 million children, with and without disabilities, are in the primary custody of an aging grandparent or other relative other than their parents. Parental substance abuse, human immunodeficiency virus (HIV)/acquired immune deficiency syndrome (AIDS), incarceration, poverty, death, or military deployment are the reasons more children are now in kinship care. Moreover, the children are likely to exhibit difficult behaviors or have disabilities themselves. Significant percentages of these grandparent caregivers are poor and have access to few resources or supports.

457

CAPTA legislation also requires that CBCAP leads take into account the special needs of parents with disabilities. An estimated ten million families in the U.S., about 15% of all U.S. families, include at least one parent who has a disability. In a national survey, 42% of parents with disabilities reported facing attitudinal barriers including discrimination, and 15% of parents with disabilities reported attempts to have their children taken away from them. A comprehensive approach to prevention necessitates that these families' special needs for respite and other supports are taken into account.

State and local surveys have shown respite to be the most frequently requested service of parents and other family caregivers. Yet respite is unused, in short supply, inaccessible, or unaffordable to many of the nation's family caregivers. In a study of a nationally representative profile of noninstitutionalized children ages 0–17 years of age who were receiving support from the supplemental security income (SSI) program because of a disability, only 8% reported using respite care, but three-quarters of families had unmet respite needs. This study suggests a myriad of barriers that prevent families from accessing the respite they need.

A variety of federal, state, and private sources provide some assistance with respite, but the degree of respite and crisis care support varies widely by state and even county. Most respite programs impose restrictive disability, age, and income eligibility criteria that exclude many families, especially families of children with emotional or mental health conditions or physical disabilities, or children with disabilities over age 18 who are still living at home.

In addition, a lack of family resources to pay for care and a reluctance to ask for help, are significant barriers to respite access. Moreover, a critically short supply of qualified or trained respite providers, too few respite options available on weekends or evenings, a lack of state and community fiscal resources to sustain or expand programs, and limited information on how and where to find and pay for respite result in long waiting lists for services, or in the case of crisis care, families turned away in the midst of a crisis.

In 2006, Congress enacted the Lifespan Respite Care Act to assist states in coordinating state and federal funding streams and approve access to respite for all families regardless of age or disability.

## Presenting the Evidence about Respite

While most families take great joy in helping their children with disabling or chronic conditions to live at home, it has been well documented that family caregivers experience physical and emotional problems and undue levels of stress directly related to their caregiving responsibilities. Respite has been shown to help alleviate the stress resulting from caring for a child with a disabling or chronic condition—the very stress that is often a precursor to abuse or neglect.

State lifespan respite programs are statewide systems up and running in Oklahoma, Oregon, Nebraska, and Wisconsin to improve respite coordination and delivery for families regardless of age or disability. These lifespan respite programs have been able to demonstrate that with increased access to respite, families have demonstrated lower levels of stress and isolation, the precursors to abuse or neglect.

- In a survey of Nebraska's family caregivers, respite was shown to reduce feelings of stress and isolation. The survey found that one out of four families with children under 21 reported that they were less likely to place their child in out-of-home care once respite services were available. In addition, 79% of the respondents reported decreased stress and 58% reported decreased isolation.

- Data from an outcomes evaluation project conducted by the Respite Care Association of Wisconsin demonstrated that provision of respite significantly reduced caregiver stress, stress-related health problems, and social isolation. Furthermore, respondents reported reduced likelihood of institutionalization of the person with special needs and reduced likelihood of divorce.

Respite and crisis care have also shown promise in helping to avoid or delay out-of-home placements for children and sustaining marriage. A study of Vermont's well-established respite care program for families with children or adolescents with serious emotional disturbance found that participating families experienced fewer out-of-home placements than nonusers and were more optimistic about their future capabilities to take care of their children. Data from an ARCH outcome-based evaluation pilot study show that respite may also reduce the likelihood of divorce and help sustain marriages.

As discussed, respite as a post-adoption service is essential to support families who have adopted children with special needs, especially medically fragile children and children with physical or emotional disorders.

Even more dramatic results were found in a study of parents who adopt children with special needs, many of whom were grandparent caregivers in a respite program in southern California. During the three years of the program, services were provided to substantially more families and children than initially intended, and these services were associated with substantially reduced stress levels among parents providing care to special-needs adopted children; improved family relationships in the adoptive families; increased ability of adoptive parents to participate in social and recreational activities; and reduction of risk factors that increase likelihood of abuse and neglect, specifically, parental stress and strain on family relationships.

In assessing the prevention of child abuse and neglect as an outcome, an evaluation of crisis nursery services for five crisis nurseries in Illinois from 2000 to 2003 based on analysis of administrative data reported to the Illinois Department of Human Services (IDHS) found that caregiver reported perception of risk of maltreatment improved during each of the three years studied. In fiscal year (FY) 2003, 98% of the 745 caregivers completing evaluations reported a reduced risk of maltreatment, up from 73% of 248 caregivers who completed evaluations in FY 2001. In FY 2003, 90% also reported a decrease in stress. An evaluation of a pilot crisis child care project in a rural midwestern state found that in comparisons of child maltreatment rates, there was a significant decrease in the reported incidence of child maltreatment in rural counties with a crisis child care program compared with counties that did not offer this intervention.

The most recent study conducted by researchers at the Access to Respite Care and Help (ARCH) National Respite Network utilized two groups of families in northern California who were compared using data from child protective services (CPS) administrative records. Families in all groups were matched prior to analysis. The comparison group, Group A, comprised families in counties without crisis respite but who would have been appropriate for services had they been available. The target group comprised families who received crisis respite. This group was further subdivided into two groups: Group B, families with previous histories with CPS; and Group C, families who received crisis respite and had no prior CPS involvement. The children who received care were at high risk for maltreatment when brought to the crisis respite facilities. The study found that the parents who received crisis respite services had an increased number of CPS referrals. It is hypothesized that this outcome occurred because families utilizing services received an increased level of scrutiny by mandated reporters than families not engaged in services. However, those reports are far less likely to be substantiated than reports on children who did not receive crisis respite, suggesting that the children are less likely to have experienced abuse or neglect than the children in a comparison group. Over a quarter of the families using crisis respite thought it was likely that their children might have been placed in foster care had the nurseries not been available.

Respite is not only effective in protecting children, it is low cost. In a joint study conducted by the Child Welfare League of America (CWLA) and ARCH, it was estimated that the costs for CWLA and ARCH agencies to provide planned respite were similar, about $10 per hour, which is less costly in both financial and social terms than placing children in out-of-home care. The national average (non-specialized) foster care maintenance payment was $4,832 per year in 1998, while ARCH estimates that providing 12 hours of respite each month costs $1,422.88 per year. The voucher program is especially cost effective. Oklahoma's Lifespan Respite Program serves approximately 2200 caregivers annually with vouchers. The average cost for the respite vouchers has been between $5.62 and $5.87 per hour, compared with $12.80 to $26.50 per hour if the caregiver had chosen a provider from a private or public agency.

## CBCAP Agencies Take the Lead in Supporting Respite

The Idaho CBCAP program uses part of its allocation to provide respite to underserved populations. Respite care was a special initiative during fiscal year 2006 with the Idaho Children's Trust Fund funding a multi-year grant to provide respite care in a rural community. In addition, CBCAP funds are used to assist Children's Mental Health and the Idaho Respite Coalition in working to provide respite care to families who are raising children with mental health diagnoses.

In Wisconsin, the Wisconsin Respite Care Association is working with the state Children's Trust Fund to prevent initial occurrences of child abuse and neglect by targeting planned or emergency respite care to families exhibiting risk factors. The organization is currently working to: establish regional partnerships to coordinate resources and deliver direct respite care services; establish guidelines and standards for programs and providers; establish evaluation protocol; and provide training and technical assistance.

Nebraska uses its CBCAP funds to support respite in several ways. The Exceptional Family Resource Center in McCook received CBCAP funding to provide respite for families of children with disabilities. CBCAP helped expand respite in an eleven county area in Western Nebraska through Lifespan Respite Subsidies for Families. A new respite program was funded through the YWCA in Lincoln to provide services for children ages six weeks to 12 years, including children with disabilities.

461

In Alabama, the Children's Trust Fund uses CBCAP funds to contract with United Cerebral Palsy–Huntsville to provide respite vouchers or home health respite in five counties through the Alabama Lifespan Respite Network. Under the voucher program, families of children with disabilities or chronic conditions up to age 19 are eligible for quarterly vouchers and may hire and train anyone of their choosing as long as they are 18 or older and do not reside in the home.

Chapter 52

# Home Visiting Programs That Reduce Child Maltreatment

Congress recognized the preventative value of home visitation in the legislation authorizing Title II of the Child Abuse Prevention and Treatment Act, the Community-Based Grants for Child Abuse and Neglect Prevention (CBCAP), when it identified home visiting as one of the core child abuse and neglect prevention services that state CBCAP lead agencies are to fund if practicable. A significant number of state CBCAP programs are funding a variety of home visitation models. The purpose of this chapter is to provide an overview of selected programs, but is not meant to be a comprehensive review of the home visitation research, which has burgeoned in recent years.

Research evidence in the late 1980s and early 1990s provided promising results for the effectiveness of home visiting programs. Such programs first received heightened national recognition in 1991 from the U.S. Advisory Board on Child Abuse and Neglect, which gave top priority to its recommendation for universal neonatal home visitation as a child abuse prevention strategy. In 2003, the Centers for Disease Control and Prevention (CDC) did a systematic review of the literature which led them to conclude that home visiting programs can be effective in reducing maltreatment.

Since the early 1990s, private and public funding for home visiting programs increased greatly and the research field has blossomed.

---

Text in this chapter is excerpted from "Home Visiting Programs: A Brief Overview of Selected Models," Fact Sheet 15, FRIENDS National Resource Center for Community-Based Grants for Child Abuse and Neglect Prevention (CBCAP), U. S. Department of Health and Human Services, December 2007.

Home visiting programs now number in the thousands. One estimate suggests that as many 400,000 children and families are being reached by home visiting programs annually across the nation at a cost of perhaps $750 million to $1 billion.

A variety of home visiting models exist and differ in many technical aspects, such as the target population, the experience and credentials of the home visitor, the duration and intensity of the visits, and the end goal or focus of the intervention. Yet, the common ground that unites home visiting program models is the importance placed on infant and child development from birth to three years, the idea that parents play a pivotal role in shaping children's lives, and that often the best way to reach families with young children is by bringing services to their front door. Home visitors can view the environments in which the families live, gain a better understanding of the families needs, and therefore tailor services to meet those needs.

### *What does the research say?*

The literature has shown that home visiting programs can produce benefits for children and parents. However, most programs, with a few exceptions, produce modest benefits. Services appear to be most beneficial for families when the initial need is greatest or where parents perceive that children need the services because of low birthweight, special needs, or behavioral problems. The most successful home visiting efforts with longer lasting results are those that are offered in conjunction with center-based early childhood education. Focusing on the intensity of services that families receive, bolstering home visitors' skills, and improving the content of the home visiting curriculum could significantly improve the quality of current home visiting services.

Employing additional characteristics that have been identified in effective home visiting programs could also improve the expected outcomes such as:

- internal consistency (do what they say they will do),
- long-term availability,
- parents approached as partners,
- well trained and well supervised program staff,
- home visitors with capacity to form relationships and model positive relationships with families,
- low caseloads (12–15), and
- linkages to other services in the community.

Though there is a large body of research evidence in support of home visiting services, the field is not without some disagreement. A randomized trial by Duggan and colleagues (2004), considered to be a well conducted study, found that the Healthy Start Hawaii program (the predecessor to Healthy Families America) was ineffective in preventing either self-reported or officially reported child maltreatment. In an invited commentary, Chaffin (2004) questioned whether child abuse prevention advocates have too eagerly accepted the effectiveness of home visiting programs based on weak research evidence.

Many prevention advocates and researchers who are well-versed in the home visiting literature responded by acknowledging that ongoing research and evaluation is critical to developing quality programs and services. Therefore, it has been recommended that home visiting programs and models strive to be learning organizations and use data to further their decision-making regarding program improvements. Some concede that home visiting programs were never intended to be a silver bullet for all that afflicts families, and must be used to help connect families to additional services if needed. Moreover, the nature and quality of program implementation has a critical impact on intervention effectiveness. The relative importance of program logistics (type of home visitor, staff retention, family retention, duration of services) is still somewhat controversial in home visiting discussions, but adherence to program fidelity is crucial to deliver desired results. All of these considerations must be taken into account when selecting a home visiting model that best serves the special needs of the local community.

### Challenges for Implementation

A myriad of challenges exist for implementation of successful home visitation efforts. It is important to note that programs are not universally successful: 20–30% families don't participate long enough for expected outcomes to emerge, especially for families with mental health, substance abuse, or domestic violence issues who are typically much harder to engage. In addition, the agencies that provide mental health, healthcare, foster care, and child protective services that must interact with families can impose their own set of barriers and challenges. The working conditions for home visitors also pose additional challenges, especially when available resources are insufficient. High turnover, low levels of compensation, and safety issues for home visitors can compromise program fidelity and the overall quality of the program.

## Models of Home Visiting

### Early Head Start
Website: http://www.ehsnrc.org

**Target population:** Infants and toddlers from low income families, 10% of enrollees are children with disabilities.

**Service intensity and duration:** Each family receives one 90-minute visit per week, totaling 52 visits per year. Visits are done by professionals who receive training in child development, family development, and community building.

**Intended outcomes:** Positive child development, school readiness, child and maternal mental health, and successful social relationships.

**Approximate cost:** In 2002, the average cost per child was $10,544.

### Healthy Families America (HFA)
Website: http://www.healthyfamiliesamerica.org

**Target population:** At risk families identified by Family Stress Checklist and Kempe Assessment. Enrollment before child reaches three months of age continuing to age five years.

**Service intensity and duration:** Weekly home visits are done by trained paraprofessionals during at least the first six months of the child's life with intensity decreasing based on family need.

**Intended outcomes:** Positive parent-child bonding, optimal child health and development, enhanced parental self-sufficiency, and prevention of child abuse and neglect.

**Approximate cost:** $3,500 per year, per family.

### Healthy Steps
Website: http://www.healthysteps.org

**Target population:** Low to medium risk parents of children ages birth to 30 months of age.

**Service intensity and duration:** The Healthy Steps protocol recommends six home visits done by a nurse, child development specialist, or a social worker.

**Intended outcomes:** Development of a close relationship between health care professionals and parents to address the physical, emotional, and intellectual growth and development of children from birth to age three, removal of environmental hazards while in the home, improvement of parents understanding of child development.

**Approximate cost:** Between $402 and $933 per family in 2000 dollars.

### Home-Based Instruction for Parents of Preschool Youngsters (HIPPY)
Website: http://www.hippyusa.org

**Target population:** Universal for children ages 3–5 years.

**Service intensity and duration:** Biweekly home visits and biweekly group meetings for two to three years. Home visitors are members of the participating communities and are also parents in the program. Visitors are supervised by a professional coordinator.

**Intended outcomes:** Early literacy, school readiness, and parental involvement.

**Approximate cost:** $1,250 per year, per family.

### Nurse-Family Partnership
Website: http://www.nursefamilypartnership.org

**Target population:** First-time, low-income mothers, early pregnancy through age two years (families must enroll in early pregnancy).

**Service intensity and duration:** Home visits occurring weekly to monthly conducted by public health nurses for approximately three years.

**Intended outcomes:** Improved prenatal health, fewer childhood injuries, fewer subsequent pregnancies, increased intervals between births, increased maternal employment, and improved school readiness.

**Approximate cost:** $5,000 per year, per family.

## Parent-Child Program
Website: http://www.parent-child.org

**Target population:** At-risk parents and children ages 16 months through age four years.

**Service intensity and duration:** Home visits twice weekly for 30 min. each visit for two years (23 weeks with 46 visits is minimum amount of weeks and visits that constitute a program year). The local sponsoring agency hires a site coordinator who is then trained by the Parent-Child Home Program's national center. These site coordinators then recruit and train home visitors.

**Intended outcomes:** Early literacy, increased school readiness, enhanced social-emotional development, and strengthened parent-child relationships.

**Approximate cost:** $2,400 per year, per family.

## Parents as Teachers
Website: http://parentsasteachers.org

**Target population:** Universal for pregnancy through age five years.

**Service intensity and duration:** Home visits weekly to monthly by trained paraprofessionals from pregnancy through age five years. Families can enroll any time during this period.

**Intended outcomes:** Increased parent knowledge of early childhood development and improved parenting practices, early detection of developmental delays and health issues, prevention of child abuse and neglect, and increased school readiness.

**Approximate cost:** $2,000 per year, per family.

# Chapter 53

# *Parent Mutual Self-Help Support Groups*

Parent mutual self-help support groups play an active role in strengthening families. In group settings, families find support and gain information, both of which help parents develop resilience and the ability to better handle life's stressful events. The premise of parent mutual self-help support groups is that they help promote protective factors.

Through its Strengthening Families Initiative, the Center for the Study of Social Policy has determined that there are five protective factors paramount in the prevention of child abuse and neglect. As adapted by the Community-Based Child Abuse Prevention Program (CBCAP), these five protective factors are:

- nurturing and attachment of the children,
- knowledge of effective parenting,
- knowledge of child and youth development,
- parental resilience, and
- social connections and solid support for parents.

Parent mutual self-help support groups adhere to these five guidelines in their core philosophy and have gained national recognition

"The Role of Parent Mutual Support," Fact Sheet 17, FRIENDS National Resource Center for Community-Based Child Abuse Prevention (CBCAP), U.S. Department of Health and Human Services (HHS), July 2008.

in the campaign to prevent child abuse and neglect. Over the past four decades, research on risk factors and conditions associated with child abuse and neglect have pointed to the need for social support and the benefits that a parent support group can provide.

There are many justifications for parent support groups. Parent self-help support groups encourage families to interact with their neighbors and within their communities which is instrumental in the prevention of child abuse and neglect. A goal of parent support groups is to empower participants and parents with a healthy mental outlook have a lower risk of child abuse and neglect. Support groups are logistically versatile because they can be offered in conjunction with other programs that focus on the prevention of child abuse and neglect, and implementation costs can be low. Parent mutual support groups are inclusive, embracing fathers, grandparents, and other relatives who help care for children. The groups can address many challenges for parents, such as caring for children with special needs, addressing substance abuse problems, or—most recently—responding constructively to the aftermath of natural disasters (Falconer, 2006; Gay, 2005).

Congress recognized the value of parent mutual support groups in the legislation authorizing CBCAP, which identifies parent mutual support as one of the core child abuse and neglect prevention services that state lead agencies are to fund. A significant number of state CBCAP programs are funding parent mutual support programs as stand-alone efforts or as part of more comprehensive strategies (FRIENDS, 2007).

## Models of Mutual Self-Help Support Groups

Nationally, two models of parent mutual self-help support groups have demonstrated that such groups can promote protective factors and reduce risk factors, helping to strengthen families and protect children: Parents Anonymous, Inc.®, and Circle of Parents, Inc. Both also promote the principles of shared leadership and parent leadership.

The Parents Anonymous® and Circle of Parents models are based on practices that are parent-centered, parent-led, and parent-driven and are guided by the following principles:

• Parent mutual self-help support that is ongoing

• Support to address current family issues during support group meetings

- Positive parenting skills and healthy parent-child relationships
- Connection to valuable community services and support for the well-being of families and children
- Effective partnerships between practitioners and parents to strengthen families and children
- Parent leadership promoted within the support group, in the community, and at state and national levels

## What the Research Shows

Current research finds a number of positive benefits of parent mutual support.

Recent research by the National Council on Crime and Delinquency, funded by the Office of Juvenile Justice and Delinquency Prevention, U.S. Department of Justice, found reduced child maltreatment, reduced risk factors, and increased protective factors among a nationally representative sample of parents who participated in Parents Anonymous® groups over a six-month period. Parents Anonymous® is the nation's oldest child abuse prevention organization; it has 267 accredited organizations and local affiliates and an evidence-based program to help prevent child abuse and neglect (NCCD, 2007).

### *Statistically Significant Results*

Reduced child maltreatment outcomes:

- 73% of parents decreased their distress;
- 65% of parents decreased their rigidity;
- 56% of parents reduced use of psychological aggression towards their children; and
- for parents who reported using physical aggression, 83% stopped physically abusing their children.

Reduced risk factors:

- 86% of high-stressed parents reduced their parental stress;
- 71% of parents reduced their life stressors;
- 40% of parents reduced any form of domestic violence; and
- 32% of parents reduced their drug/alcohol use.

Increased protective factors:

- 67% of parents improved their quality of life;
- for parents starting out needing improvement, 90% improved in emotional and instrumental support;
- 88% improved in parenting sense of competence;
- 84% improved in general social support;
- 69% improved in use of non-violent discipline tactics; and
- 67% improved in family functioning.

Additionally, a qualitative study conducted with Hispanic/Latino parents confirmed these results. In summary, parents who continued to attend Parents Anonymous® groups over time showed improvement in child maltreatment outcomes and risk and protective factors compared to those who dropped out. Strong evidence suggests that parents benefit and strengthen their families through Parents Anonymous® regardless of the participant's race, gender, education, or income.

Ongoing evaluations also have been conducted with parents attending Circle of Parents support groups in Florida, Minnesota, and Washington. In Florida, participants in most parent support groups are surveyed each quarter using a retrospective pretest methodology. All measures are based on self-reports by parent participants. In Minnesota, Circle of Parent participants are surveyed once a year. The research design is longitudinal and allows measurement of changes in parenting behaviors across multiple years. In Washington, as in Florida, the surveys are "slice-in-time" surveys that combine pre-measures and post-measures in one tool (Falconer, 2006)

In one overall assessment, similar performance outcomes were compared.

**Table 53.1.** Performance Outcomes of Parent Support Groups

|  | Florida | Washington |
|---|---|---|
| Percentage of participants who improved the quality of the parent/child relationship | 67.6% | 72% |
| Percentage of participants who improved their parenting skills | 74.5% | 78% |
| Percentage of participants who improved their support system awareness and use | 70.1% | 71% |

In Florida's 2005–2006 evaluation of the Florida Ounce of Prevention's Circle of Parents program, 79.9% of participants improved their self-management skills (Minnesota and Washington did not assess this outcome in their latest evaluation). Minnesota reported statistically significant improvements among participants in their quality of the parent/child relationships, and in parenting skills. In both Florida and Washington, as the number of support group sessions attended increased, the percentage of participants who improved for each protective factor outcome measure also increased.

Finally, additional research conducted at Wichita State University in collaboration with the Kansas Children's Service League found that Latino families living in rural areas where they face language barriers, isolation, and few support systems benefit from parent mutual self-help support groups. A hundred and eighteen members of Parents Helping Parents (PHP) groups in seven rural counties in Kansas were surveyed. Their responses indicate they rely on the support group for information and support for parenting. Among protective factors, 78% of participants said they received information on child development, 74% indicated an increase in positive parenting skills, and 86% gained information on how to cope with difficult life situations (Wituk, et al, 2001).

Additional small-scale evaluations have been conducted on other free-standing programs. For example, a New York City program for grandparent caregivers of children with disabilities held six group sessions for study participants. A wait-list control group was offered the intervention post-test assessment three months after the intervention for the treatment group. Compared with the control group, the experimental group recorded a decrease in depressive symptoms, an increase in family empowerment, and an improvement in grandparents' sense of caregiving (McCallion, Janicki, and Kolomer, 2004).

## Conclusion

Overall, parent mutual self-help support groups are effective in helping to increase protective factors in the prevention of child abuse and neglect. Through the concepts of shared leadership and parent leadership, parents become empowered to actively promote the well-being of their families and to seek out and advocate for resources in their communities. Through parent involvement in support groups, parents begin to develop relationships in their communities, which connect them to the support and services they need to enhance the quality of life for themselves and their children.

# References

Falconer, M. K. 2006. *Mutual Self-Help Parent Support Groups in the Prevention of Child Abuse and Neglect.* The Ounce of Prevention Fund of Florida. Available at http://www.ounce.org/pdf/Mutual_Self_Help_Support_Group_White_Paper.pdf. Accessed October 22, 2007.

FRIENDS National Resource Center. 2007. *FY06 Performance Report Summaries: Reports submitted by states in December of 2006 and reflect activities from Federal Fiscal Year 2005 CBCAP Grant Award.* Chapel Hill, NC: Author. Available at http://www.friendsnrc.org/resources/06sum.htm. Accessed October 22, 2007.

Gay, K. D. (2005). The Circle of Parents Program: Increasing Social Support for Parents and Caregivers. *North Carolina Medical Journal,* 66 (5).

McCallion, P, Janicki, M.P., and Kolomer, S. 2004. Controlled evaluation of support groups for grandparent caregivers of children with developmental disabilities and delays. *American Journal on Mental Retardation,* 109(5), 352–361.

Parents Anonymous, Inc. 2007. *Parents Anonymous, Inc. Prevents Child Abuse and Neglect: New Research Demonstrates Evidence-Based Programs, Strengthening Families around the World.* Available at http:// www.parentsanonymous.org/pahtml/eviBased1a.html. Accessed October 22, 2007.

Pion-Berlin, L. and Polinsky, M. L. 2000. *Research Profiles.* Parents Anonymous, Inc., Research Series: No. 1.

Wituk, S, Commer, A, Lindstrom, J, and Meisen, Greg. 2001. The Benefits of Parenting Self-Help Groups for Rural Latino Parents. *Journal of Rural Community Psychology,* Vol. E4(1). Available at http://www.marshall.edu/jrcp/WituckSI.htm. Accessed October 22, 2007.

## For More Information

**Parents Anonymous, Inc.**
675 W. Foothill Blvd., Suite 220
Claremont, CA 91711-3475
Phone: 909-621-6184
Fax: 909-625-6304

Website: http://www.parentsanonymous.org
E-mail: parentsanonymous@parentsanonymous.org

## *Circle of Parents*

500 N. Michigan Ave., Suite 200
Chicago, IL 60611
Phone: 312-334-6837
Fax: 312-334-6852
Website: http://www.circleofparents.org

Chapter 54

# Parent Education That Helps Prevent Child Maltreatment

Parent education is designed to strengthen and support families and communities to prevent child abuse and neglect. The Child Abuse Prevention and Treatment Act, as reauthorized by the Keeping Children and Families Safe Act of 2003, identifies parent education as a core prevention service. A significant number of Community-Based Child Abuse and Neglect Prevention (CBCAP) grants are funding parent education programs as stand-alone efforts or as part of more comprehensive strategies.

Successful parent education programs help parents acquire and internalize parenting and problem-solving skills necessary to build a healthy family. Research has shown that effective parent training and family interventions promote protective factors and lead to positive outcomes for both parents and children (Lundahl and Harris, 2006). Protective factors include nurturing and attachment, knowledge of parenting and of child and youth development, parental resilience, social connections, and concrete supports for parents (Child Welfare Information Gateway, U.S. Department of Health and Human Services Children's Bureau, and FRIENDS National Resource Center For Community-Based Child Abuse Prevention, 2008).

---

Text in this chapter is excerpted from "Parent Education," Fact Sheet 16, FRIENDS National Resource Center for Community-Based Child Abuse and Neglect Prevention (CBCAP), U.S. Department of Health and Human Services (HHS), April 2008.

This chapter provides an overview of research regarding some key characteristics and training strategies of successful parent education programs.

## What the Research Shows

Program characteristics and specific training strategies are both key considerations when selecting a parent education program. Program characteristics refer to broader aspects of a program, such as theoretical grounding or how the program is structured, staffed, and evaluated. Training strategies refer to specific teaching methods that have been found to be effective in working directly with parents.

## Key Program Characteristics

The following characteristics have been found to be strong predictors of program effectiveness:

- **Strength-based focus:** A large body of research supports the emphasis on family interventions and education programs that focus on family strengths and resilience instead of family weaknesses. This approach reinforces existing protective factors to prevent the occurrence or reoccurrence of child abuse and neglect (Center for the Study of Social Policy, 2003).

- **Family-centered practice:** Family-centered parent training programs include family skills training and family activities to help children and parents communicate effectively and take advantage of concrete social supports. Family-centered programs also seek to develop training strategies that are culturally appropriate and consistent with the beliefs and principles of families and their communities (Colosi and Dunifon, 2003).

- **Individual and group approaches:** Evidence suggests that a combination of individual and group parent training is the most effective approach when building skills that emphasize social connections and parents' ability to access social supports. However, the individual approach was found to be more effective when serving families in need of specific or tailored services (Lundahl, Nimer, and Parsons, 2006).

- **Qualified staff:** Program success is in large part dependent on qualified staff. Program staff should have a sound theoretical grounding as well as hands-on experience in the classroom or working with families and groups in different settings. Staff should also be able to provide culturally competent services consistent with the values of the family and the community.

- **Targeted service groups:** Learning is enhanced when the participants of each program include a clearly defined group of people with common needs or identifying characteristics (Colosi and Dunifon, 2003). Group characteristics, such as high risk families or working versus nonworking parents, can also help determine the appropriate program duration and intensity (Brown, 2005).

- **Clear program goals and continuous evaluation:** Successful programs maintain individualized and group plans developed in partnership with participants. Progress toward program goals is routinely and effectively evaluated by aggregate analyses using both quantitative and qualitative research methods consistent with the services offered. In addition, these programs have an effective process for gathering consumer feedback and use this information, along with outcome-based evaluation efforts, for continuous quality improvement.

## *Parent Training Strategies*

The following parent training strategies may be employed in a variety of service settings and with multiple target populations. These strategies reinforce protective factors and can be adapted as appropriate to fit program and participant needs.

- **Encourage peer support:** Programs that offer opportunities for parental peer support have a positive impact on children's cognitive outcomes. Peer support also strengthens family bonds and gives parents an opportunity to share their experiences in constructive settings (Layzer, Goodson, Bernstein, and Price, 2001).

- **Involve fathers:** Research indicates that father involvement in parent training leads to better outcomes and promotes family cooperation and cohesion. Excluding fathers from parent training programs decreases the likelihood of success (Lundahl, Tollefson, Risser, and Lovejoy, 2007).

- **Promote positive family interaction:** Promoting family relationships is a key component of parent education programs and involves strategies to improve family interaction, communication, and parental supervision. Increasing positive parent-child interactions has been found to be associated with larger effects on measures of enhanced parenting behaviors (Kaminski, Valle, Filene, and Boyle, 2007). Strengthening marriages also plays a part in achieving positive family interaction (Brown, 2005).

- **Use interactive training techniques:** Interactive methods, as opposed to didactic lecturing, are a key aspect of successful education programs and include activities such as group discussion, role playing, active modeling, homework exercises, and reviewing videos of effective parenting approaches (Brown, 2005).

- **Provide opportunities to practice new skills:** Requiring parents to practice new skills with their children during parent training sessions is consistently associated with greater effectiveness of parent education programs. Specific skills associated with larger effects on parent and child behavior include emotional communication skills, the use of time-out, and parenting consistency. These were found to be more effective than other common strategies, such as teaching parents problem-solving skills or ways to promote children's cognitive, academic, or social skills (Kaminski et al., 2007; Lundahl, and Harris, 2006).

## Evidence-Based and Evidence-Informed Programs

This section lists selected parent education curricula that have been included on various registries of evidence-based and evidence-informed programs. Each focuses on specific risk and protective factors. Curriculum availability will vary, and some programs require specific training for group facilitators.

The following list is by no means all-inclusive. It does not constitute an endorsement of any particular program and is provided only as a descriptive tool.

### Guiding Good Choices®
Toll-Free: 800-477-4776
Website: http://www.channing-bete.com/prevention-programs/
guiding-good-choices

**Program objectives:** Give parents the skills they need to help reduce their children's risk for using alcohol and other drugs by enhancing family management and communication skills.

**Target population:** Parents of children ages 9–14. Delivery setting and format: Conducted at convenient locations once per week; take-home self-study program or family workshops available.

**Duration:** Five 2-hour workshops.

**Training resources:** Workshop guide, video, family guide, and visual aids.

## The Incredible Years
1411 8ᵗʰ Ave. W.
Seattle, WA 98119
Toll-Free: 888-506-3562
Phone: 206-285-7565
Fax: 888-506-3562
Website: http://www.incredibleyears.com
E-mail: incredibleyears@incredibleyears.com

**Program objectives:** Strengthen parenting competencies (monitoring, positive discipline, confidence) and foster parents' involvement in children's school experiences in order to promote children's academic, social, and emotional competencies and reduce conduct problems.

**Target population:** Parents, teachers, and children ages 3–12 (individual curricula may be used separately or in combination).

**Delivery setting and format:** Conducted in a community agency, outpatient clinic, or school in groups of 12–16 parents or groups of six children.

**Duration:** The basic parent training program is 12–14 weeks. The child training program is 18–22 weeks. The advanced parent program is a supplemental program. Basic training plus advanced training takes 18–22 weeks.

**Training resources:** Program manual and staff training available.

## Nurturing Parenting Programs®
Family Development Resources
Toll-Free: 800-688-5822
Website: http://www.nurturingparenting.com

**Program objectives:** Build nurturing parenting skills as an alternative to abusive and neglectful parenting and childrearing practices, in order to prevent recidivism in families receiving social services, lower the rate of teenage pregnancies, reduce the rate of juvenile delinquency and alcohol abuse, and stop the intergenerational cycle of child abuse.

**Target population:** Parents with children birth to five years old, 5–11 years old, and 12–18 years old. Programs for school-age children 5–11 years old and teens 12–18 years old are also offered.

**Delivery setting and format:** Conducted in birth family homes, community agencies, departments of mental health, departments of social services, parent education programs, prisons, residential care facilities, and schools, in groups of 8–12 adults. Children meet in a separate group.

**Duration:** 12–48 weeks.

**Training resources:** Training manual available.

### *Parent-Child Interaction Therapy (PCIT)*
Child Study Laboratory
Department of Clinical and Health Psychology
University of Florida
P.O. Box 100165
Gainesville, FL 32610
Phone: 352-273-5239
Website: http://www.pcit.org

**Program objectives:** Strengthen the parent-child bond, decrease harsh and ineffective discipline-control tactics, improve child social skills and cooperation, and reduce child negative or maladaptive behaviors.

**Target population:** Children ages 3–6 years with parent-child relationship and behavior problems and may be conducted with parents, foster parents, or other caretakers. Program adaptation available for physically abusive parents with children ages 4–12 years.

**Delivery setting and format:** Conducted in a community agency or outpatient clinic in groups of three or four families during a 90-minute session. It allows time for individual coaching of each parent-child group while the other groups observe and provide feedback.

**Duration:** Average number of sessions is 14, but varies from 10–20 sessions.

**Training resources:** 40 hours of direct training, with ongoing supervision and consultation for approximately 4–6 months; a manual is used during sessions with families.

### *ParentMagic, Inc.*
800 Roosevelt Rd., B-309
Glen Ellyn, IL 60137
Toll-Free: 800-442-4453
Fax: 800-635-8301
Website: http://www.parentmagic.com

**Program objectives:** Help parents learn effective methods of controlling negative behavior, encouraging good behavior, and strengthening the child-parent relationship. The program seeks to encourage gentle but firm discipline without arguing, yelling, or spanking.

**Target population:** Parents, grandparents, teachers, baby sitters, and caretakers working with children.

**Delivery setting and format:** Conducted in adoptive homes, birth family homes, community agencies, foster homes, hospitals, outpatient clinics, residential care facilities, and schools in groups of 6–25 parents of children approximately 2–12 years of age.

**Duration:** 1.5 hours per session for 4–8 weeks.

**Training resources:** Training manual available.

### *STEP (Systematic Training for Effective Parenting)*
STEP Publishers, LLC
P.O. Box 51722
Bowling Green, KY 42102-6722
Toll-Free: 800-720-1286
Website: http://www.parentingeducation.com

**Program objectives:** Help parents learn effective ways to relate to their children, how to encourage cooperative behavior in their children, and how not to reinforce unacceptable behaviors. STEP also helps parents change dysfunctional and destructive relationships with their children by offering concrete alternatives to abusive and ineffective methods of discipline and control.

**Target population:** Parents of children ages 0–6 years, and parents of teenagers.

**Delivery setting and format:** Conducted in adoptive homes, birth family homes, community agencies, foster homes, hospitals, outpatient clinics, residential care facilities, and schools in small discussion groups to promote better interaction.

**Duration:** Seven weeks.

**Training resources:** Training and program manuals available.

*Triple P-Positive Parenting Program*
P.O. Box 12755
Columbia, SC 29211
Phone: 803-451-2278
Fax: 803-451-2277
Website: http://www.TripleP-America.com
E-mail: contact.us@triplep.net

**Program objectives:** Prevent severe behavioral, emotional, and developmental problems in children by enhancing the knowledge, skills, and confidence of parents.

**Target population:** Parents and caregivers of children from birth through age 16 years.

**Delivery setting and format:** Conducted in adoptive homes, birth family homes, community agencies, foster homes, hospitals, outpatient clinics, residential care facilities, and schools in groups of 10–12 parents of children and adolescents from birth to age 16 years.

**Duration:** Varies depending on the type of intervention required.

**Training resources:** Training manual available.

## References

Brown, M. (2005). *USDA Parent Education and Support Literature Review*. University of Delaware Cooperative Extension. Retrieved

February 11, 2008, from: http://ag.udel.edu/extension/fam/professional resources/parentEd/2005litreview.htm.

Center for the Study of Social Policy. (2003). *Protective Factors Literature Review: Early Care and Education Programs and the Prevention of Child Abuse and Neglect.* Retrieved February 11, 2008, from: www.cssp.org/uploadFiles/horton.pdf.

Child Welfare Information Gateway, U.S. Department of Health and Human Services Children's Bureau, and FRIENDS National Resource Center for Community-Based Child Abuse Prevention. (2008). *Promoting Healthy Families in Your Community: 2008 Resource Packet.* Retrieved February 20, 2008, from: www.childwelfare.gov/pubs/res %5Fpacket%5F2008.

Colosi, L. and Dunifon, R. (2003). Effective Parent Education Programs. Cornell University College of Human Ecology: Parenting in Context. Retrieved February 11, 2008, from: www.parenting.cit .cornell.edu/Effective%20Parent%20Education%20Programs.pdf.

Kaminski, J. W., Valle, L. A., Filene, J. H., and Boyle, C. L. (2008). A Meta-Analytic Review of Components Associated with Parent Training Program Effectiveness. *Journal of Abnormal Child Psychology,* 36(4), 567–589.

Layzer, J. I., Goodson, B. D., Bernstein, L., and Price, C. (2001). National Evaluation of Family Support Programs Volume A: The Meta-Analysis. Cambridge, MA: Abt Associates, Inc. Retrieved February 11, 2008, from: www.acf.hhs.gov/programs/ opre/abuse_neglect/fam_sup/ reports/famsup/ fam_sup_vol_a.pdf.

Lundahl, B. W., Tollefson, D., Risser, H., and Lovejoy, M. C. (2007). A Meta-Analysis of Father Involvement in Parent Training. *Research on Social Work Practice,* 18, 1–10.

Lundahl, B. W., Nimer, J., and Parsons, B. (2006). Preventing Child Abuse: A Meta-Analysis of Parent Training Programs. *Research on Social Work Practice,* 16, 251–62.

Lundahl, B. W., and Harris, N. (2006). *Delivering parent training to families at risk to abuse: lessons from three meta-analyses.* Columbus, OH: American Professional Society on the Abuse of Children. April 2008.

## Additional Resources

The following resources include additional research and information on model parent education programs and curricula.

### Child Trends
4301 Connecticut Ave., NW, Suite 350
Washington, DC 20008
Phone: 202-572-6000
Fax: 202-362-8420
Website: http://www.childtrends.org

### Find Youth Info
Website: http://www.findyouthinfo.gov

This federal government website offers interactive tools and other resources to help support youth. Included are many tools and resources and information about evidence-based youth programs.

### Promising Practices Network on Children, Families, and Communities
Website: http://www.promisingpractices.net/programs_alpha.asp

The Office of Juvenile Justice and Delinquency Prevention's Promising Practices Network features descriptions of evaluated programs that improve outcomes for children.

Chapter 55

# Protect Your Family from Sex Offenders in Your Community

## Concerned about Sex Offenders in Your Neighborhood

A neighbor tells you about a "pedophile down the street," you learn of a "sexual predator" who is a member of your faith community, the local paper reports on "child molesters hanging around" at your kid's school. What can you do?

You thought your neighborhood was pretty safe. Suddenly, your sense of security is shaken. Media stereotypes about people who sexually abuse children can make it all seem overwhelming. You needn't be overwhelmed. Start by learning the facts. Accurate information about the situation can help you turn fear into confidence that you really can keep your family safe. Here are some other things you can do to help make you feel secure again.

## What You Can Do

### Don't Panic, Respond Calmly

Act with thought. Many people with a history of sexually offending are motivated to succeed when they re-enter society. Contrary to conventional wisdom, counseling can be very effective. Re-arrest rates for sexual offenses are actually very low. When given steady support, counseling, and supervision, they often pose little threat to anyone in the neighborhood.

## Create a Family Safety Plan

Your children and your family need to know what to do if anyone—family, friend, acquaintance, neighbor, or stranger—is approaching a child sexually. Remember, abuse is most likely to happen with someone you already know. If there was a public notice, ask the contact person or organization on the notice for more information. There may be a public meeting, local resources, or other materials that would help you and your family. Information may be available on the state's sex offender registry.

*Building Blocks of Your Family Safety Plan*

1. Educate everyone in the family.

   • Understand healthy sexual development in children as well as the sexual behaviors that may be of concern to you as a parent or caregiver.

   • Learn the warning signs of a child who may have been hurt by sexual abuse as well as the warning signs in an adult, adolescent, or child who may be touching a child in a sexual way. Your concerns may be about non-touching behaviors as well (for example, showing pornography to a child).

   • Teach children the proper names for body parts and what to do if someone tries to touch them in a sexual way. Remember to let young children know that no one has the right to touch their private parts (unless for medical reasons) and that they should not touch anyone else's private parts.

2. Open the lines of communication.

   • Whether talking with a child, adolescent, or adult, about sexualized behaviors or your concerns, the conversation is just a beginning and not a one-time event.

   • Let everyone in the family know it is okay to ask questions. It is important for adults to set the tone for everyone by talking about the range of healthy sexual behaviors and speaking up about sexual abuse.

3. Set clear family boundaries.

- Talk about and set clear family boundaries with family members and with other adults who spend time around or supervise the children (for example, if a child does not want to hug or kiss someone hello or goodbye, then he or she can shake hands instead).

- If a child is not comfortable with a particular adult or older child, then you or some other adult must let that person know (for example, tell him or her that you don't want your child to sit on his or her lap).

- As a child matures, boundaries within the home may need to change as well (for example, knock on the door before entering the room of an adolescent).

4. Get safe adults involved.

- Be sure that no one in your family is isolated. Identify one or more support people for every member of the family.

- Research shows that one of the key factors in a child's resilience (ability to bounce back after stressful events) is that he or she had someone to talk with and confide in. Be a safe, responsible, and consistent resource person for a child or adolescent.

- If someone is "too good to be true" then ask more questions—this friend or family member may not be a safe person for your child. Unfortunately, unconditional trust cannot protect children from harm.

5. Know your local resources and how to use them.

- List who to call for advice, information, and help. National resources are listed on the Stop It Now! website at www .stopitnow.org/resources.

- Learn about the agencies in your area. Know who to call to make a report if you learn that a child has been sexually abused.

6. Care enough to reach out for help.

- If you are concerned about the sexualized behaviors in a parent, cousin, sibling, friend, or neighbor, care enough to talk with them. If you are concerned about your own thoughts and feelings towards children, help is available.

- Call the Stop It Now! helpline at 888-773-8368 to learn more about the resources in your community.

- Make sure everyone knows that it's okay to talk with you about what may have already happened—that you love them and will help them.

### Attend the Public Community Notification Meeting

If there is community notification meeting, go to learn more about this person, their risk level, and how they will be supervised in the community. Learn about the restrictions that have been placed on this person so that if you see them doing something inappropriate you know how to report it.

### Find Out If the Person Convicted of a Sexual Offense Is Being Supervised

Ask the person or organization who has notified you whether the person who sexually abused in the past is being supervised by a probation or parole officer. You should be able to get the name and telephone number of the probation or parole officer. This officer may be able to answer more complex questions about the risk this person may pose to your family.

### Consider Joining with Another Neighbor to Meet the Offender

Consider approaching the person with an offer of support, perhaps through the probation or parole office. Remember, you may already know this person or know their family and friends. Even if they are new in your community, they are a part of it now. If the person who sexually abused is open and honest about the past, they may really be trying to change and live a different life. Show your support for their willingness to live a different life that keeps children safe. Your support and watchfulness can help in their recovery. It is also a chance to alert them that you know about their past and are aware of their actions today.

### Notify the Police If You See This Person in a Suspicious Situation

Avoid a hostile confrontation. Making threats or taking revenge may put you at legal risk. It's also important to avoid any action that may just push the person who has sexually abused into hiding, where normal life is almost impossible and it's easier to go back to old abusive ways. No matter how you feel about this person, if you see him or her in a suspicious or dangerous situation, call the police or probation/parole officer. Many people who have sexually abused go on to live productive, abuse-free lives. But not all will make the needed changes in their lives. Your supportive watchfulness may help the person who has abused keep under control.

## Don't Wait to Take Action for Prevention

What we do know is that there are people who have abused in our communities, some already identified, some not. Don't just wait to be notified about someone who has been convicted of a sexual offense. Talk to your family and friends now. Make the sexual safety of children a priority all the time with everyone in your community.

- **Remember: 88% of sexual abuse is never reported:** Authorities can't notify you about most people who sexually abuse because they've never been identified.

- **Your safety action plan does not change:** Whether or not you've been notified about someone with an offense in your community, you still need to be concerned about safety. Think about those who may abuse in the same way that you stay aware of possible speeding cars, children in the streets, or drug dealers near your child's school.

- **You can limit access:** If you know what to look for and how to take action, people who sexually abuse children will not have access to them. Their abusive behavior can be stopped when we are all aware. They can get help to prevent any further abuse.

## For More Information

### Dru Sjodin National Sex Offender Public Website
U.S. Department of Justice
Website: http://www.nsopw.gov/Core/PublicRegistrySites.aspx

### Stop It Now!
351 Pleasant Street, Suite B-319
Northampton, MA 01060
Toll-Free Helpline: 888-PREVENT (888-773-8368)

Phone: 413-587-3500
Fax: 413-587-3505
Website: http://www.stopitnow.org

# Part Six

# Strategies for
# Positive Parenting

Chapter 56

# Age-Appropriate Guidelines for Child Discipline

## Child Discipline

### What is discipline?

As part of their natural development, children sometimes challenge or test parental and adult expectations and authority. Sometimes, children simply choose to misbehave in order to gain something (for example, attention, an object, power, peer approval). This is a significant part of the growth process of children, yet it should not be without consequence. Discipline is how children learn right from wrong, acceptable from unacceptable.

Parental or adult discipline of children should be designed to help children engage better with others and to modify or control their behavior. Providing appropriate discipline to children is one of the most essential responsibilities of a parent. And providing consistent and positive discipline helps children grow into responsible adults.

According to the Committee for Children (2004), the purpose of discipline is "to encourage moral, physical, and intellectual development and a sense of responsibility in children. Ultimately, older children will do the right thing, not because they fear external reprisal, but because they have internalized a standard initially presented by

This chapter begins with an excerpt from "Child Discipline," © 2004 American Humane Association (www.americanhumane.org). Reprinted with permission. Reviewed in March 2009 by David A. Cooke, MD, FACP. Additional information from The Nemours Foundation is cited separately within the text.

parents and other caretakers. In learning to rely on their own resources rather than their parents, children gain self-confidence and a positive self-image."

### How can I discipline positively?

American Humane encourages parents and other caregivers to use techniques that constitute a positive and appropriate discipline of children, such as the following:

- Discipline with love
- Listen and communicate
- Focus on the behavior, not the child
- Respond immediately
- Relate the discipline to the offending behavior in duration and severity
- Be realistic
- Remain calm
- Be fair
- Do not harm or injure
- Set boundaries
- Make it a learning opportunity
- Be consistent
- Be creative
- Develop rules and expectations in advance
- Use time-outs
- Reward or praise desirable behaviors
- Model desired behavior
- Encourage the child's cooperation and understanding
- Develop behavioral contracts and incentive charts

### What else can I do?

Be a role model. This can help you teach your children appropriate behavior, self-control, responsibility, and accountability, while increasing their self-esteem. If you need help managing your own behavior or want to learn better parenting techniques, contact your local child protective services agency, community center, church, physician, mental health facility, or school for a referral or assistance.

## Age-Appropriate Discipline Guidelines

*Source: "Disciplining Your Child," October 2008, reprinted with permission from www.kidshealth.org. Copyright © 2008 The Nemours Foundation. This information was provided by KidsHealth, one of the largest resources online for medically reviewed health information written for parents, kids, and teens. For more articles like this one, visit www.KidsHealth.org, or www.TeensHealth.org.*

How do you keep a 1-year-old from heading toward the digital video disc (DVD) player? What should you do when your preschooler throws a fit? How can you get a teenager to respect your authority?

Whatever the age of your child, it's important to be consistent when it comes to discipline. If parents don't stick to the rules and consequences they set up, their kids aren't likely to either.

Here are some ideas about how to vary your approach to discipline to best fit your family.

### Ages Birth to Two

Babies and toddlers are naturally curious. So it's wise to eliminate temptations and no-nos—items such as televisions and video equipment, stereos, jewelry, and especially cleaning supplies and medications should be kept well out of reach.

When your crawling baby or roving toddler heads toward an unacceptable or dangerous play object, calmly say "No" and either remove your child from the area or distract him or her with an appropriate activity.

Time-outs can be effective discipline for toddlers. A child who has been hitting, biting, or throwing food, for example, should be told why the behavior is unacceptable and taken to a designated time-out area—a kitchen chair or bottom stair—for a minute or two to calm down (longer time-outs are not effective for toddlers).

It's important to not spank, hit, or slap a child of any age. Babies and toddlers are especially unlikely to be able to make any connection between their behavior and physical punishment. They will only feel the pain of the hit.

And don't forget that kids learn by watching adults, particularly their parents. Make sure your behavior is role-model material. You'll make a much stronger impression by putting your own belongings away rather than just issuing orders to your child to pick up toys while your stuff is left strewn around.

### Ages Three to Five

As your child grows and begins to understand the connection between actions and consequences, make sure you start communicating the rules of your family's home.

Explain to kids what you expect of them before you punish them for a certain behavior. For instance, the first time your 3-year-old uses crayons to decorate the living room wall, discuss why that's not allowed and what will happen if your child does it again (for instance, your child will have to help clean the wall and will not be able to use the crayons for the rest of the day). If the wall gets decorated again a few days later, issue a reminder that crayons are for paper only and then enforce the consequences.

The earlier that parents establish this kind of "I set the rules and you're expected to listen or accept the consequences" standard, the better for everyone. Although it's sometimes easier for parents to ignore occasional bad behavior or not follow through on some threatened punishment, this sets a bad precedent. Consistency is the key to effective discipline, and it's important for parents to decide (together, if you are not a single parent) what the rules are and then uphold them.

While you become clear on what behaviors will be punished, don't forget to reward good behaviors. Don't underestimate the positive effect that your praise can have—discipline is not just about punishment but also about recognizing good behavior. For example, saying "I'm proud of you for sharing your toys at playgroup" is usually more effective than punishing a child for the opposite behavior—not sharing. And be specific when doling out praise; don't just say, "Good job!"

If your child continues an unacceptable behavior no matter what you do, try making a chart with a box for each day of the week. Decide how many times your child can misbehave before a punishment kicks in or how long the proper behavior must be displayed before it is rewarded. Post the chart on the refrigerator and then track the good and unacceptable behaviors every day. This will give your child (and you) a concrete look at how it's going. Once this begins to work, praise your child for learning to control misbehavior and, especially, for overcoming any stubborn problem.

Time-outs also can work well for kids at this age. Establish a suitable time-out place that's free of distractions and will force your child to think about how he or she has behaved. Remember, getting sent to your room doesn't have an impact if a computer, television, and video games are there. Don't forget to consider the length of time that will best suit your child. Experts say one minute for each year of age is a good rule of thumb; others recommend using the time-out until the child is calmed down (to teach self-regulation).

It's important to tell kids what the right thing to do is, not just to say what the wrong thing is. For example, instead of saying "Don't jump on the couch," try "Please sit on the furniture and put your feet on the floor."

### Ages Six to Eight

Time-outs and consequences are also effective discipline strategies for this age group.

Again, consistency is crucial, as is follow-through. Make good on any promises of discipline or else you risk undermining your authority. Kids have to believe that you mean what you say. This is not to say you can't give second chances or allow a certain margin of error, but for the most part, you should act on what you say.

Be careful not to make unrealistic threats of punishment ("Slam that door and you'll never watch television again!") in anger, since not following through could weaken all your threats. If you threaten to turn the car around and go home if the squabbling in the backseat doesn't stop, make sure you do exactly that. The credibility you'll gain with your kids is much more valuable than a lost beach day.

Huge punishments may take away your power as a parent. If you ground your son or daughter for a month, your child may not feel motivated to change behaviors because everything has already been taken away.

### Ages Nine to Twelve

Kids in this age group—just as with all ages—can be disciplined with natural consequences. As they mature and request more independence and responsibility, teaching them to deal with the consequences of their behavior is an effective and appropriate method of discipline.

For example, if your fifth grader's homework isn't done before bedtime, should you make him or her stay up to do it or even lend a hand yourself? Probably not—you'll miss an opportunity to teach a key life lesson. If homework is incomplete, your child will go to school the next day without it and suffer the resulting bad grade.

It's natural for parents to want to rescue kids from mistakes, but in the long run they do kids a favor by letting them fail sometimes. Kids see what behaving improperly can mean and probably won't make those mistakes again. However, if your child does not seem to be learning from natural consequences, set up some of your own to help modify the behavior.

## Ages Thirteen and Up

By now you've laid the groundwork. Your child knows what's expected and that you mean what you say about the penalties for bad behavior. Don't let down your guard now—discipline is just as important for teens as it is for younger kids. Just as with the 4-year-old who needs you to set a bedtime and enforce it, your teen needs boundaries, too.

Set up rules regarding homework, visits by friends, curfews, and dating and discuss them beforehand with your teenager so there will be no misunderstandings. Your teen will probably complain from time to time, but also will realize that you're in control. Believe it or not, teens still want and need you to set limits and enforce order in their lives, even as you grant them greater freedom and responsibility.

When your teen does break a rule, taking away privileges may seem the best plan of action. While it's fine to take away the car for a week, for example, be sure to also discuss why coming home an hour past curfew is unacceptable and worrisome.

Remember to give a teenager some control over things. Not only will this limit the number of power struggles you have, it will help your teen respect the decisions that you do need to make. You could allow a younger teen to make decisions concerning school clothes, hair styles, or even the condition of his or her room. As your teen gets older, that realm of control might be extended to include an occasional relaxed curfew.

It's also important to focus on the positives. For example, have your teen earn a later curfew by demonstrating positive behavior instead of setting an earlier curfew as punishment for irresponsible behavior.

## A Word about Spanking

Perhaps no form of discipline is more controversial than spanking. Here are some reasons why the American Academy of Pediatrics (AAP) discourages spanking:

- Spanking teaches kids that it's okay to hit when they're angry.

- Spanking can physically harm children.

- Rather than teaching kids how to change their behavior, spanking makes them fearful of their parents and merely teaches them to avoid getting caught.

- For kids seeking attention by acting out, spanking may inadvertently "reward" them—negative attention is better than no attention at all.

Chapter 57

# Anger Management Tips for Parents

## Chapter Contents

# Section 57.1

# *Strategies for Coping with a Crying Baby*

## *Anger Management: Parent Coping Strategies*

Being a parent or caretaker is not easy. A baby's constant crying can be stressful and can be a dangerous trigger for you.

If a caretaker or parent feels overwhelmed and frustrated with a crying baby, it is vital they get help before they reach the point of shaking an infant. Ways to cope:

- Put the baby down in a crib or safe place.
- Walk out of the room, take a deep breath, count to twenty.
- Call someone close who can come over and give you a break.

Try to remember it is a good idea to take breaks from the demands of child care, particularly if your baby is acting overly fussy.

- Ask a family member or friend to help.
- Hire a baby sitter.
- Take deep breaths.
- Write in a journal.
- Call a friend to talk.
- Draw or paint.
- Listen to soothing music.
- Exercise.
- Vent your frustration by beating a pillow or throwing eggs in the shower.
- Nearly anything that does not harm a child is better than shaking your baby.

If you parent or care for young children, try to remember that babies fuss and cry because they are uncomfortable and have no better way to express themselves. They are not doing it to make you angry or unhappy. Some tips for coping with a crying baby include the following:

- Feed slowly and burp often

- Offer a pacifier

- Hold against your chest and walk or rock

- Put on soft music or sing

- Take the baby for a ride in a stroller or car or put your baby in a baby swing

- If you breast feed, avoid eating onions, beans, or drinking coffee, tea, or cola

If the baby is still crying and is not hungry, wet, or feverish, here are some things you can try:

- A pacifier chilled for teething

- Wrap the baby snugly in a blanket

- Hold the baby close, walk or rock the baby while talking or singing softly

- While sitting, lay your baby face down across your knees, gently pat his or her back

- Take the baby for a ride in the stroller or car

- Lay your baby down in her crib for a few minutes and walk away, perhaps he or she will calm down on his or her own

The next time everyday pressures build up to the point where you feel like striking out—stop! Try any of these simple alternatives. You'll feel better, and so will your child.

- Take a deep breath, and another. Then remember you're an adult.

- Close your eyes and imagine you're hearing what your child is about to hear.

- Press your lips together and count to ten—better yet, count to twenty.

505

- If someone can watch the children, go outside and take a walk.

- Take a hot bath or splash cold water on your face.

- Hug a pillow or stuffed animal.

- Turn on some music. Maybe even sing along.

- Pick up a pencil and write down as many helpful words you can think of. Save the list.

- Put your child in a time-out chair. Remember the rule: one time-out minute for each year of age.

- Put yourself in a time-out chair.

- Think about why you are angry: Is it your child, or is your child simply a convenient target for your anger?

- Call for prevention information: 866-243-BABY (2229).

## Stop Using Words That Hurt: Use Words That Help

Here are some expressions that can give children confidence and raise their self-esteem:

- I love you.
- That's great!
- Let's talk about you.
- I believe you can do it.
- Believe in yourself as I believe in you.
- You're doing just fine.
- You're very special.
- Good job.

# Section 57.2

# *Taming Your Child's Temper*

"Taming Tempers," April 2006, reprinted with permission from www
.kidshealth.org. © The Nemours Foundation. This information was provided by KidsHealth, one of the largest resources online for medically
reviewed health information written for parents, kids, and teens. For more
articles like this one, visit www.KidsHealth.org, or www.TeensHealth.org.

Parents expect temper tantrums from 2-year-olds, but angry outbursts don't necessarily stop after the toddler years. Older kids sometimes have trouble handling anger and frustration, too.

Some kids only lose their cool on occasion. But others seem to have
a harder time when things don't go their way. Kids who tend to have
strong reactions by nature will need more help from parents to manage their tempers.

Controlling outbursts can be difficult for kids—and helping them
learn to do so is a tough job for the parents who love them. Try to be
patient and positive, and know that these skills take time to develop
and that just about every child can improve with the right coaching.

## *A Parent's Role*

Managing kids—whether it's one or more—can be a challenge.
Some days keeping the peace while keeping your cool seems impossible. But whether you're reacting to an occasional temper flare-up
or a pattern of outbursts, managing your own anger when things get
heated will make it easier to teach kids to do the same.

To help tame a temper, try to be your child's ally—you're both root-
ing for your child to triumph over the temper that keeps getting him
or her into trouble.

While your own patience may be frayed by angry outbursts, opposition, defiance, arguing, and talking back, it's during these episodes
that you need your patience most. Of course you feel angry, but what
counts is how you handle that.

Reacting to your child's meltdowns with yelling and outbursts of
your own will only teach your child to do the same. But keeping your

cool and calmly working through a frustrating situation lets you show—and teach—your child appropriate ways to handle anger and frustration.

Let's say you hear your kids fighting over a toy in the other room. You have ignored it, hoping that they would work it out themselves. But the arguing turns into screaming, and soon you hear doors slamming, the thump of hitting, and an eruption into tears. You decide to get involved before someone gets hurt.

By the time you arrive at the scene of the fight, you may be at the end of your own rope. After all, the sound of screaming is upsetting, and you may be frustrated that your kids aren't sharing or trying to get along. (And you know that this toy they're fighting over is going to be lost, broken, or ignored before long anyway!)

So what's the best way for you to react? With your own self-control intact. Teaching by example is your most powerful tool. Speak calmly, clearly, and firmly—not with anger, blame, harsh criticisms, threats, or putdowns. Of course, that's easier said than done. But remember that you're trying to teach your child how to handle anger. If you yell or threaten, you'll model and ingrain the exact kinds of behavior you want to discourage. Your child sees you so angry and so incapable of controlling your own temper that you can't help but scream—and that won't help your child learn not to scream.

## What You Can Do

Regulating emotions and managing behavior are skills that develop slowly over time during childhood. Just like any other skills, your child will need to learn and practice them, with your help.

If it's uncharacteristic for your child to have a tantrum, on the rare occasion that it happens all you may need to do is clearly but calmly review the rules. "I know you're upset, but no yelling and no name-calling, please" may be all your child needs to gain composure. Follow up by clearly, calmly, and patiently giving an instruction like "tell me what you're upset about" or "please apologize to your brother for calling him that name." In this way, you're guiding your child back to acceptable behavior and encouraging self-control.

Kids whose temper outbursts are routine may lack the necessary self-control to deal with frustration and anger, and may need more help managing those emotions. These steps may help:

**Help your child put it into words.** If your child is in the midst of an outburst, find out what's wrong. If necessary, use a time-out to get your child to settle down, or calmly issue a reminder about house rules and expectations—"There's no yelling or throwing stuff; please stop that right now and cool your jets." Remind your child to talk to you without whining, sulking, or yelling. Once your child calms down, ask what got him or her so upset. You might say, "Use your words to tell me what's wrong and what you're mad about." By doing this you help your child put emotions into words and figure out what, if anything, needs to be done to solve the problem.

**Listen and respond.** Once your child puts the feelings into words, it's up to you to listen and say that you understand. If your child is struggling for words, offer some help: "so that made you angry," "you must have felt frustrated," or "that must have hurt your feelings." Offer to help find an answer if there's a problem to be solved, a conflict to be mended, or if an apology is required. Many times, feeling listened to and understood is all kids need to regain their composure. But while acknowledging your child's feelings, it's important to make it clear that strong emotions aren't an excuse for unacceptable behavior. "I know you're mad, but it's still not okay to hit." Then tell your child some things to try instead.

**Create clear ground rules and stick to them.** Set and maintain clear expectations for what is and what is not acceptable. You can do this without using threats, accusations, or putdowns. Your child will get the message if you make clear, simple statements about what's off limits and explain what you want him or her to do. You might say: "There's no yelling in this house. Use your words to tell me what's upsetting you." Or try these:

- In this family, we don't hit or push or shove.
- There's no screaming allowed.
- There's no door-slamming in our house.
- There's no name calling.
- We don't do that in this family.
- You may not throw things or break things on purpose.

## *Coping Strategies for Your Child*

Kids who've learned that it's not okay to yell, hit, and throw stuff when they're upset need other strategies for calming down when they're angry. Offer some ideas to help your child learn safe ways to get the anger out or to find other activities that can create a better mood.

**Take a break from the situation.** Tell your child that it's okay to walk away from a conflict to avoid an angry outburst. By moving to another part of the house or the backyard, your child can get some space and work on calming down.

**Find a way to (safely) get the anger out.** There may be no punching walls or even pillows, but you can suggest some good ways for a child to vent. Doing a bunch of jumping jacks, dancing around the bedroom, or going outside and doing cartwheels are all good choices. Or your child can choose to write about or draw a picture of what is so upsetting.

**Learn to shift.** This one is tough for kids—and adults, too. Explain that part of calming down is moving from a really angry mood to a more in-control mood. Instead of thinking of the person or situation that caused the anger, encourage your son or daughter to think of something else to do. Suggest things to think of or do that might bring about a better mood. Your child may feel better after a walk around the block, a bike ride, playing a game, reading a favorite book, digging in the garden, or listening to a favorite song. Try one of these things together so you both experience how doing something different can change the way a person feels.

## *Building a Strong Foundation*

Fortunately, really angry episodes don't happen too often for most kids. Those with temper troubles often have an active, strong-willed style and extra energy that needs to be discharged. Try these steps during the calm times—they can prevent problems before they start by helping your child learn and practice skills needed to manage the heat of the moment:

**Help your child label emotions.** Help your child get in the habit of saying what he or she is feeling and why—for example, "I'm mad because I have to clean my room while my friends are playing." Using words doesn't get your child out of doing a chore, but having the discussion can defuse the situation. You're having a conversation instead of an argument. Praise your child for talking about it instead of slamming the door, for instance.

**See that your child gets a lot of physical activity.** Active play can really help kids who have big tempers. Encourage outside play and sports your child likes. Karate, wrestling, and running can be especially good for kids who are trying to get their tempers under control. But any activity that gets the heart pumping can help burn off energy and stress.

**Encourage your child to take control.** Compare a temper to a puppy that hasn't yet learned to behave and that's running around all over the place getting into things. Puppies might not mean to be bad—but they need to be trained so that they can learn that there's no eating shoes, no jumping on people or certain furniture, and so forth. The point is that your child's temper—like a puppy—needs to be trained to learn when it's okay to play, how to use all that rambunctious energy, and how to follow rules.

**Try to be flexible.** Parenting can be a fatiguing experience, but try not to be too rigid. Hearing a constant chorus of "no" can be disheartening for kids. Sometimes, of course, "no" is absolutely the only answer—"no, you can't ride your bike without your helmet!" But other times, you might let the kids win one. For instance, if your child wants to keep the wiffleball game going a little longer, maybe give it 15 more minutes.

As anyone who's been really angry knows, following sensible advice can be tough when emotions run high. Give your child responsibility for getting under control, but be there to remind him or her of how to do it.

Most kids can learn to get better at handling anger and frustration. But if your child frequently gets into fights and arguments with friends, siblings, and adults, additional help might be needed. Talk with the other adults in your child's life—teachers, school counselors, and coaches might be able to help, and your child's doctor can recommend a counselor or psychologist.

Chapter 58

# Fostering Good Sportsmanship in Children

Emily was crying by the time the softball game ended. It wasn't because her team had lost. It wasn't because she was unhappy about her own playing. It wasn't even because of anything the other team had said or done. Emily's tears came after her dad yelled at her—in front of all her teammates—for missing the fly ball that could have saved the game. Emily is just eight years old.

If your child has ever participated in a sport, you've undoubtedly met people like Emily's dad, parents who behave inappropriately and upset their kids. These parents get so wrapped up in winning and losing or how well their own kids perform that they lose sight of what's really important. They forget that one of the most important goals of kids' sports is to promote a sense of good sportsmanship.

## What Is Good Sportsmanship?

Good sportsmanship is when teammates, opponents, coaches, and officials treat each other with respect. Kids learn the basics of sportsmanship from the adults in their lives, especially their parents and their coaches. Kids who see adults behaving in a sportsmanlike way

"Sportsmanship," October 2008, reprinted with permission from www .kidshealth.org. Copyright © 2008 The Nemours Foundation. This information was provided by KidsHealth, one of the largest resources online for medically reviewed health information written for parents, kids, and teens. For more articles like this one, visit www.KidsHealth.org, or www.TeensHealth.org.

gradually come to understand that the real winners in sports are those who know how to persevere and to behave with dignity—whether they win or lose a game.

Parents can help their kids understand that good sportsmanship includes both small gestures and heroic efforts. It starts with something as simple as shaking hands with opponents before a game and includes acknowledging good plays made by others and accepting bad calls gracefully.

Displaying good sportsmanship isn't always easy: It can be tough to congratulate the opposing team after losing a close or important game. But the kids who learn how to do it will benefit in many ways.

Kids who bully or taunt others on the playing field aren't likely to change their behavior when in the classroom or in social situations. In the same way, a child who practices good sportsmanship is likely to carry the respect and appreciation of other people into every other aspect of life.

## Good Sports Are Winners

Ask first- or second-graders who won a game and they may answer, "I think it was a tie." It's likely the question isn't of any real interest at that age. Kids may be more eager to talk about the hits they got or the catches they almost made.

But as they move into older and more competitive leagues, kids become more focused on winning. They often forget to have fun. Without constant reminders and good examples, they may also forget what behavior is appropriate before, during, and after a sporting event.

Kids who have coaches who care only about being in first place and say that anything goes as long as they win, pick up the message that it's okay to be ruthless on the field. If parents constantly pressure them to play better or second-guess their every move, kids get the message that they're only as good as their last good play—and they'll try anything to make one.

Adults who emphasize good sportsmanship, however, see winning as just one of several goals they'd like their kids to achieve. They help young athletes take pride in their accomplishments and in their improving skills, so that the kids see themselves as winners, even if the scoreboard doesn't show the numbers going in their favor.

The best coaches—and parents—encourage their kids to play fair, to have fun, and to concentrate on helping the team while polishing their own skills.

## *Fostering Good Sportsmanship*

Remember the saying "Actions speak louder than words"? That's especially true when it comes to teaching your kids the basics of good sportsmanship. Your behavior during practices and games will influence them more than any pep talk or lecture you give them.

Here are some suggestions on how to build sportsmanship in your kids:

- Unless you're coaching your child's team, you need to remember that you're the parent. Shout words of encouragement, not directions, from the sidelines (there is a difference).

- If you are your kid's coach, don't expect too much out of your own child. Don't be harder on him or her than on anyone else on the team, but don't play favorites either.

- Keep your comments positive. Don't bad-mouth coaches, players, or game officials. If you have a serious concern about the way that games or practices are being conducted, or if you're upset about other parents' behavior, discuss it privately with the coach or with a league official.

- After a competition, it's important not to dwell on who won or lost. Instead, try asking, "How did you feel you did during the game?" If your child feels weak at a particular skill, like throwing or catching, offer to work on it together before the next game.

- Applaud good plays no matter who makes them.

- Set a good example with your courteous behavior toward the parents of kids on the other team. Congratulate them when their kids win.

- Remember that it's your kids, not you, who are playing. Don't push them into a sport because it's what you enjoyed. As kids get older, let them choose what sports they want to play and decide the level of commitment they want to make.

- Keep your perspective. It's just a game. Even if the team loses every game of the season, it's unlikely to ruin your child's life or chances of success.

- Look for examples of good sportsmanship in professional athletes and point them out to your kids. Talk about the bad examples, too, and why they upset you.

- Finally, don't forget to have fun. Even if your child isn't the star, enjoy the game while you're thinking of all the benefits your child is gaining—new skills, new friends, and attitudes that can help all through life.

Chapter 59

# Leaving Your
# Child Home Alone

Whether it's a snow day home from school, an unexpected business appointment, or a child care arrangement that fell through at the last minute, situations are likely to arise where you feel you have little choice but to leave your child home alone.

It's natural to be a bit anxious when you first leave your child without any supervision. But it doesn't have to be something for which you and your child feel unprepared. With some planning—and trial runs where you remain close by—you can approach the situation with confidence.

Handled well, staying home alone can be a positive experience for your child, too—one that helps him or her gain a sense of self-assurance and independence.

### Is Your Child Ready?

It's obvious that a 5-year-old can't go it alone, and that a 16-year-old can probably handle it. But what about those school-aged kids in

This chapter begins with "Leaving Your Child Home Alone," May 2006 reprinted with permission from www.kidshealth.org. Copyright © 2006 The Nemours Foundation. This information was provided by KidsHealth, one of the largest resources online for medically reviewed health information written for parents, kids, and teens. For more articles like this one, visit www.KidsHealth .org., or www.TeensHealth.org. The chapter concludes with an excerpt titled, "Legal Considerations when Leaving Your Child Home Alone," from "Leaving Your Child Home Alone," Child Welfare Information Gateway, U.S. Department of Health and Human Services (HHS) 2007.

the middle? It can be difficult to know when kids are ready to handle being home alone. Ultimately, it comes down to your judgment about what your child is ready for.

You'll want to know how your child feels about the prospect, of course. But often kids insist that they'll be fine long before you feel comfortable with the idea. And then there are older kids who seem afraid even when you're pretty confident that they would be just fine. So how do you know?

In general, it's probably not a good idea to leave a child younger than ten years old home alone. Every child is different, but at that age, most kids don't have the maturity and skills to respond to an emergency if they're alone.

But there are other factors to consider too.

Think about the area where you live. Are there neighbors nearby you know and trust to help your child in case of an emergency? Or is it mostly strangers? Do you live on a busy street with lots of traffic? Or is it a quiet area? Is there a lot of crime in your area?

It's also important to consider how your child handles various situations. Here are a few questions to think about:

- Does your child show signs of responsibility with things like homework, household chores, and following directions?

- How does your child handle unexpected situations? How calm does your child stay when things don't go his or her way?

- Does your child understand and follow rules?

- Can your child understand and follow safety measures?

- Does your child make good judgments about what kinds of risks to take?

- Does your child know basic first-aid procedures?

- Does your child follow your instructions about staying away from strangers?

Even if you're confident that your child does well with all of the above, it's wise to make some practice runs, or home-alone trials, before the big day. Let your child stay home alone for 30 minutes to an hour while you remain nearby and easily reachable. When you return, discuss how it went and talk about things that you might want to change or skills that your child may need to learn for the next time.

## *Handling the Unexpected*

You can feel more confident about your absence if your child learns some basic skills that might come in handy during an emergency. Organizations such as the American Red Cross offer courses in first aid and cardiopulmonary resuscitation (CPR) in local places like schools, hospitals, and community centers.

Before you leave your child home alone, be sure he or she can complete certain tasks and safety precautions, such as:

- knowing when and how to call 911 and what address information to give the dispatcher;

- knowing how to work the home security system, if you have one, and what to do if the alarm is accidentally set off;

- locking and unlocking doors;

- working the phone or cell phone (in some areas, you have to dial 1 or the area code to dial out);

- turning lights off and on;

- operating the microwave;

- knowing what to do if:
  - there's a small fire in the kitchen,
  - the smoke alarm goes off,
  - there's a tornado or other severe weather,
  - a stranger comes to the door,
  - someone calls for a parent who isn't home,
  - there's a power outage.

Try to regularly discuss some emergency scenarios—ask what your child would do if, for example, he or she smelled smoke, a stranger knocked at the door, or someone called for you while you're gone.

## *Before You Leave*

Even after you decide that your child is ready to stay home alone, you're bound to feel a little anxious when the time comes. But some practical steps taken in advance can make it easier for you both:

- **Schedule time to get in touch.** Set up a schedule for calling. You might have your child call as soon as he or she walks in the

519

door (if coming home to an empty house), or set up a time when you'll call home to check in. Figure out something that's convenient for both of you. Make sure your child understands when you'll be able to get in touch and when you might not be able to answer a call.

- **Set ground rules.** Try to set up some special rules for when you're away and make sure that your child knows and understands them. Consider rules about:
  - having a friend or friends over while you're not there;
  - rooms of the house that are off limits, especially with friends;
  - television time and types of shows;
  - internet and computer rules;
  - kitchen and cooking (you may want to make the oven and utensils like sharp knives off limits);
  - opening the door for strangers;
  - answering the phone;
  - getting along with siblings;
  - not telling anyone he or she is alone.

- **Stock up.** Make sure your house has everyday goods and emergency supplies. Stock the kitchen with healthy foods your child can eat, and leave a dose of any medication that your child needs to take. In addition, leave flashlights in an accessible place in case there's a power outage. Post important phone numbers—yours and those of friends, family members, the doctor, police, and fire department—that your child might need in an emergency.

- **Be sure that you:**
  - create a list of friends your child can call or things your child can do when he or she is lonely;
  - leave a snack or a note so your child knows you're thinking of him or her;
  - make up a schedule for your child to follow while you're away;
  - make sure the parental controls and filtering systems, if you have any, are programmed for the internet on your computer and on your television.

- **Childproof your home.** No matter how well your child follows rules, be sure to secure anything that could be a health or safety risk. Lock them up and put them in a place where your child cannot get to them or, when possible, remove them from your home. These items include:

  - alcohol;

  - prescription medications;

  - over-the-counter medications that could cause problems if taken in excess: sleeping pills, cough medicine, and so forth;

  - guns (if you do keep one, make sure it is locked up and leave it unloaded and stored away from ammunition);

  - tobacco;

  - car keys;

  - lighters and matches.

### *Ready to Go*

When you're ready to leave your child home alone for the first time, there are other things you can do to help both of you get comfortable with the transition.

You might have an older teen or a friend of the family come over to stay with your child. Don't call that person a "baby sitter"—tell your child that the person is there to keep him or her company.

You may also want to let your child invite a trusted friend of the same age to come over, and propose this as a trial run for later solo stays. Be sure to let the friend's parents know that you won't be home.

And don't forget that pets can be great company for kids who are home alone. Many kids feel safer with a pet around—even a small one, like a hamster, can make them feel like they have a companion.

So cover your bases and relax. With the right preparation, and some practice, you and your child will get comfortable with home-alone days in no time!

## Legal Considerations when Leaving Your Child Home Alone

Depending on the laws and child protective policies in your area, leaving a young child unsupervised may be considered neglect, especially if doing so places the child in danger. If you are concerned about a child who appears to be neglected or inadequately supervised, contact your local child protective services (CPS) agency. If you need help contacting your local CPS agency, call the Childhelp® National Child Abuse Hotline at 800-4-A-CHILD (800-422-4453). Find more information on their website at http://www.childhelp.org.

### *What to Consider Before Leaving Your Child Home Alone*

When deciding whether to leave a child home alone, you will want to consider your child's physical, mental, and emotional well-being, as well as laws and policies in your state regarding this issue.

### *Legal Guidelines*

Some parents look to the law for help in deciding when it is appropriate to leave a child home alone. According to the National Child Care Information Center, only Illinois and Maryland currently have laws regarding a minimum age for leaving a child home alone. Even in those states, other factors such as concern for a child's well-being and the amount of time the child is left alone, are considered. States that do not have laws may still offer guidelines for parents. For information on laws and guidelines in your state, contact your local CPS agency.

### *Circumstances*

When and how a child is left home alone can make a difference to his or her safety and success. You may want to consider the following questions:

- How long will your child be left home alone at one time? Will it be during the day, evening, or night? Will the child need to fix a meal?

- How often will the child be expected to care for him- or herself?

- How many children are being left home alone? Children who seem ready to stay home alone may not necessarily be ready to care for younger siblings.

- Is your home safe and free of hazards?

- How safe is your neighborhood?

Chapter 60

# What to Do If Your Child Is Being Bullied

## What Is Bullying?

Bullying among children is aggressive behavior that is intentional and that involves an imbalance of power or strength. A child who is being bullied has a hard time defending himself or herself. Usually, bullying is repeated over time. Bullying can take many forms, such as hitting or punching (physical bullying); teasing or name-calling (verbal bullying); intimidation using gestures or social exclusion (non-verbal bullying or emotional bullying); and sending insulting messages by phone or computer e-mail (cyberbullying).

## Effects of Bullying

Bullying can have serious consequences. Children and youth who are bullied are more likely than other children to:

- be depressed, lonely, anxious;
- have low self-esteem;
- be absent from school;
- feel sick; or
- think about suicide.

---

"What to Do If Your Child Is Being Bullied," Health Resources and Services Administration (HRSA), 2004. Reviewed in March, 2009 by David A. Cooke, MD, FACP.

## Reporting Bullying to Parents

Children frequently do not tell their parents that they are being bullied because they are embarrassed, ashamed, frightened of the children who are bullying them, or afraid of being seen as a tattler. If your child tells you about being bullied, it has taken a lot of courage to do so. Your child needs your help to stop the bullying.

## What You Can Do

1. First, focus on your child. Be supportive and gather information about the bullying.

   • Never tell your child to ignore the bullying. What the child may "hear" is that you are going to ignore it. If the child were able to simply ignore it, he or she likely would not have told you about it. Often, trying to ignore bullying allows it to become more serious.

   • Don't blame the child who is being bullied. Don't assume that your child did something to provoke the bullying. Don't say, "What did you do to aggravate the other child?"

   • Listen carefully to what your child tells you about the bullying. Ask him or her to describe who was involved and how and where each bullying episode happened.

   • Learn as much as you can about the bullying tactics used, and when and where the bullying happened. Can your child name other children or adults who may have witnessed the bullying?

   • Empathize with your child. Tell him or her that bullying is wrong, not their fault, and that you are glad he or she had the courage to tell you about it. Ask your child what he or she thinks can be done to help. Assure him or her that you will think about what needs to be done and you will let him or her know what you are going to do.

   • If you disagree with how your child handled the bullying situation, don't criticize him or her.

   • Do not encourage physical retaliation ("Just hit them back") as a solution. Hitting another student is not likely to end the problem, and it could get your child suspended or expelled or escalate the situation.

- Check your emotions. A parent's protective instincts stir strong emotions. Although it is difficult, a parent is wise to step back and consider the next steps carefully.

2. Contact your child's teacher or principal.

    - Parents are often reluctant to report bullying to school officials, but bullying may not stop without the help of adults.

    - Keep your emotions in check. Give factual information about your child's experience of being bullied including who, what, when, where, and how.

    - Emphasize that you want to work with the staff at school to find a solution to stop the bullying, for the sake of your child as well as other students.

    - Do not contact the parents of the student(s) who bullied your child. This is usually a parent's first response, but sometimes it makes matters worse. School officials should contact the parents of the child or children who did the bullying.

    - Expect the bullying to stop. Talk regularly with your child and with school staff to see whether the bullying has stopped. If the bullying persists, contact school authorities again.

3. Help your child become more resilient to bullying.

    - Help to develop talents or positive attributes of your child. Suggest and facilitate music, athletics, and art activities. Doing so may help your child be more confident among his or her peers.

    - Encourage your child to make contact with friendly students in his or her class. Your child's teacher may be able to suggest students with whom your child can make friends, spend time, or collaborate on work.

    - Help your child meet new friends outside of the school environment. A new environment can provide a fresh start for a child who has been bullied repeatedly.

    - Teach your child safety strategies. Teach him or her how to seek help from an adult when feeling threatened by a bully. Talk about whom he or she should go to for help and role-play what he or she should say. Assure your child that reporting bullying is not the same as tattling.

- Ask yourself if your child is being bullied because of a learning difficulty or a lack of social skills? If your child is hyperactive, impulsive, or overly talkative, the child who bullies may be reacting out of annoyance. This doesn't make the bullying right, but it may help to explain why your child is being bullied. If your child easily irritates people, seek help from a counselor so that your child can better learn the informal social rules of his or her peer group.

- Home is where the heart is. Make sure your child has a safe and loving home environment where he or she can take shelter, physically and emotionally. Always maintain open lines of communication with your child.

Chapter 61

# Protecting Your Child from Electronic Aggression

## A Parent's Guide to Internet Safety

While online computer exploration opens a world of possibilities for children, expanding their horizons and exposing them to different cultures and ways of life, they can be exposed to dangers as they hit the road exploring the information highway. There are individuals who attempt to sexually exploit children through the use of online services and the internet. Some of these individuals gradually seduce their targets through the use of attention, affection, kindness, and even gifts. These individuals are often willing to devote considerable amounts of time, money, and energy in this process. They listen to and empathize with the problems of children. They will be aware of the latest music, hobbies, and interests of children. These individuals attempt to gradually lower children's inhibitions by slowly introducing sexual context and content into their conversations.

There are other individuals, however, who immediately engage in sexually explicit conversation with children. Some offenders primarily collect and trade child-pornographic images, while others seek face-to-face meetings with children via online contacts. It is important for parents to understand that children can be indirectly victimized through conversation, for example "chat," as well as the transfer

This chapter includes text from "A Parent's Guide to Internet Safety," Federal Bureau of Investigation (FBI); and text from "Technology and Youth: Protecting Your Child from Electronic Aggression," Centers for Disease Control and Prevention (CDC), 2008.

of sexually explicit information and material. Computer-sex offenders may also be evaluating children they come in contact with online for future face-to-face contact and direct victimization. Parents and children should remember that a computer-sex offender can be any age or sex the person does not have to fit the caricature of a dirty, unkempt, older man wearing a raincoat to be someone who could harm a child.

Children, especially adolescents, are sometimes interested in and curious about sexuality and sexually explicit material. They may be moving away from the total control of parents and seeking to establish new relationships outside their family. Because they may be curious, children or adolescents sometimes use their online access to actively seek out such materials and individuals. Sex offenders targeting children will use and exploit these characteristics and needs. Some adolescent children may also be attracted to and lured by online offenders closer to their age who, although not technically child molesters, may be dangerous. Nevertheless, they have been seduced and manipulated by a clever offender and do not fully understand or recognize the potential danger of these contacts.

This information was prepared from actual investigations involving child victims, as well as investigations where law enforcement officers posed as children.

## What are signs that your child might be at risk online?

**Your child spends large amounts of time online, especially at night.** Most children that fall victim to computer-sex offenders spend large amounts of time online, particularly in chat rooms. They may go online after dinner and on the weekends. They may be latchkey kids whose parents have told them to stay at home after school. They go online to chat with friends, make new friends, pass time, and sometimes look for sexually explicit information. While much of the knowledge and experience gained may be valuable, parents should consider monitoring the amount of time spent online.

Children online are at the greatest risk during the evening hours. While offenders are online around the clock, most work during the day and spend their evenings online trying to locate and lure children or seeking pornography.

**You find pornography on your child's computer.** Pornography is often used in the sexual victimization of children. Sex offenders often supply their potential victims with pornography as a means of opening sexual discussions and for seduction. Child pornography may be used to show the child victim that sex between children and adults is "normal." Parents should be conscious of the fact that a child may hide the pornographic files on diskettes from them. This may be especially true if the computer is used by other family members.

**Your child receives phone calls from men you don't know or is making calls,** sometimes long distance, to numbers you don't recognize. While talking to a child victim online is a thrill for a computer-sex offender, it can be very cumbersome. Most want to talk to the children on the telephone. They often engage in "phone sex" with the children and often seek to set up an actual meeting for real sex.

While a child may be hesitant to give out his or her home phone number, the computer-sex offenders will give out theirs. With Caller ID, they can readily find out the child's phone number. Some computer-sex offenders have even obtained toll-free 800 numbers, so that their potential victims can call them without their parents finding out. Others will tell the child to call collect. Both of these methods result in the computer-sex offender being able to find out the child's phone number.

**Your child receives mail, gifts, or packages from someone you don't know.** As part of the seduction process, it is common for offenders to send letters, photographs, and all manner of gifts to their potential victims. Computer-sex offenders have even sent plane tickets in order for the child to travel across the country to meet them.

**Your child turns the computer monitor off or quickly changes the screen on the monitor when you come into the room.** A child looking at pornographic images or having sexually explicit conversations does not want you to see it on the screen.

**Your child becomes withdrawn from the family.** Computer-sex offenders will work very hard at driving a wedge between a child and their family or at exploiting their relationship. They will accentuate any minor problems at home that the child might have. Children may also become withdrawn after sexual victimization.

**Your child is using an online account belonging to someone else.** Even if you don't subscribe to an online service or internet service, your child may meet an offender while online at a friend's house or the library. Most computers come preloaded with online and/or internet software. Computer-sex offenders will sometimes provide potential victims with a computer account for communications with them.

***What should you do if you suspect your child is communicating with a sexual predator online?***

- Consider talking openly with your child about your suspicions. Tell them about the dangers of computer-sex offenders.

- Review what is on your child's computer. If you don't know how, ask a friend, coworker, relative, or other knowledgeable person. Pornography or any kind of sexual communication can be a warning sign.

- Use the Caller ID service to determine who is calling your child. Most telephone companies that offer Caller ID also offer a service that allows you to block your number from appearing on someone else's Caller ID. Telephone companies also offer an additional service feature that rejects incoming calls that you block. This rejection feature prevents computer-sex offenders or anyone else from calling your home anonymously.

- Devices can be purchased that show telephone numbers that have been dialed from your home phone. Additionally, the last number called from your home phone can be retrieved provided that the telephone is equipped with a redial feature. You will also need a telephone pager to complete this retrieval.

- Monitor your child's access to all types of live electronic communications (for example: chat rooms, instant messages, and so forth), and monitor your child's e-mail. Computer-sex offenders almost always meet potential victims via chat rooms. After meeting a child online, they will continue to communicate electronically often via e-mail.

Should any of the following situations arise in your household, via the internet or online service, you should immediately contact your local or state law enforcement agency, the Federal Bureau of Investigation (FBI), and the National Center for Missing and Exploited Children:

1. Your child or anyone in the household has received child pornography.

2. Your child has been sexually solicited by someone who knows that your child is under 18 years of age.

3. Your child has received sexually explicit images from someone that knows your child is under the age of 18.

If one of these scenarios occurs, keep the computer turned off in order to preserve any evidence for future law enforcement use. Unless directed to do so by the law enforcement agency, you should not attempt to copy any of the images or text found on the computer.

### What can you do to minimize the chances of an online exploiter victimizing your child?

- Communicate, and talk to your child about sexual victimization and potential online danger.

- Spend time with your children online. Have them teach you about their favorite online destinations.

- Keep the computer in a common room in the house, not in your child's bedroom. It is much more difficult for a computer-sex offender to communicate with a child when the computer screen is visible to a parent or another member of the household.

- Utilize parental controls provided by your service provider or blocking software. While electronic chat can be a great place for children to make new friends and discuss various topics of interest, it is also prowled by computer-sex offenders. Use of chat rooms, in particular, should be heavily monitored. While parents should utilize these mechanisms, they should not totally rely on them.

- Always maintain access to your child's online account and randomly check his or her e-mail. Be aware that your child could be contacted through the U.S. mail. Be up front with your child about your access and reasons why.

- Teach your child the responsible use of the resources online. There is much more to the online experience than chat rooms.

- Find out what computer safeguards are utilized by your child's school, the public library, and at the homes of your child's friends. These are all places, outside your normal supervision, where your child could encounter an online predator.

- Understand, even if your child was a willing participant in any form of sexual exploitation, that he or she is not at fault and is the victim. The offender always bears the complete responsibility for his or her actions.

- Instruct your children:

  - to never arrange a face-to-face meeting with someone they met online;

  - to never upload (post) pictures of themselves onto the internet or online service to people they do not personally know;

  - to never give out identifying information such as their name, home address, school name, or telephone number;

  - to never download pictures from an unknown source, as there is a good chance there could be sexually explicit images;

  - to never respond to messages or bulletin board postings that are suggestive, obscene, belligerent, or harassing; and

  - that whatever they are told online may or may not be true.

## Electronic Aggression

New technology has many potential benefits for youth. With the help of new technology, young people can interact with others across the United States and throughout the world on a regular basis. Social networking sites like Facebook and MySpace also allow youth to develop new relationships with others, some of whom they have never even met in person. New technology also provides opportunities to make rewarding social connections for those youth who have difficulty developing friendships in traditional social settings or because of limited contact with same-aged peers. In addition, regular internet access allows teens and pre-teens to quickly increase their knowledge on a wide variety of topics.

However, the recent explosion in technology does not come without possible risks. Youth can use electronic media to embarrass, harass, or threaten their peers. Increasing numbers of adolescents are becoming victims of this new form of violence—electronic aggression. Research suggests that 9% to 35% of young people report being victims of this type of violence. Like traditional forms of youth violence, electronic aggression is associated with emotional distress and conduct problems at school. Electronic aggression is any type of harassment or bullying that occurs through e-mail, a chat room, instant messaging, a website (including blogs), or text messaging. Examples of electronic aggression include the following:

- Disclosing someone else's personal information in a public area (such as a website) in order to cause embarrassment

- Posting rumors or lies about someone in a public area (for example, a discussion board)

- Distributing embarrassing pictures of someone by posting them in a public area (a website) or sending them via e-mail

- Assuming another person's electronic identity to post or send messages about others with the intent of causing the other person harm

- Sending mean, embarrassing, or threatening text messages, instant messages, or e-mails

## *Tips for Parents and Caregivers*

**Talk to your child:** Parents and caregivers often ask children where they are going and who they are going with when they leave the house. You should ask these same questions when your child goes on the internet. Because children are reluctant to disclose victimization for fear of having their internet and cellular phone privileges revoked; develop solutions to prevent or address victimization that do not punish the child.

**Develop rules:** Together with your child, develop rules about acceptable and safe behaviors for all electronic media. Make plans for what they should do if they become a victim of electronic aggression or know someone who is being victimized. The rules should focus on ways to maximize the benefits of technology and decrease its risks.

**Explore the internet:** Visit the websites your child frequents, and assess the pros and cons. Remember, most websites and online activities are beneficial. They help young people learn new information, interact with others, and connect with people who have similar interests.

**Talk with other parents and caregivers:** Talk to other parents and caregivers about how they have discussed technology use with their children. Ask about the rules they have developed and how they stay informed about their child's technology use.

**Connect with the school:** Parents and caregivers are encouraged to work with their child's school and school district to develop a class for parents and caregivers that educates them about school policies on electronic aggression, recent incidents in the community involving electronic aggression, and resources available to parents and caregivers who have concerns. Work with the school and other partners to develop a collaborative approach to preventing electronic aggression.

**Educate yourself:** Stay informed about the new devices and websites your child is using. Technology changes rapidly, and many developers offer information to keep people aware of advances. Continually talk with your child about "where they are going" and explore the technology yourself. Technology is not going away, and forbidding young people to access electronic media may not be a good long-term solution. Together, parents and children can come up with ways to maximize the benefits of technology and decrease its risks.

Chapter 62

# *Parenting a Child Who Has Been Sexually Abused*

Note: Although the term "parents" is used throughout this chapter, the information and strategies provided may be equally helpful for kinship care providers, guardians, and other caregivers.

## *Educating Yourself*

The first step to helping a child who may have been a victim of sexual abuse is to understand more about how sexual abuse is defined, behaviors that may indicate abuse has occurred, how these behaviors may differ from typical sexual behaviors in children, and how sexual abuse may affect children.

### *Signs of Sexual Abuse*

If you are a foster or adoptive parent to a child from the foster care system, you may not know whether he or she has been sexually abused. Child welfare agencies usually share all known information about your child's history with you; however, many children do not disclose past abuse until they feel safe. For this reason, foster or adoptive parents are sometimes the first to learn that sexual abuse has occurred. Even when there is no documentation of prior abuse, you may suspect abuse because of the child's behavior.

Excerpted from "Parenting a Child Who Has Been Sexually Abused: A Guide for Foster and Adoptive Parents," Child Welfare Information Gateway, U.S. Department of Health and Human Services (HHS), April 2008.

Determining whether a child has been abused requires a careful evaluation by a trained professional. While it is normal for all children to have and express sexual curiosity, children who have been sexually abused may demonstrate behaviors that are outside of the range of what might be considered normal. There is no one specific sign or behavior that can be considered proof that sexual abuse has occurred.

### Factors Affecting the Impact of Sexual Abuse

If you suspect, or a professional has determined, that a child in your care has been a victim of sexual abuse, it is important to understand how children may be affected.

All children who have been sexually abused have had their physical and emotional boundaries violated and crossed. With this violation often comes a breach of the child's sense of security and trust. Abused children may come to believe that the world is not a safe place and that adults are not trustworthy.

However, children who have experienced sexual abuse are not all affected the same way. As with other types of abuse, many factors influence how children think and feel about the abuse, how the abuse affects them, and how their recovery progresses. Some factors that can affect the impact of abuse include the following:

- The relationship of the abuser to the child and how much the abuse caused a betrayal of trust

- The abuser's use of friendliness or seduction

- The abuser's use of threats of harm or violence, including threats to pets, siblings, or parents

- The abuser's use of secrecy

- How long the abuse occurred

- Gender of the abuser being the same as or different from the child

- The age (developmental level) of the child at the time of the abuse (younger children are more vulnerable)

- The child's emotional development at the time of the abuse

- The child's ability to cope with his or her emotional and physical responses to the abuse (for example, fear and arousal)

- How much responsibility the child feels for the abuse

It is very important for children to understand that they are not to blame for the abuse they experienced. Your family's immediate response to learning about the sexual abuse and ongoing acceptance of what the child has told you will play a critical role in your child's ability to recover and go back to a healthy life.

## Establishing Family Guidelines for Safety and Privacy

There are things you can do to help ensure that any child visiting or living in your home experiences a structured, safe, and nurturing environment. Some sexually abused children may have a heightened sensitivity to certain situations. Making your home a comfortable place for children who have been sexually abused can mean changing some habits or patterns of family life. Incorporating some of these guidelines may also help reduce foster or adoptive parents' vulnerability to abuse allegations by children living with them. Consider whether the following tips may be helpful in your family's situation:

- **Make sure every family member's comfort level with touching, hugging, and kissing is respected:** Do not force touching on children who seem uncomfortable being touched. Encourage children to respect the comfort and privacy of others.

- **Be cautious with playful touch, such as play fighting and tickling:** These may be uncomfortable or scary reminders of sexual abuse to some children.

- **Help children learn the importance of privacy:** Remind children to knock before entering bathrooms and bedrooms, and encourage children to dress and bathe themselves if they are able. Teach children about privacy and respect.

- **Keep adult sexuality private:** Teenage siblings may need reminders about what is permitted in your home when boyfriends and girlfriends are present.

- **Be aware of and limit sexual messages received through the media:** Children who have experienced sexual abuse can find sexual content overstimulating or disturbing. It may be helpful to monitor music and music videos, as well as television programs, video games, and movies containing nudity, sexual activity, or sexual language. Limit access to grown-up magazines and monitor children's internet use.

If your child has touching problems (or any sexually aggressive behaviors), you may need to take additional steps to help ensure safety for your child as well as his or her peers. Consider how these tips may apply to your own situation:

- **With friends:** If your child has issues with touching other children, you may want to ensure supervision when he or she is playing with friends, whether at your home or theirs. Sleep-overs may not be a good idea when children have touching problems.

- **At school:** You may wish to inform your child's school of any inappropriate sexual behavior, to ensure an appropriate level of supervision. Often this information can be kept confidential by a school counselor or other personnel.

- **In the community:** Supervision becomes critical any time children with sexual behavior problems are with groups of children, for example at day camp or after-school programs.

In any case, keep the lines of communication open, so children feel more comfortable turning to you with problems and talking with you about anything—not just sexual abuse. Remember however, that sexual abuse is difficult for most children to disclose even to a trusted adult.

## Seeking Help

Responding to the needs of a child who has been sexually abused may involve the whole family and will likely have an impact on all family relationships. Mental health professionals (for example, counselors, therapists, or social workers) can help you and your family cope with reactions, thoughts, and feelings about the abuse.

### Impact of Sexual Abuse on the Family

Being an adoptive or foster parent to sexually abused children can be stressful to marriages and relationships. Parenting in these situations may require some couples to be more open with each other and their children about sexuality than in the past. If one parent is more involved in addressing the issue than another, the imbalance can create difficulties in the parental relationship. A couple's sexual relationship can also be affected, if sex begins to feel like a troubled area of the family's life. When these problems emerge, it is often helpful to get professional advice.

Your child's siblings (birth, foster, or adoptive) may be exposed to new or focused attention on sexuality that can be challenging for them. If one child is acting out sexually, you may need to talk with siblings about what they see, think, and feel, as well as how to respond. Children may also need to be coached on what (and how much) to say about their sibling's problems to their friends. If your children see that you are actively managing the problem, they will feel more secure and will worry less.

When one child has been sexually abused, parents often become very protective of their other children. It is important to find a balance between reasonable worry and overprotectiveness. Useful strategies to prevent further abuse may include teaching children to stand up for themselves, talking with them about being in charge of their bodies, and fostering open communication with your children.

## Counseling for Parents and Children

Talking with a mental health professional who specializes in child sexual abuse as soon as problems arise can help parents determine if their children's behavior is cause for concern. Specialists can also provide parents with guidance in responding to their children's difficulties and offer suggestions for how to talk with their children. A mental health professional may suggest special areas of attention in family life and offer specific suggestions for creating structured, safe, and nurturing environments.

To help a child who has been abused, many mental health professionals will begin with a thorough assessment to explore how the child functions in all areas of life. The specialist will want to know about:

- past stressors (history of abuse, frequent moves and other losses);
- current stressors (a medical problem or learning disability);
- emotional state (Is the child usually happy or anxious?);
- coping strategies (Does the child withdraw or act out when angry or sad?);
- the child's friendships;
- the child's strengths (Is the child creative, athletic, organized?);
- the child's communication skills; and
- the child's attachments to adults in his or her life.

After a thorough assessment, the mental health professional will decide if the child and family could benefit from therapy. Not all abused children require therapy. For those who do, the mental health professional will develop a plan tailored to the child and family's strengths and needs. This plan may include one or more of the following types of therapy:

- **Individual therapy:** The frequency and duration of therapy can vary tremendously. The style of therapy will depend on the child's age and the therapist's training. Some therapists use creative techniques (for example, art, play, and music therapy) to help children who are uncomfortable talking about their experiences. Other therapists use traditional talk therapy or a combination of approaches.

- **Group therapy:** Meeting in groups with other children who have been sexually abused can help children understand themselves; feel less alone (by interacting with others who have had similar experiences); and learn new skills through role plays, discussion, games, and play.

- **Family therapy:** Many therapists will see children and parents together to support positive parent-child communication and to guide parents in learning new skills that will help their children feel better and behave appropriately. Whether or not family therapy is advised, it is vital for parents to stay involved in their child's therapy or other kinds of treatment. Skilled mental health professionals will always seek to involve the parents by asking for and sharing information.

## *Your Child Welfare Agency*

If you are a foster parent or seeking to adopt a child, you may wish to talk with your social worker about what you discover about your child's history and any behaviors that worry you. Sharing your concerns will help your social worker help you and your family. If your child exhibits problematic sexual behaviors, be aware that you may also be required to report these to child protective services in order to comply with mandated reporting laws in your jurisdiction.

Many adoptive parents also call their local child welfare agency to seek advice if their child shows troubling behaviors. Child welfare workers are often good sources of information, can offer advice, and are familiar with community resources. Adoption agencies may also be able to provide additional post-adoption services or support to adoptive parents who find out about their child's history of sexual abuse after the adoption is finalized.

## What to Look for in a Mental Health Professional

Finding a knowledgeable and experienced mental health professional is key to getting the help your family needs. Some communities have special programs for treating children who have been sexually abused, such as child protection teams and child advocacy centers. You may also find qualified specialists in your community through the following organizations.

- Child advocacy centers

- Rape crisis or sexual assault centers

- Local psychological or psychiatric association referral services

- Child abuse hotlines

- Child protective services (CPS) agencies

- Nonprofit service providers serving families of missing or exploited children

- University departments of social work, psychology, or psychiatry

- Crime victim assistance programs in the law enforcement agency, prosecutor's, or district attorney's office

- Family court services, including court appointed special advocate (CASA) groups or guardians ad litem

Therapy for children who have been sexually abused is specialized work. When selecting a mental health professional, look for the following:

- An advanced degree in a recognized mental health specialty such as psychiatry, psychology, social work, counseling, or psychiatric nursing

- Licensure to practice as a mental health professional in your state (Some mental health services are provided by students under the supervision of licensed professionals.)

- Special training in child sexual abuse, including the dynamics of abuse, how it affects children and adults, and the use of goal-oriented treatment plans

- Knowledge about the legal issues involved in child sexual abuse, especially the laws about reporting child sexual victimization, procedures used by law enforcement and protective services, evidence collection, and expert testimony in your state

## *Conclusion*

Many people want to help children who have been sexually abused, but many struggle with feelings of anger and disgust as they learn more about the abuse. You may need help to resolve these struggles and to move toward acceptance of your child's background.

If you were (or suspect you may have been) sexually abused as a child, dealing with your own child's difficulties may be particularly challenging. Your courage in facing these issues and tackling a personally difficult and painful subject can actually be helpful to your children by demonstrating to them that sexual abuse experiences can be managed and overcome.

Creating a structured, safe, and nurturing home is the greatest gift that you can give to all of your children. Seek help when you need it, share your successes with your social worker, and remember that a healthy relationship with your children allows them to begin the recovery process. It is in the parent-child relationship that your child learns trust and respect, two important building blocks of your children's safety and well-being.

Chapter 63

# Parents Can Help Children Cope with Violence

Parents and family members play important roles. They help children who experience violence or disaster. They help children cope with trauma. They help protect children from further trauma. They help children get medical care and counseling. They also help young people avoid or overcome emotional problems. These problems can result from trauma.

## Coping with Trauma after Violence and Disasters

Children face many traumas. Each year, they are injured. They see others harmed by violence. They suffer sexual abuse. They lose loved ones. Or, they witness other tragic events.

Children are very sensitive. They struggle to make sense of trauma. They also respond differently to traumas. They may have emotional reactions. They may hurt deeply. They may find it hard to recover from frightening experiences. They need support. Adult helpers can provide this support. This may help children resolve emotional problems.

## What Is Trauma?

There are two types of trauma—physical and mental. Physical trauma includes the body's response to serious injury and threat. Mental trauma includes frightening thoughts and painful feelings.

This chapter includes text from "Helping Children and Adolescents Cope with Violence and Disasters: What Parents Can Do," National Institute of Mental Health (NIMH), January 2009.

They are the mind's response to serious injury. Mental trauma can produce strong feelings. It can also produce extreme behavior; such as intense fear or helplessness, withdrawal or detachment, lack of concentration, irritability, sleep disturbance, aggression, hyper-vigilance (intensely watching for more distressing events), or flashbacks (sense that event is reoccurring).

A response could be fear. It could be fear that a loved one will be hurt or killed. It is believed that more direct exposures to traumatic events causes greater harm. For instance, in a school shooting, an injured student will probably be more severely affected emotionally than a student who was in another part of the building. However, second-hand exposure to violence can also be traumatic. This includes witnessing violence such as seeing or hearing about death and destruction after a building is bombed or a plane crashes.

## Helping Young Trauma Survivors

Helping children begins at the scene of the event. It may need to continue for weeks or months. Most children recover within a few weeks. Some need help longer. Grief (a deep emotional response to loss) may take months to resolve. It could be for a loved one or a teacher. It could be for a friend or pet. Grief may be re-experienced or worsened by news reports or the event's anniversary.

Some children may need help from a mental health professional. Some people may seek other kinds of help. They may turn to religious leaders. They may turn to community leaders. It is important to identify children who need the most support. Help them obtain it. Monitor their healing.

Identify children who exhibit the following:

- Refuse to go places that remind them of the event

- Seem numb emotionally

- Show little reaction to the event

- Behave dangerously

These children may need extra help.

In general, adult helpers should do the following:

- Attend to children:
  - Listen to them

- Accept and do not argue about their feelings
- Help them cope with the reality of their experiences
- Reduce effects of other sources of stress:
  - Frequent moving or changes in place of residence
  - Long periods away from family and friends
  - Pressures at school
  - Transportation problems
  - Fighting within the family
  - Being hungry
- Monitor healing:
  - It takes time
  - Do not ignore severe reactions
  - Attend to sudden changes in behaviors, speech, language use, or in emotional and feeling states
- Remind children that adults love them, support them, and will be with them when possible

## How Parents Can Help

After violence or a disaster parents and family should help with the following:

- Identify and address their own feelings—this will allow them to help others
- Explain to children what happened
- Let children know:
  - You love them
  - The event was not their fault
  - You will take care of them, but only if you can; be honest
  - It's okay for them to feel upset
- Do:
  - Allow children to cry
  - Allow sadness

- Let children talk about feelings
- Let them write about feelings
- Let them draw pictures
- Do not:
  - Expect children to be brave or tough
  - Make children discuss the event before they are ready
  - Get angry if children show strong emotions
  - Get upset if they begin bed-wetting, acting out, or thumb-sucking
- If children have trouble sleeping:
  - Give them extra attention
  - Let them sleep with a light on
  - Let them sleep in your room (for a short time)
- Try to keep normal routines (such routines may not be normal for some children):
  - Bedtime stories
  - Eating dinner together
  - Watching television together
  - Reading books, exercising, playing games
- If you can't keep normal routines, make new ones together
- Help children feel in control:
  - Let them choose meals, if possible
  - Let them pick out clothes, if possible
  - Let them make some decisions for themselves, when possible

## Help for all People in the First Days and Weeks

Key steps after a disaster can help adults cope. Adults can then provide better care for children. Create an environment of safety. Be calm. Be hopeful. Be friendly, even if people are difficult. Connect to others. Listen to their stories. But, listen only if they want to share. Encourage respect for adult decision-making.

In general, help people to do the following:

- Get food
- Get a safe place to live
- Get help from a doctor or nurse if hurt
- Contact loved ones or friends
- Keep children with parents or relatives
- Become aware of available help
- Become aware of where to get help
- Understand what happened
- Understand what is being done
- Move towards meeting their own needs

Avoid certain things such as the following:

- Don't force people to tell their stories
- Don't probe for personal details
- Do not say:
  - "Everything will be okay"
  - "At least you survived"
  - What you think people should feel
  - How people should have acted
  - People suffered for personal behaviors or beliefs
  - Negative things about available help
- Don't make promises that you can't keep (for example: "You will go home soon.")

## How Children React to Trauma

Children's reactions to trauma can be immediate. Reactions may also appear much later. Reactions differ in severity. They also cover a range of behaviors. People from different cultures may have their own ways of reacting. Other reactions vary according to age.

One common response is loss of trust. Another is fear of the event reoccurring. Some children are more vulnerable to trauma's effects. Children with existing mental health problems may be more affected. Children who have experienced other traumatic events may be more affected.

## Children Age Five and Under

Children under five can react in a number of ways:

- Facial expressions of fear
- Clinging to parent or caregiver
- Crying or screaming
- Whimpering or trembling
- Moving aimlessly
- Becoming immobile
- Returning to behaviors common to being younger such as thumb-sucking, bedwetting, being afraid of the dark

Young children's reactions are strongly influenced by parent reactions to the event.

## Children Age Six to Eleven

Children between six and eleven have a range of reactions. They may react in the following ways:

- Isolate themselves
- Become quiet around friends, family, and teachers
- Have nightmares or other sleep problems
- Become irritable or disruptive
- Have outbursts of anger
- Start fights
- Be unable to concentrate
- Refuse to go to school
- Complain of unfounded physical problems
- Develop unfounded fears
- Become depressed
- Become filled with guilt
- Feel numb emotionally
- Do poorly with school and homework.

### *Adolescents Age Twelve to Seventeen*

Children between twelve and seventeen have various reactions:

- Flashbacks to the traumatic event (flashbacks are the mind reliving the event)
- Avoiding reminders of the event
- Drug, alcohol, tobacco use and abuse
- Antisocial behavior, i.e., disruptive, disrespectful, or destructive behavior
- Physical complaints
- Nightmares or other sleep problems
- Isolation or confusion
- Depression
- Suicidal thoughts

Adolescents may feel guilty about the event. They may feel guilt for not preventing injury or deaths. They may also have thoughts of revenge.

## *More about Trauma and Stress*

Some children will have prolonged problems after a traumatic event. These may include grief, depression, anxiety, and post-traumatic stress disorder (PTSD). Children may show a range of symptoms including the following:

- Re-experiencing the event through play, trauma-specific nightmares, in flashbacks and unwanted memories, or by distress over events that remind them of the trauma
- Avoidance of reminders of the event
- Lack of responsiveness
- Lack of interest in things that used to interest them
- A sense of having no future
- Increased sleep disturbances
- Irritability
- Poor concentration

- Be easily startled

- Behavior from earlier life stages

Children experience trauma differently. It is difficult to tell how many will develop mental health problems. Some trauma survivors get better with only good support. Others need counseling by a mental health professional.

If, after a month in a safe environment, children are not able to perform normal routines or new symptoms develop, then contact a health professional.

Some people are more sensitive to trauma. Factors that may influence how someone may respond include the following:

- Being directly involved in the trauma, especially as a victim

- Severe or prolonged exposure to the event

- Personal history of prior trauma

- Family or personal history of mental illness and severe behavioral problems

- Lack of social support

- Lack of caring family and friends

- Ongoing life stressors such as moving to a new home, or new school, divorce, job change, financial troubles

Some symptoms may require immediate attention. Contact a mental health professional if these symptoms occur:

- Flashbacks

- Racing heart and sweating

- Being easily startled

- Being emotionally numb

- Being very sad or depressed

- Thoughts or actions to end life

# Part Seven

# Additional Help
# and Information

Chapter 64

# Glossary of Terms Related to Child Abuse and Neglect

**adjudicatory hearings:** Held by the juvenile and family court to determine whether a child has been maltreated or whether another legal basis exists for the state to intervene to protect the child. [2]

**Adoption and Safe Families Act (ASFA):** Signed into law November 1997 and designed to improve the safety of children, to promote adoption and other permanent homes for children who need them, and to support families. The law requires child protective services (CPS) agencies to provide more timely and focused assessment and intervention services to the children and families that are served within the CPS system. [2]

**alleged victim:** Child about whom a report regarding maltreatment has been made to a CPS agency. [1]

**assessment:** A process by which the CPS agency determines whether the child and/or other persons involved in the report of alleged maltreatment is in need of services. [1]

**Child Abuse Prevention and Treatment Act (CAPTA):** See Keeping Children and Families Safe Act. [2]

---

Terms in this chapter that are marked with a [1] are excerpted from "National Child Abuse and Neglect Data System Glossary," Administration for Children and Families, updated February 10, 2009. Terms marked with a [2] are excerpted from "Working with the Courts in Child Protection: Appendix A," Child Welfare Information Gateway, U.S. Department of Health and Human Services (HHS), updated September 18, 2008.

**child protective services (CPS):** The designated social services agency (in most states) to receive reports, investigate, and provide intervention and treatment services to children and families in which child maltreatment has occurred. [2]

**child victim:** A child for whom an incident of abuse or neglect has been substantiated or indicated by an investigation or assessment. [1]

**court-appointed representative:** A person required to be appointed by the court to represent a child in a neglect or abuse proceeding. May be an attorney or a court-appointed special advocate (or both) and is often referred to as a guardian ad litem. Makes recommendations to the court concerning the best interests of the child. [1]

**court-appointed special advocates (CASA):** Individuals (usually volunteers) who serve to ensure that the needs and interests of a child in child protection judicial proceedings are fully protected. [2]

**dependent child:** As used in statues providing for the care of dependent, neglected, and delinquent children, the term means dependent upon the public support. This includes any child under the age of 18 who is destitute, or whose home by reason of neglect by the parents is an unfit place for such child, or whose father, mother, guardian, or custodian does not properly provide for such a child. [2]

**differential response:** An area of CPS reform that offers greater flexibility in responding to allegations of abuse and neglect. Also referred to as dual track or multi-track response, it permits CPS agencies to respond differentially to children's needs for safety, the degree of risk present, and the family's needs for services and support. [2]

**dispositional hearings:** Held by the juvenile and family court to determine the legal resolution of cases after adjudication, such as whether placement of the child in out-of-home care is necessary, and what services the children and family will need to reduce the risk and to address the effects of maltreatment. [2]

**emotional abuse:** See psychological maltreatment.

**family assessment:** The stage of the child protection process when the CPS caseworker, community treatment provider, and the family reach a mutual understanding regarding the behaviors and conditions that must change to reduce or eliminate the risk of maltreatment, the most critical treatment needs that must be addressed, and the strengths on which to build. [2]

**family drug court:** A drug court that deals with cases involving parental rights in which an adult is the litigant (for example, any party to a lawsuit, which means plaintiff, defendant, petitioner, respondent, cross-complainant and cross-defendant, but not a witness or attorney); the case comes before the court through either a criminal or civil proceeding; and the case arises out of the substance abuse of a parent. [2]

**family preservation services:** Activities designed to protect children from harm and to assist families at risk or in crisis, including services to prevent placement, to support the reunification of children with their families, or to support the continued placement of children in adoptive homes or other permanent living arrangements. [1]

**family support services:** Community-based preventative activities designed to alleviate stress and promote parental competencies and behaviors that will increase the ability of families to successfully nurture their children, enable families to use other resources and opportunities available in the community, and create supportive networks to enhance child-rearing abilities of parents. [1]

**foster care:** Twenty-four-hour substitute care for children placed away from their parents or guardians and for whom the state agency has placement and care responsibility. This includes, but is not limited to, family foster homes, foster homes of relatives, group homes, emergency shelters, residential facilities, child care institutions, and pre-adoptive homes regardless of whether the facility is licensed and whether payments are made by the state or local agency for the care of the child, or whether there is federal matching of any payments made. [1]

**guardian ad litem:** A lawyer or layperson who represents a child in juvenile or family court. Usually this person considers the "best interest" of the child and may perform a variety of roles, including those of independent investigator, advocate, advisor, and guardian for the child. A layperson who serves in this role is sometimes known as a court-appointed special advocate or CASA. [2]

**immunity:** Established in all child abuse laws to protect reporters from civil law suits and criminal prosecution resulting from filing a report of child abuse and neglect. [2]

**initial assessment or investigation:** The stage of the CPS case process where the CPS caseworker determines the validity of the child maltreatment report, assesses the risk of maltreatment, determines if the child is safe, develops a safety plan if needed to assure the child's protection, and determines services needed. [2]

**juvenile and family courts:** Established in most states to resolve conflict and to otherwise intervene in the lives of families in a manner that promotes the best interest of children. These courts specialize in areas such as child maltreatment, domestic violence, juvenile delinquency, divorce, child custody, and child support. [2]

**Keeping Children and Families Safe Act:** The Keeping Children and Families Safe Act of 2003 (P.L. 108-36) included the reauthorization of the Child Abuse Prevention and Treatment Act (CAPTA) in its Title I, Sec. 111. CAPTA provides minimum standards for defining child physical abuse and neglect and sexual abuse that states must incorporate into their statutory definitions in order to receive federal funds. CAPTA defines child abuse and neglect as "at a minimum, any recent act or failure to act on the part of a parent or caretaker, which results in death, serious physical or emotional harm, sexual abuse or exploitation, or an act or failure to act which presents an imminent risk of serious harm." [2]

**kinship care:** Formal child placement by the juvenile court and child welfare agency in the home of a child's relative. [2]

**maltreatment:** An act or failure to act by a parent, caretaker, or other person as defined under state law which results in physical abuse, neglect, medical neglect, sexual abuse, emotional abuse, or an act or failure to act which presents an imminent risk of serious harm to a child. [1]

**maltreatment death:** Death of a child as a result of abuse or neglect, because either: (a) an injury resulting from the abuse or neglect was the cause of death; or (b) abuse and/or neglect were contributing factors to the cause of death. [1]

**maltreatment type:** A particular form of child maltreatment determined by investigation to be substantiated or indicated under state law. Types include physical abuse, neglect or deprivation of necessities, sexual abuse, psychological or emotional maltreatment, and other forms included in state law. [1]

**mandated reporter:** Individuals required by state statutes to report suspected child abuse and neglect to the proper authorities (usually CPS or law enforcement agencies). Mandated reporters typically include professionals, such as educators and other school personnel, health care and mental health professionals, social workers, childcare providers, and law enforcement officers. Some states identify all citizens as mandated reporters. [2]

**neglect:** The failure to provide for a child's basic needs. Neglect can be physical, educational, or emotional. Physical neglect can include not providing adequate food or clothing, appropriate medical care, supervision, or proper weather protection (heat or coats). Educational neglect includes failure to provide appropriate schooling, special educational needs, or allowing excessive truancies. Psychological neglect includes the lack of any emotional support and love, chronic inattention to the child, exposure to spouse abuse, or drug and alcohol abuse. [2]

**not substantiated:** Investigation disposition that determines that there is not sufficient evidence under state law or policy to conclude that the child has been maltreated or is at risk of being maltreated. [1]

**parent or caretaker:** Person responsible for the care of the child. [2]

**perpetrator:** The person who has been determined to have caused or knowingly allowed the maltreatment of the child. [1]

**physical abuse:** The inflicting of a nonaccidental physical injury upon a child. This may include, burning, hitting, punching, shaking, kicking, beating, or otherwise harming a child. It may, however, have been the result of over-discipline or physical punishment that is inappropriate to the child's age. [2]

**preventive services:** Beneficial activities aimed at preventing child abuse and neglect. Such activities may be directed at specific populations identified as being at increased risk of becoming abusive and may be designed to increase the strength and stability of families, to increase parents' confidence and competence in their parenting abilities, and to afford children a stable and supportive environment. [1]

**psychological or emotional maltreatment:** Type of maltreatment that refers to acts or omissions, other than physical abuse or sexual abuse, that caused, or could have caused, conduct, cognitive, affective, or other mental disorders. It includes emotional neglect, psychological abuse and mental injury. Frequently occurs as verbal abuse or excessive demands on a child's performance and may cause the child to have a negative self-image and disturbed behavior. [1]

**report:** Notification to the CPS agency of suspected child maltreatment; can include one or more children. [1]

**respite care services:** Beneficial activities involving temporary care of the child(ren) to provide relief to the caretaker. It may involve care of the children outside of the caretaker's own home for a brief period of time, such as overnight or for a weekend. Not considered by the state to be foster care or other placement. [1]

**risk assessment:** To assess and measure the likelihood that a child will be maltreated in the future, frequently through the use of checklists, matrices, scales, and other methods of measurement. [2]

**risk factors:** Behaviors and conditions present in the child, parent, or family that likely will contribute to child maltreatment occurring in the future. [2]

**safety plan:** A casework document developed when it is determined that the child is in imminent or potential risk of serious harm. In the safety plan, the caseworker targets the factors that are causing or contributing to the risk of imminent serious harm to the child, and identifies, along with the family, the interventions that will control the safety factors and ensure the child's protection. [2]

**sexual abuse:** A type of maltreatment that refers to the involvement of the child in sexual activity to provide sexual gratification or financial benefit to the perpetrator, including contacts for sexual purposes, molestation, statutory rape, prostitution, pornography, exposure, incest, or other sexually exploitative activities. [1]

**substantiated:** A type of investigation disposition that concludes that the allegation of maltreatment or risk of maltreatment was supported or founded by state law or state policy. This is the highest level of finding by a state agency. [1]

**treatment:** The stage of the child protection case process when specific services are provided by CPS and other providers to reduce the risk of maltreatment, support families in meeting case goals, and address the effects of maltreatment. [2]

Chapter 65

# State Telephone Numbers for Reporting Child Abuse and Neglect

**Note:** If a child is in danger or a life-threatening situation, call 911 immediately.

Following is an alphabetical listing of state toll-free numbers for specific agencies designated to receive and investigate reports of suspected child abuse and neglect.

**Alabama**
Phone: 334-242-9500
Website: http://
www.dhr.state.al.us/
page.asp?pageid=304
E-mail: fsd@dhr.alabama.gov

**Alaska**
Toll-Free: 800-478-4444
Website: http://www.hss.state
.ak.us/ocs/default.htm

**Arizona**
Toll-Free: 888-767-2445
Website: https://www.azdes.gov/
dcyf/cps/reporting.asp

**Arkansas**
Toll-Free: 800-482-5964
Toll-Free TDD: 800-843-6349
Website: http://www.arkansas
.gov/reportARchildabuse

---

This chapter includes text from "Child Abuse Reporting Numbers," Child Welfare Information Gateway, U.S. Department of Health and Human Services (HHS). All contact information was current as of May 1, 2009.

## California
Toll-Free: Phone numbers for all 58 counties can be found online at: http://www.childsworld.ca.gov/res/pdf/CPSEmergNumbers.pdf
Website: http://www.dss.cahwnet.gov/cdssweb/PG20.htm

## Colorado
Phone: 303-866-5932
Website: http://www.cdhs.state.co.us/childwelfare/FAQ.htm

## Connecticut
Toll-Free: 800-842-2288
Toll-Free TDD: 800-624-5518
Website: http://www.state.ct.us/dcf/HOTLINE.htm

## Delaware
Toll-Free: 800-292-9582
Website: http://kids.delaware.gov/services/crisis.shtml

## District of Columbia
Phone: 202-671-SAFE (7233)
Website: http://cfsa.dc. gov/cfsa/cwp/view.asp?a=3&q=520663&cfsaNav=|31319|

## Florida
Toll-Free: 800-96-ABUSE (22873)
Website: http://www.dcf.state.fl.us/abuse

## Georgia
Phone: 404-651-9361
Website: http://dfcs.dhr.georgia.gov/portal/site

## Hawaii
Phone: 808-832-5300
Website: http://www.hawaii.gov/dhs/protection/social_services/child_welfare

## Idaho
Toll-Free: 800-926-2588
Toll-Free TDD: 208-332-7205
Website: http://www.healthandwelfare.idaho.gov/site/3333/default.aspx

## Illinois
Toll-Free: 800-25-ABUSE (22873)
Phone: 217-524-2606
Website: http://www.state.il.us/dcfs/child/index.shtml

## Indiana
Toll-Free: 800-800-5556
Website: http://www.in.gov/dcs/protection/dfcchi.html

## Iowa
Toll-Free: 800-362-2178
Website: http://www.dhs.state.ia.us/dhs2005/dhs_homepage/children_family/abuse_reporting/child_abuse.html

## Kansas
Toll-Free: 800-922-5330
Website: http://www.srskansas.org/services/child_protective_services.htm

## Kentucky
Toll-Free: 800-752-6200
Website: http://chfs.ky.gov/dcbs/dpp/childsafety.htm

## Louisiana
Phone: Website lists hotline
numbers by parish
Website: http://www.dss.state.la
.us/index.cfm?md=pagebuilder
&tmp=home&pid=181

## Maine
Toll-Free: 800-452-1999
Toll-Free TTY: 800-963-9490
Website: http://www.maine.gov/
dhhs/bcfs/abusereporting.htm

## Maryland
Toll-Free: 800-332-6347
Toll-Free Spanish: 800-732-7850
Toll-Free TTY: 800-925-4434
Website: http://www.dhr.state
.md.us/cps/report.htm

## Massachusetts
Toll-Free: 800-792-5200
Website: http://mass.gov/?pageID
=eohhs2terminal&L=5&L0
=Home&L1=Consumer&L2
=Family+Services&L3=Violence
%2c+Abuse+or+Neglect&L4
=Child+Abuse+and+Neglect&sid
=Eeohhs2&b=terminalcontent
&f=dss_c_can_reporting&csid
=Eeohhs2

## Michigan
Toll-Free: 800-942-4357
Website: http://www.michigan
.gov/dhs/0,1607,7-124-5452
_7119_7193-15252—,00.html

## Minnesota
Phone: Numbers found for each
county online at: http://www
.state.mn.us/portal/mn/jsp/
content.do?az_type=description
&subchannel=-536879913
&programid=536879800 &sc3
=null&sc2=null&id=-8494
&agency=NorthStar
Website: http://www.dhs.state.mn
.us/main/idcplg?IdcService =GET
_DYNAMIC_C ONVERSION
&RevisionSelectionMethod
=LatestReleased&dDocName
=id_000152

## Mississippi
Toll-Free: 800-222-8000
Phone: 601-359-4991
Website: http://www.mdhs.state
.ms.us/fcs_prot.html

## Missouri
Toll-Free: 800-392-3738
Phone: 573-751-3448
Website: http://www.dss.mo.gov/
cd/rptcan.htm

## Montana
Toll-Free: 866-820-5437
Website: http://www.dphhs.mt
.gov/cfsd/index.shtml

## Nebraska
Toll-Free: 800-652-1999
Website: http://www.hhs.state
.ne.us/cha/chaindex.htm

## Nevada
Toll-Free: 800-992-5757
Website: http://dcfs.state.nv.us/
DCFS_ReportSuspectedChild
Abuse.htm

## New Hampshire
Toll-Free: 800-894-5533
Phone: 603-271-6556
Website: http://www.dhhs.state
.nh.us/DHHS/BCP/default.htm

## New Jersey
Toll-Free: 877-NJ-ABUSE
(65-22873)
Toll-Free TTY: 800-835-5510
Website: http://www.state.nj.us/
dcf/abuse/how

## New Mexico
Toll-Free: 800-797-3260
Website: http://www.cyfd.org/
node/26

## New York
Toll-Free: 800-342-3720
Toll-Free TDD: 800-638-5163
Phone: 518-474-8740
Website: http://www.ocfs.state
.ny.us/main/cps

## North Carolina
Phone: 919-733-4622
Website: http://www.dhhs.state
.nc.us/dss/cps/index.htm

## North Dakota
Toll-Free: 800-245-3736
Website: http://www.nd.gov/
dhs/services/childfamily/cps/
#reporting

## Ohio
Toll-Free: 866-635-3748
Website: http://jfs.ohio.gov/
county/cntydir.stm

## Oklahoma
Toll-Free: 800-522-3511
Website: http://www.okdhs.org/
programsandservices/cps/
default.htm

## Oregon
Phone: A list of county numbers
can be found at website.
Website: http://www.oregon.gov/
DHS/children/abuse/cps/report
.shtml
E-mail for non-emergency re-
ports: dhs.info@state.or.us

## Pennsylvania
Toll-Free: 800-932-0313
Toll-Free TDD: 866-872-1677
Website: http://www.dpw.state
.pa.us/ServicesPrograms/
ChildWelfare/003671030.htm

## Rhode Island
Toll-Free: 800-RI-CHILD
(74-24453)
Website: http://www.dcyf.ri.gov/
child_welfare/index.php

## South Carolina
Phone: 803-898-7318
Website: http://www.state.sc.us/
dss/cps/index.html

## South Dakota
Phone: 605-773-3227
Website: http://dss.sd.gov/cps/
protective/reporting.asp

## Tennessee
Toll-Free: 877-237-0004; or
877-54-ABUSE (22873)
Website: http://state.tn.us/youth/
childsafety.htm

## Texas
Toll-Free: 800-252-5400
Website: https://www.dfps.state
.tx.us/Child_Protection/About
_Child_Protective_Services/
reportChildAbuse.asp

## Utah
Toll-Free: 800-678-9399
Website: http://www.hsdcfs.utah
.gov

## Vermont
Toll-Free: 800-649-5285
Website: http://www.dcf.state
.vt.us/fsd/reporting_child_abuse

## Virginia
Toll-Free: 800-552-7096
Phone (out of state): 804-786-8536
Website: http://www.dss.virginia
.gov/family/cps/index.html

## Washington
Toll-Free: 866-END-HARM
(363-4276)
Toll-Free (after hours):
800-562-5624
Toll-Free TTY: 800-624-6186
Website: http://www1.dshs.wa
.gov/ca/safety/abuseReport.asp?2

## West Virginia
Toll-Free: 800-352-6513
Website: http://www.wvdhhr.org/
bcf/children_adult/cps/report.asp

## Wisconsin
Phone: 608-266-3036
Website: http://dcf.wisconsin.gov/
children/CPS/cpswimap.HTM

## Wyoming
Phone: 307-777-3663
Website: http://dfsweb.state.wy
.us/menu.htm

Chapter 66

# Organizations with Information for Victims and Survivors of Child Sexual Abuse

*Adult Survivors of Child Abuse (ASCA)*
Morris Center for Healing from Child Abuse
P.O. Box 14477
San Francisco, CA 94114
Phone: 415-928-4576
Website: http://www.ascasupport.org
E-mail: ascaoutreach@yahoo.com

Adult Survivors of Child Abuse (ASCA) supports and assists survivors of child abuse to move on with their lives. In addition, ASCA was created with the intention of guaranteeing that all survivors of childhood abuse, regardless of their financial situation, have access to a program focused on recovery from childhood abuse, including physical, sexual, and/or emotional abuse or neglect.

*American Psychological Association (APA)*
750 First St. NE
Washington, DC 20002-4242
Toll-Free: 800-374-2721
Phone: 202-336-5500
Website: http://www.apa.org

Excerpted from "Adult Survivors Resources List," Child Welfare Information Gateway, U.S. Department of Health and Human Services (HHS), 2008. This information was current as of April 27, 2009.

The American Psychological Association is a national scientific and professional organization representing the field of psychology. The APA offers a wide range of programs and services including a consumer help center, media information, a research office, and a section on public interest topics such as disabilities, ethnic minorities, and issues involving children, youth, and families.

## Child Welfare Information Gateway
Children's Bureau/ACYF
1250 Maryland Ave., SW, 8th Fl.
Washington, DC 20024
Toll-Free: 800-394-3366
Phone: 703-385-7565
Fax: 703-385-3206
Website: http://www.childwelfare.gov
E-mail: info@childwelfare.gov

Child Welfare Information Gateway connects professionals and the general public to information and resources targeted to the safety, permanency, and well-being of children and families. A service of the Children's Bureau, Administration for Children and Families, U.S. Department of Health and Human Services, Child Welfare Information Gateway provides access to programs, research, laws and policies, training resources, statistics, and much more.

## Childhelp®
15757 N. 78th St.
Scottsdale, AZ 85260
Toll-Free: 800-4-A-CHILD (2-24453)
Phone: 480-922-8212
Fax: 480-922-7061
Website: http://www.childhelp.org

Childhelp® is dedicated to helping victims of child abuse and neglect. Childhelp's approach focuses on prevention, intervention, and treatment. The Childhelp National Child Abuse Hotline operates 24 hours a day, seven days a week, and receives calls from throughout the United States, Canada, the U.S. Virgin Islands, Puerto Rico, and Guam. Childhelp's programs and services also include residential treatment services; children's advocacy centers; therapeutic foster care; group homes; child abuse prevention, education and training; and the National Day of Hope®, part of National Child Abuse Prevention Month every April.

## Darkness to Light
7 Radcliffe St., Suite 200
Charleston, SC 29403
Toll-Free: 866-FOR-LIGHT (367-5444)
Phone: 843-965-5444
Fax: 843-965-5449
Website: http://www.darkness2light.org
E-mail: stewards@d2l.org

Darkness to Light is a primary prevention program whose mission is to engage adults in the prevention of child sexual abuse; to reduce the incidence of child sexual abuse nationally through education and public awareness aimed at adults; and to provide adults with information to recognize and react responsibly to child sexual abuse. A link to local resources in all states is provided at http://www.darkness2light .org/GetHelp/helplines.asp.

## FaithTrust Institute
2400 N. 45th St., No. 101
Seattle, WA 98103
Toll-Free: 877-860-2255
Phone: 206-634-1903 (ext. 10)
Fax: 206-634-0115
Website: http://www.faithtrustinstitute.org
E-mail: info@faithtrustinstitute.org

The FaithTrust Institute is an interreligious educational resource that addresses issues of sexual and domestic violence. The Institute's goals are to engage religious leaders in the task of ending abuse, and to serve as a bridge between the religious and secular communities.

## National Institute of Mental Health (NIMH)
6001 Executive Blvd.
Rm. 8184, MSC 9663
Bethesda, MD 20892-9663
Toll-Free: 866-615-6464
Toll-Free TTY: 866-415-8051
Phone: 301-443-4513
Phone TTY: 301-443-8431
Fax: 301-443-4279
Website: http://www.nimh.nih.gov
E-mail: nimhinfo@nih.gov

The National Institute of Mental Health (NIMH) works to diminish the burden of mental illness through research. NIMH seeks to achieve better understanding, treatment, and eventually prevention of mental illness.

### National Sexual Violence Resource Center (NSVRC)

123 N. Enola Dr.
Enola, PA 17025
Toll-Free: 877-739-3895
Phone: 717-909-0710
Fax: 717-909-0714
TTY: 717-909-0715
Website: http://www.nsvrc.org
E-mail: resources@nsvrc.org

The National Sexual Violence Resource Center (NSVRC) serves as an information and resource center regarding all aspects of sexual violence. It provides national leadership, consultation, and technical assistance by generating and facilitating the development and flow of information on sexual violence intervention and prevention strategies. The NSVRC works to address the causes and impact of sexual violence through collaboration, prevention efforts, and the distribution of resources. It also has a relief fund for sexual assault survivors with information available online at http://www.relieffundforsexual assaultvictims.org.

### Office for Victims of Crime (OVC)

U.S. Department of Justice
810 7th St. NW
Washington, DC 20531
Toll-Free: 800-851-3420
Phone: 202-307-5983
Website: http://www.ovc.gov
E-mail: askovc@ncjrs.gov

The Office for Victims of Crimes was established by the 1984 Victims of Crime Act (VOCA) to oversee diverse programs that benefit victims of crime. OVC provides substantial funding to state victim assistance and compensation programs, the lifeline services that help victims to heal. The agency also supports training designed to educate criminal justice and allied professionals on the rights and needs of crime victims. OVC is one of five bureaus and four offices with grant-making authority within the Office of Justice Programs of the U.S. Department of Justice.

### *Rape, Abuse & Incest National Network (RAINN)*
2000 L St. NW, Suite 406
Washington, DC 20036
Toll-Free: 800-656-HOPE (4673)
Phone: 202-544-3064
Fax: 202-544-3556
Website: http://www.rainn.org
E-mail: info@rainn.org

The Rape, Abuse & Incest National Network (RAINN) is an anti-sexual assault organization. RAINN operates the National Sexual Assault Hotline (800-656-HOPE), which provides victims of sexual assault with free, confidential services around the clock, and it carries out programs to prevent sexual assault and to help victims.

### *Safer Society Foundation, Inc.*
P.O. Box 340
Brandon, VT 05733-0340
Phone: 802-247-3132
Fax: 802-247-4233
Website: http://www.safersociety.org
E-mail: ssfi@sover.net

The Safer Society Foundation, Inc., a nonprofit agency, is a national research, advocacy, and referral center on the prevention and treatment of sexual abuse. The Foundation provides training and consultation, research, sex offender treatment referrals, a computerized program network, and a resource library. It also publishes materials for the prevention and treatment of sexual abuse.

### *Sidran Institute*
200 E. Joppa Rd., Suite 207
Baltimore, MD 21286-3107
Phone: 410-825-8888
Fax: 410-337-0747
Website: http://www.sidran.org

The Sidran Institute, a leader in traumatic stress education and advocacy, is a nationally focused nonprofit organization devoted to helping people who have experienced traumatic life events. The Institute promotes improved understanding of the early recognition and treatment of trauma-related stress in children, the long-term effects of trauma on adults, and strategies that lead to the greatest success in self-help recovery for trauma survivors. The Sidran Institute also advocates clinical practices considered successful in aiding trauma victims and the development of public policy initiatives that are responsive to the needs of adult and child survivors of traumatic events.

## Stop It Now!
351 Pleasant St., Suite B-319
Northampton, MA 01060
Toll-Free: 888-PREVENT (773-8368)
Phone: 413-587-3500
Fax: 413-587-3505
Website: http://www.stopitnow.org

Stop It Now! is a national, nonprofit working to prevent and ultimately eradicate child sexual abuse. Stop It Now! challenges adults to take action by calling on abusers, adults at risk to abuse, and their friends and family, to come forward, learn the warning signs, and seek help. Services are available from 9 a.m.–6 p.m., eastern standard time (EST), Mon.–Fri. The toll-free number is a confidential hotline.

## Survivors of Incest Anonymous (SIA)
World Service Office
P.O. Box 190
Benson, MD 21018-9998
Phone: 410-893-3322
Website: http://www.siawso.org

Survivors of Incest Anonymous (SIA) is a 12-step, self-help recovery program modeled after Alcoholics Anonymous. There are no dues or fees. Confidentiality and anonymity are essential to the program. SIA is for men and women, 18 years and older, who were sexually abused as children.

Chapter 67

# Organizations with Information and Referrals for Adults and Juveniles with Sexual Behavior Problems

**Association for the Treatment of Sexual Abusers (ATSA)**
4900 SW Griffith Dr.
Suite 274
Beaverton, OR, 97005
Phone: 503-643-1023
Fax: 503-643-5084
Website: http://www.atsa.com
E-mail: atsa@atsa.com

**Child Molestation Research and Prevention Institute**
1401 Peachtree St.
Suite 120
Atlanta, GA 30309
Phone: 404-872-5152
Website: http://www
.childmolestationprevention.org
E-mail: contact@cmrpi.org

**Croga.org–You Can Stop!**
Website: http://www.croga.org

**Cybersexualaddiction.com**
http://www.cybersexualaddiction
.com

**National Adolescent Perpetration Network**
Kempe Center and Foundation
Gary Pavilion at Children's Hospital
Anschutz Medical Campus
13123 E. 16th Ave. B390
Aurora, CO 80045
Phone: 303-864-5300
Website: http://www.kempe.org/
index.php?s=25
E-mail: questions@kempe.org

---

Information in this chapter was compiled from many sources deemed accurate. All contact information was updated and verified in May 2009. Inclusion does not constitute endorsement.

*Recovery from Child Pornography Use*
1040 North J. St.
Richmond, IN 47374
Website: http://www.childlustrecovery.org

*Safer Society Foundation, Inc.*
P.O. Box 340
Brandon, VT 05733
Phone: 802-247-3132
Fax: 802-247-4233
Website: http://www.safersociety.org

*Self-Help for Sexual Addictions*
P.O. Box 70949
Houston, TX 77270
Toll-Free: 800-477-8191
Website: http://www.sexaa.org
E-mail: info@ssa-recovery.org

*Sex Abuse Treatment Alliance*
P.O. Box 761
Milwaukee, WI 53201
Phone: 517-482-2085
Website: http://www.satasort.org
E-mail: info@satasort.org

*Sexaholics Anonymous International*
Central Office
P.O. Box 3565
Brentwood, TN 37024
Toll-Free: 866-424-8777
Phone: 615-370-6062
Fax: 615-370-0882
Website: http://www.sa.org
E-mail: saico@sa.org

*Sexual Compulsives Anonymous (SCA)*
P.O. Box 1585
Old Chelsea Station
New York, NY 10011
Toll-Free: 800-977-HEAL (4325)
Website: http://www.sca-recovery.org

*Society for the Advancement of Sexual Health*
P.O. Box 433
Royston, GA 30662
Phone: 706-356-7031
Fax: 866-389-3974
Website: http://www.sash.net
E-mail: sash@sash.net

*Stop It Now!*
351 Pleasant St., Suite B-319
Northampton, MA 01060
Toll-Free: 888-PREVENT (773-8368)
Phone: 413-587-3500
Fax: 413-587-3505
Website: http://www.stopitnow.org

Chapter 68

# Directory of Child Abuse Prevention Organizations

**American Humane Association Children's Division**
63 Inverness Dr. E.
Englewood, CO 80112-5117
Toll-Free: 800-227-4645
Phone: 303-792-9900
Fax: 303-792-5333
Website: http://
www.americanhumane.org
E-mail:
info@americanhumane.org

**American Professional Society on the Abuse of Children**
350 Poplar Ave.
Elmhurst, IL 60126
Phone: 630-941-1235
Toll-Free: 877-402-7722
Fax: 630-359-4274
Website: http://www.apsac.org
E-mail: apsac@apsac.org

**Center for Faith-Based and Community Initiatives**
U. S. Department of Health and
Human Services
200 Independence Ave., SW
Washington, DC 20201
Toll-Free: 877-696-6775
Phone: 202-619-0257
Website: http://www.dhhs.gov/
fbci

**Child Molestation Research and Prevention Institute**
1401 Peachtree St.
Suite 120
Atlanta, GA 30309
Phone: 404-872-5152
Website: http://www
.childmolestationprevention.org
E-mail: contact@cmrpi.org

---

Information in this chapter was compiled from many sources deemed accurate. All contact information was updated and verified in May 2009. Inclusion does not constitute endorsement.

**Child Trends**
4301 Connecticut Ave., NW
Suite 350
Washington, DC 20008
Phone: 202-572-6000
Fax: 202-362-8420
Website: http://
www.childtrends.org

**Child Welfare Information Gateway**
1250 Maryland Ave., SW, 8th Fl.
Washington, DC 20024
Toll-Free: 800-394-3366
Phone: 703-385-7565
Fax: 703-385-3206
Website: http://
www.childwelfare.gov
E-mail: info@childwelfare.gov

**Child Welfare League of America**
2345 Crystal Dr., Suite 250
Arlington, VA 22202
Phone: 703-412-2400
Fax: 703-412-2401
Website: http://www.cwla.org

**Childhelp USA**
15757 N. 78th St.
Scottsdale, AZ 85260
Toll-Free: 800-4-A-CHILD
(2-24453)
Phone: 480-922-8212
Fax: 480-922-7061
Website: http://
www.childhelp.org

**Circle of Parents**
500 N. Michigan Ave.
Suite 200
Chicago, IL 60611
Phone: 312-334-6837
Fax: 312-334-6852
Website: http://
www.circleofparents.org

**Family Support America**
(formerly Family Resource
Coalition of America)
307 W. 200 S., Suite 2004
Salt Lake City, UT 84101
Website: http://
www.familysupportamerica.org
E-mail: admin
@familysupportamerica.org

**Find Youth Info**
Toll-Free: 888-600-4777
Website: http://
www.findyouthinfo.gov
E-mail: FindYouthInfo
_Support@kitsolutions.net

**National Association of Counsel for Children**
13123 E. 16th Ave., B390
Aurora, CO 80045
Toll-Free: 888-828-NACC (6222)
Phone: 303-864-5359
Fax: 303-864-5351
Website: http://
www.naccchildlaw.org
E-mail:
advocate@naccchildlaw.org

### National Black Child Development Institute
1313 L St., NW, Suite 110
Washington, DC 20005-4110
Phone: 202-833-2220
Fax: 202-833-8222
Website: http://www.nbcdi.org
E-mail: moreinfo@nbcdi.org

### National Center for Missing and Exploited Children
Charles B. Wang International Children's Bldg.
699 Prince St.
Alexandria, VA 22314-3175
Toll-Free: 800-THE-LOST (843-5678)
Phone: 703-274-3900
Fax: 703-274-2220
Website: http://www.missingkids.com

### National Center for Victims of Crime (NCVC)
2000 M St., NW, Suite 480
Washington, DC 20036
Toll-Free: 800-FYI-CALL (394-2255)
Toll-Free TDD: 800-211-7996
Phone: 202-467-8700
Fax: 202-467-8701
Website: http://www.ncvc.org
E-mail: webmaster@ncvc.org or gethelp@ncvc.org

### National Child Welfare Resource Center on Legal and Judicial Issues
American Bar Association
Center on Children and the Law
740 15th St., NW
Washington, DC 20005-1019
Toll-Free: 800-285-2221
Phone: 202-662-1720
Fax: 202-662-1755
Website: http://www.abanet.org/child/rclji/home.html

### National Children's Advocacy Center
210 Pratt Ave.
Huntsville, AL 35801
Phone: 256-533-KIDS (5437)
Fax: 256-534-6883
Website: http://www.nationalcac.org

### National Council of Juvenile and Family Court Judges
Permanency Planning for Children Dept.
P.O. Box 8970
Reno, NV 89507
Phone: 775-784-6012
Fax: 775-784-6628
Website: http://www.ncjfcj.org
E-mail: staff@ncjfcj.org

## National Court Appointed Special Advocate Association

100 W. Harrison St.,
North Tower, Suite 500
Seattle, WA 98119-4123
Toll-Free: 800-628-3233
Fax: 206-270-0078
Website: http://
www.nationalcasa.org
E-mail: staff@nationalcasa.org

## National Domestic Violence Hotline

P.O. Box 161810
Austin, TX 78716
Toll-Free Hotline:
800-799-SAFE (7233)
Toll-Free TTY: 800-787-3224
Phone: 512-794-1133
Website: http://www.ndvh.org

## National Exchange Club Foundation for the Prevention of Child Abuse

3050 Central Ave.
Toledo, OH 43606-1700
Toll-Free: 800-XCHANGE
(924-2643)
Phone: 419-535-3232
Fax: 419-535-1989
Website: http://www
.nationalexchangeclub.com
E-mail: info@
nationalexchangeclub.org

## National Fatherhood Initiative

101 Lake Forest Blvd., Suite 360
Gaithersburg, MD 20877
Phone: 301-948-0599
Fax: 301-948-4325
Website: http://
www.fatherhood.org

## National Indian Child Welfare Association

5100 SW Macadam Ave.
Suite 300
Portland, OR 97239
Phone: 503-222-4044
Fax: 503-222-4007
Website: http://www.nicwa.org

## National Resource Center for Adoption

16250 Northland Dr.
Suite 120
Southfield, MI 48075
Phone: 248-443-0306
Fax: 248-443-7099
Website: http://
www.nrcadoption.org
E-mail: nrc@nrcadoption.org

## National Sexual Violence Resource Center

123 N. Enola Dr.
Enola, PA 17025
Toll-Free: 877-739-3895
Phone: 717-909-0710
Fax: 717-909-0714
TTY: 717-909-0715

*Parents Anonymous, Inc.*
675 W. Foothill Blvd., Suite 220
Claremont, CA 91711-3475
Phone: 909-621-6184
Fax: 909-625-6304
Website: http://
www.parentsanonymous.org
E-mail: Parentsanonymous
@parentsanonymous.org

*Prevent Child Abuse America*
500 N. Michigan Ave., Suite 200
Chicago, IL 60611
Toll-Free: 800-244-5373
Phone: 312-663-3520
Fax: 312-939-8962
Website: http://
www.preventchildabuse.org
E-mail:
mailbox@preventchildabuse.org

*Rape, Abuse & Incest National Network (RAINN)*
2000 L St., NW, Suite 406
Washington, DC 20036
Toll-Free National Sexual
Assault Hotline: 800-656-HOPE
(4673)
Phone: 202-544-3064
Fax: 202-544-3556
Website: http://www.rainn.org
E-mail: info@rainn.org

*Safer Society Foundation*
P.O. Box 340
Brandon, VT 05733-0340
Phone: 802-247-3132
Fax: 802-247-4233
Website: http://
www.safersociety.org

*Shaken Baby Syndrome Prevention Plus*
649 Main St., Suite B
Groveport, OH 43125
Toll-Free: 800-858-5222
Phone: 614-836-8360
Fax: 614-836-8359
Website: http://www.sbsplus.com
E-mail: sbspp@aol.com

*Stop It Now!*
351 Pleasant St., Suite B-319
Northampton, MA 01060
Toll-Free Helpline:
888-PREVENT (773-8368)
Phone: 413-587-3500
Fax: 413-587-3505
Website:
http:www.stopitnow.com

*Texas Association Against Sexual Assault (TAASA)*
6200 La Calma, Suite 110
Austin, TX 78752
Phone: 512-474-7190
Fax: 512-474-6490
Website: http://www.taasa.org

*Youth Law Center*
Children's Legal Protection
Center
1010 Vermont Ave., NW
Suite 310
Washington, DC 20005-4902
Phone: 202-637-0377
Fax: 202-379-1600
Website: http://www.ylc.org
E-mail:
info@youthlawcenter.com

# *Index*

Index

# *Index*

581

guardian ad litem (GAL)
child maltreatment legislation 272
defined 555
see also court appointed
special advocates
guardianship, kinship care 312
see also caregivers; caretakers
"Guidelines for Helping Children
Experiencing Abuse or Neglect"
(American Humane Association) 265n
"Guide to Effective Programs for
Children and Youth: Parent-Child
Interaction Therapy (PCIT)" (Child
Trends) 410n
"Guide to Effective Programs for
Children and Youth: Trauma-
Focused Cognitive-Behavioral
Therapy (TF-CBT)" (Child
Trends) 412n
Guiding Good Choices program,
contact information 480

# H

Hanson, R.F. 417n
harassment
electronic aggression 194–95
sexual abuse 230–31
youth sports 175–79
Harm Standard, described 52
Hawaii
child abuse reporting
contact information 560
clergy, child abuse reporting *292*
differential response policy *326*
health care delay, described 7
health care denial, described 7
health insurance *see* insurance
coverage
Health Resources and Services
Administration (HRSA), bullying
publications 181n, 523n
Healthy Families America (HFA)
program, website address 466
"Healthy Marriage and the Legacy
of Child Maltreatment: A Child
Welfare Perspective" (Conway;
Hutson) 125n

Healthy Steps program,
website address 466
"Helping Children and Adolescents
Cope with Violence and Disasters:
What Parents Can Do" (NIMH)
543n
"Helping St. Louis County Families:
A Guide for Court Professionals"
(Litton) 111n
"Helping Your Foster Child
Transition to Your Adopted Child:
Factsheet for Families" (Child
Welfare Information Gateway) 387n
HFA *see* Healthy Families America
HHS *see* US Department of Health
and Human Services
HIPPY *see* Home-Based Instruction
for Parents of Preschool Youngsters
Home-Based Instruction for Parents
of Preschool Youngsters (HIPPY)
program, website address 467
home visitation programs,
overview 463–68
"Home Visiting Programs: A Brief
Overview of Selected Models"
(DHHS) 463n
hospitalizations, child abuse
financial considerations *53*
"How the Child Welfare System
Works" (Child Welfare Information
Gateway) 295n
HRSA *see* Health Resources
and Services Administration
Hutson, Rutledge Q. 125n

# I

Idaho
child abuse reporting
contact information 560
clergy, child abuse reporting *292*
differential response policy *326*
Illinois
child abuse reporting
contact information 560
clergy, child abuse reporting *292*
respite care services 460
immunity, defined 555

statistics, continued
  domestic violence, children 112
  electronic aggression 191–92
  female genital mutilation 257, 259
  foster care 364–70
  physical abuse 137–38
  prenatal substance abuse
    exposure 100
  youth violence 187–88
STEP (Systematic Training for
  Effective Parenting) program,
  contact information 483
stereotyping, sexual abuse 234
Stop It Now!
  contact information 222, 249,
    491–92, 570, 572, 577
  publications
    children abusing children 237n
    child sexual abuse 205n
    child sexual abuse prevention
      443n
    child sexual abuse
      warning signs 213n
    sex offenders 487n
stress
  child abuse risk 23
  disabled children 77–78
  long-term effects 91–98
  trauma coping
    strategies 543–50
substance abuse
  child abuse 5
  child abuse risk 25–26
  described 9
  long-term child abuse
    consequences 88–89
  parents, treatments 429–33
  prenatal exposure 63, 102–4
  youth violence 188
"Substance Abuse and Child
  Welfare: Promising Practices
  and Ethical Dilemmas" (National
  Resource Center for Family-
  Centered Practice and
  Permanency Planning) 429n
substantiated
  defined 558
  described 45
  *see also* not substantiated

suicide attempts, maltreatment
  statistics 97
*Summary Report: Violence against
  Disabled Children* (Groce) 75n
Supplemental Security Income
  (SSI), kinship care 311
"Supporting the Social-Emotional
  Development of Infants and
  Toddlers in Foster Care" (Centre of
  Excellence for Child Welfare) 375n
surgical procedures, female genital
  mutilation 258
Survivors of Incest Anonymous
  (SIA), contact information 570

**T**

"Taming Tempers" (Nemours
  Foundation) 507n
TANF *see* Temporary Assistance
  to Needy Families
technology, electronic
  aggression 191–97, 532–34
"Technology and Youth: Protecting
  Your Child from Electronic
  Aggression" (CDC) 527n
temperament, child abuse risk 27–29
temper tantrums, overview 507–11
Temporary Assistance to Needy
  Families (TANF), kinship care 310
Tennessee
  child abuse reporting
    contact information 563
  clergy, child abuse reporting *292*
  differential response policy *327*
termination of parental
  rights (TPR)
  court system 348
  described 359–61
tests
  child abuse 145–47
  shaken baby syndrome 155
  *see also* assessments
Texas
  child abuse reporting
    contact information 563
  clergy, child abuse reporting *292*
  differential response policy *327*

Virgin Islands, clergy, child abuse
reporting *292*
voluntary kinship care, described
304–5, 307–8

# W

"Warning Signs" (Stop It Now!) 213n
"Warning Signs in Children and
Adolescents of Possible Child
Sexual Abuse" (Stop It Now!) 213n
"Warning Signs That a Child Is
Being Bullied" (HRSA) 181n
Washington, DC *see* District of
Columbia
Washington state
child abuse reporting
contact information 563
clergy, child abuse reporting *292*
differential response policy *327*
welfare system, overview 295–301
West Virginia
child abuse reporting
contact information 563
clergy, child abuse reporting *292*
differential response policy *327*
"What Is Child Abuse and Neglect"
(Child Welfare Information
Gateway) 3n
"What is child physical abuse?"
(SECASA) 133n
"What to Do If Your Child Is
Being Bullied" (HRSA) 523n
WHO *see* World Health Organization
WHO Media Centre, contact
information 261
Wisconsin
child abuse reporting
contact information 563
clergy, child abuse reporting *292*

Wisconsin, continued
differential response policy *327*
respite care services 459, 461
"Working with the Courts in Child
Protection: Appendix A" (Child
Welfare Information Gateway) 553n
"Working with the Courts in Child
Protection User Manual Series:
Chapter 2" (Child Welfare
Information Gateway) 348n
"Working with the Courts in Child
Protection User Manual Series:
Chapter 3" (Child Welfare
Information Gateway) 272n
"Working with the Courts in Child
Protection User Manual Series:
Chapter 4" (Child Welfare
Information Gateway) 352n
World Health Organization (WHO),
female genital mutilation
publication 257n
Wyoming
child abuse reporting
contact information 563
clergy, child abuse reporting *292*
differential response policy *327*

# Y

Youth Law Center, contact
information 577
youth sports
good sportsmanship 513–16
harassment 175–79
youth violence, overview 187–90

# Z

Zolotor, Adam J. 164–65

600

# Health Reference Series

## Complete Catalog

List price $93 per volume. School and library price $84 per volume.

## Adolescent Health Sourcebook, 2nd Edition

*Basic Consumer Health Information about the Physical, Mental, and Emotional Growth and Development of Adolescents, Including Medical Care, Nutritional and Physical Activity Requirements, Puberty, Sexual Activity, Acne, Tanning, Body Piercing, Common Physical Illnesses and Disorders, Eating Disorders, Attention Deficit Hyperactivity Disorder, Depression, Bullying, Hazing, and Adolescent Injuries Related to Sports, Driving, and Work*

*Along with Substance Abuse Information about Nicotine, Alcohol, and Drug Use, a Glossary, and Directory of Additional Resources*

Edited by Joyce Brennfleck Shannon. 655 pages. 2007. 978-0-7808-0943-7.

"A particularly good resource for both parents and teens. The concise presentation of the material in brief and well-organized chapters creates an easy volume to browse."
—*School Library Journal, Jun '07*

"I don't believe there are any other books written in such easy to understand language that encompass such a breadth of topics. This is a complete revision of the book and is an excellent resource for parents and teens."
—*Doody's Review Service, 2007*

## Adult Health Concerns Sourcebook

*Basic Consumer Health Information about Medical and Mental Concerns of Adults, Including Facts about Choosing Healthcare Providers, Navigating Insurance Options, Maintaining Wellness, Preventing Cancer, Heart Disease, Stroke, Diabetes, and Osteoporosis, and Understanding Aging-Related Health Concerns, Including Menopause, Cognitive Changes, and Changes in the Coronary and Vascular Systems*

*Along with Tips on Caring for Aging Parents and Dealing with Health-Related Work and Travel Issues, a Glossary, and a Directory of Resources for Additional Help and Information*

Edited by Sandra J. Judd. 648 pages. 2008. 978-0-7808-0999-4.

"Provides a thorough list of topics that are important to adult health and for caregivers."
—*CHOICE, Nov '08*

"Written in easy-to-understand language . . . the content is well-organized and is intended to aid adults in making health care-related decisions."
—*AORN Journal, Dec '08*

## AIDS Sourcebook, 4th Edition

*Basic Consumer Health Information about Human Immunodeficiency Virus (HIV) and Acquired Immunodeficiency Syndrome (AIDS), Featuring Updated Statistics and Facts about Risks, Prevention, Screening, Diagnosis, Treatments, Side Effects, and Complications, and Including a Section about the Impact of HIV/AIDS on the Health of Women, Children, and Adolescents*

*Along with Tips on Managing Life with AIDS, Reports on Current Research Initiatives and Clinical Trials, a Glossary of Related Terms, and Resource Directories for Further Help and Information*

Edited by Ivy L. Alexander. 680 pages. 2008. 978-0-7808-0997-0.

**SEE ALSO** *Contagious Diseases Sourcebook, 2nd Edition*

## Alcoholism Sourcebook, 2nd Edition

*Basic Consumer Health Information about Alcohol Use, Abuse, and Dependence, Featuring Facts about the Physical, Mental, and Social Health Effects of Alcohol Addiction, Including Alcoholic Liver Disease, Pancreatic Disease, Cardiovascular Disease, Neurological Disorders, and the Effects of Drinking during Pregnancy*

*Along with Information about Alcohol Treatment, Medications, and Recovery Programs, in Addition to Tips for Reducing the Prevalence of Underage Drinking, Statistics about Alcohol Use, a Glossary of Related Terms,* and Directories of Resources for More Help and Information

Edited by Amy L. Sutton. 625 pages. 2007. 978-0-7808-0942-0.

"A comprehensive look at the adverse effects of alcohol on people of all ages . . . It serves to whet the reader's appetite to continue learning using other resources. It is practical, easy to read, and enlightening, and is the first book a lay person should consult to learn about alcoholism."
—Doody's Review Service, 2007

"Should be a basic acquisition for any serious public or college-level library including health reference titles for general-interest readers."
—California Bookwatch, Feb '07

SEE ALSO Drug Abuse Sourcebook, 2nd Edition

## Allergies Sourcebook, 3rd Edition

Basic Consumer Health Information about Allergic Disorders, Such as Anaphylaxis, Hives, Eczema, Rhinitis, Sinusitis, and Conjunctivitis, and Their Triggers, Including Pollen, Mold, Dust Mites, Animal Dander, Insects, Chemicals, Food, Food Additives, and Medications

Along with Advice about the Diagnosis and Treatment of Allergy Symptoms, a Glossary of Related Terms, a Directory of Resources for Help and Information, and Suggestions for Additional Reading

Edited by Amy L. Sutton. 588 pages. 2007. 978-0-7808-0950-5.

SEE ALSO Asthma Sourcebook, 2nd Edition

## Alzheimer Disease Sourcebook, 4th Edition

Basic Consumer Health Information about Alzheimer Disease, Other Dementias, and Related Disorders, Including Multi-Infarct Dementia, Dementia with Lewy Bodies, Frontotemporal Dementia (Pick Disease), Wernicke-Korsakoff Syndrome (Alcohol-Related Dementia), AIDS Dementia Complex, Huntington Disease, Creutzfeldt-Jacob Disease, and Delirium

Along with Information about Coping with Memory Loss and Forgetfulness, Maintaining Skills, and Long-Term Planning for People with Dementia, and Suggestions Addressing Common Caregiver Concerns, Updated Information about Current Research Efforts, a Glossary of Related Terms, and Directories of Sources for Additional Help and Information

Edited by Karen Bellenir. 603 pages. 2008. 978-0-7808-1001-3.

"An invaluable resource for persons who have received a diagnosis, for caregivers, and for family members dealing with this insidious disease. It is recommended for public, community college, and ready-reference sections in academic libraries."
—ARBAonline, Jul '08

SEE ALSO Brain Disorders Sourcebook, 2nd Edition

## Arthritis Sourcebook, 2nd Edition

Basic Consumer Health Information about Osteoarthritis, Rheumatoid Arthritis, Other Rheumatic Disorders, Infectious Forms of Arthritis, and Diseases with Symptoms Linked to Arthritis, Featuring Facts about Diagnosis, Pain Management, and Surgical Therapies

Along with Coping Strategies, Research Updates, a Glossary, and Resources for Additional Help and Information

Edited by Amy L. Sutton. 567 pages. 2004. 978-0-7808-0667-2.

"This easy-to-read volume is recommended for consumer health collections within public or academic libraries."
—E-Streams, May '05

"As expected, this updated edition continues the excellent reputation of this series in providing sound, usable health information. . . . Highly recommended."
—American Reference Books Annual, 2005

## Asthma Sourcebook, 2nd Edition

Basic Consumer Health Information about the Causes, Symptoms, Diagnosis, and Treatment of Asthma in Infants, Children, Teenagers, and Adults, Including Facts about Different Types of Asthma, Common Co-Occurring Conditions, Asthma Management Plans, Triggers, Medications, and Medication Delivery Devices

*Along with Asthma Statistics, Research Updates, a Glossary, a Directory of Asthma-Related Resources, and More*

Edited by Karen Bellenir. 581 pages. 2006. 978-0-7808-0866-9.

---

# Attention Deficit Disorder Sourcebook

*Basic Consumer Health Information about Attention Deficit/Hyperactivity Disorder in Children and Adults, Including Facts about Causes, Symptoms, Diagnostic Criteria, and Treatment Options Such as Medications, Behavior Therapy, Coaching, and Homeopathy*

*Along with Reports on Current Research Initiatives, Legal Issues, and Government Regulations, and Featuring a Glossary of Related Terms, Internet Resources, and a List of Additional Reading Material*

Edited by Dawn D. Matthews. 447 pages. 2002. 978-0-7808-0624-5.

"Recommended reference source."
*—Booklist, Jan '03*

***SEE ALSO*** *Learning Disabilities Sourcebook, 3rd Edition*

---

# Autism and Pervasive Developmental Disorders Sourcebook

*Basic Consumer Health Information about Autism Spectrum and Pervasive Developmental Disorders, Such as Classical Autism, Asperger Syndrome, Rett Syndrome, and Childhood Disintegrative Disorder, Including Information about Related Genetic Disorders and Medical Problems and Facts about Causes, Screening Methods, Diagnostic Criteria, Treatments and Interventions, and Family and Education Issues*

*Along with a Glossary of Related Terms, Tips for Evaluating the Validity of Health Claims, and a Directory of Resources for Additional Help and Information*

Edited by Sandra J. Judd. 603 pages. 2007. 978-0-7808-0953-6.

"Recommended for public libraries"
*—SciTech Book News, Mar '08*

***SEE ALSO*** *Learning Disabilities Sourcebook, 3rd Edition*

---

# Back and Neck Disorders Sourcebook, 2nd Edition

*Basic Consumer Health Information about Spinal Pain, Spinal Cord Injuries, and Related Disorders, Such as Degenerative Disk Disease, Osteoarthritis, Scoliosis, Sciatica, Spina Bifida, and Spinal Stenosis, and Featuring Facts about Maintaining Spinal Health, Self-Care, Pain Management, Rehabilitative Care, Chiropractic Care, Spinal Surgeries, and Complementary Therapies*

*Along with Suggestions for Preventing Back and Neck Pain, a Glossary of Related Terms, and a Directory of Resources*

Edited by Amy L. Sutton. 607 pages. 2004. 978-0-7808-0738-9.

"Recommended. ...An easy to use, comprehensive medical reference book."
*—E-Streams, Sep '05*

"For anyone who has back or neck problems, this book is ideal. Its easy-to-understand language and variety of topics makes this sourcebook a worthwhile read. The price...is reasonable for the amount of information contained in the book"
*—Occupational Therapy in Health Care, 2007*

---

# Blood and Circulatory Disorders Sourcebook, 2nd Edition

*Basic Consumer Health Information about the Blood and Circulatory System and Related Disorders, Such as Anemia and Other Hemoglobin Diseases, Cancer of the Blood and Associated Bone Marrow Disorders, Clotting and Bleeding Problems, and Conditions That Affect the Veins, Blood Vessels, and Arteries, Including Facts about the Donation and Transplantation of Bone Marrow, Stem Cells, and Blood and Tips for Keeping the Blood and Circulatory System Healthy*

*Along with a Glossary of Related Terms and Resources for Additional Help and Information*

Edited by Amy L. Sutton. 634 pages. 2005. 978-0-7808-0746-4.

"Highly recommended pick for basic consumer health reference holdings at all levels."
*—The Bookwatch, Aug '05*

# Brain Disorders Sourcebook, 2nd Edition

Basic Consumer Health Information about Acquired and Traumatic Brain Injuries, Infections of the Brain, Epilepsy and Seizure Disorders, Cerebral Palsy, and Degenerative Neurological Disorders, Including Amyotrophic Lateral Sclerosis (ALS), Dementias, Multiple Sclerosis, and More

Along with Information on the Brain's Structure and Function, Treatment and Rehabilitation Options, Reports on Current Research Initiatives, a Glossary of Terms Related to Brain Disorders and Injuries, and a Directory of Sources for Further Help and Information

Edited by Sandra J. Judd. 600 pages. 2005. 978-0-7808-0744-0.

"This easy-to-read volume provides up-to-date health information... Recommended for consumer health collections within public or academic libraries."

—E-Streams, Feb '06

*SEE ALSO* Alzheimer Disease Sourcebook, 4th Edition

# Breast Cancer Sourcebook, 3rd Edition

Basic Consumer Health Information about Breast Health and Breast Cancer, Including Facts about Environmental, Genetic, and Other Risk Factors, Prevention Efforts, Screening and Diagnostic Methods, Surgical Treatment Options and Other Care Choices, Complementary and Alternative Therapies, and Post-Treatment Concerns

Along with Statistical Data, News about Research Advances, a Glossary of Related Terms, and Directories of Resources for Additional Information and Support

Edited by Karen Bellenir. 606 pages. 2009. 978-0-7808-1030-3.

*SEE ALSO* Cancer Sourcebook for Women, 3rd Edition, Women's Health Concerns Sourcebook, 3rd Edition

# Breastfeeding Sourcebook

Basic Consumer Health Information about the Benefits of Breastmilk, Preparing to Breastfeed, Breastfeeding as a Baby Grows, Nutrition, and More, Including Information on Special Situations and Concerns Such as Mastitis, Illness, Medications, Allergies, Multiple Births, Prematurity, Special Needs, and Adoption

Along with a Glossary and Resources for Additional Help and Information

Edited by Jenni Lynn Colson. 367 pages. 2002. 978-0-7808-0332-9.

*SEE ALSO* Pregnancy and Birth Sourcebook, 2nd Edition

# Burns Sourcebook

Basic Consumer Health Information about Various Types of Burns and Scalds, Including Flame, Heat, Cold, Electrical, Chemical, and Sun Burns

Along with Information on Short-Term and Long-Term Treatments, Tissue Reconstruction, Plastic Surgery, Prevention Suggestions, and First Aid

Edited by Allan R. Cook. 604 pages. 1999. 978-0-7808-0204-9.

**"This is an exceptional addition to the series and is highly recommended for all consumer health collections, hospital libraries, and academic medical centers."**

—E-Streams, Mar '00

**"This key reference guide is an invaluable addition to all health care and public libraries in confronting this ongoing health issue."**

—American Reference Books Annual, 2000

*SEE ALSO* Dermatological Disorders Sourcebook, 2nd Edition

# Cancer Sourcebook, 5th Edition

Basic Consumer Health Information about Major Forms and Stages of Cancer, Featuring Facts about Head and Neck Cancers, Lung Cancers, Gastrointestinal Cancers, Genitourinary Cancers, Lymphomas, Blood Cell Cancers, Endocrine Cancers, Skin Cancers, Bone Cancers, Metastatic Cancers, and More

Along with Facts about Cancer Treatments, Cancer Risks and Prevention, a Glossary of Related Terms, Statistical Data, and a Directory of Resources for Additional Information

Edited by Karen Bellenir. 1105 pages. 2007. 978-0-7808-0947-5.

604

"The 5th, updated edition of *Cancer Sourcebook* should be in every public and health lending library collection... An unparalleled discussion essential for any health collections considering an all-in-one basic general reference."

—*California Bookwatch*, Aug '07

SEE ALSO Breast Cancer Sourcebook, 3rd Edition, Cancer Sourcebook for Women, 3rd Edition, Cancer Survivorship Sourcebook, Leukemia Sourcebook

# Cancer Sourcebook for Women, 3rd Edition

*Basic Consumer Health Information about Leading Causes of Cancer in Women, Featuring Facts about Gynecologic Cancers and Related Concerns, Such as Breast Cancer, Cervical Cancer, Endometrial Cancer, Uterine Sarcoma, Vaginal Cancer, Vulvar Cancer, and Common Non-Cancerous Gynecologic Conditions, in Addition to Facts about Lung Cancer, Colorectal Cancer, and Thyroid Cancer in Women*

*Along with Information about Cancer Risk Factors, Screening and Prevention, Treatment Options, and Tips on Coping with Life after Cancer Treatment, a Glossary of Cancer Terms, and a Directory of Resources for Additional Help and Information*

Edited by Amy L. Sutton. 687 pages. 2006. 978-0-7808-0867-6.

"This excellent book provides the general public with information compiled in a way that will help them to gain the knowledge they need. 4 Stars!"

—*Doody's Review Service*, Dec '06

"An indispensable reference for health consumers and cancer patients. Recommended for public libraries and academic libraries with a medical department."

—*E-Streams*, Sep '08

# Cancer Survivorship Sourcebook

*Basic Consumer Health Information about the Physical, Educational, Emotional, Social, and Financial Needs of Cancer Patients from Diagnosis, through Cancer Treatment, and Beyond, Including Facts about Researching Specific Types of Cancer and Learning about Clinical Trials and Treatment Options, and*

*Featuring Tips for Coping with the Side Effects of Cancer Treatments and Adjusting to Life after Cancer Treatment Concludes*

*Along with Suggestions for Caregivers, Friends, and Family Members of Cancer Patients, a Glossary of Cancer Care Terms, and Directories of Related Resources*

Edited by Karen Bellenir. 633 pages. 2007. 978-0-7808-0985-7.

"Well organized and comprehensive in coverage, the book speaks to issues encountered both during and after cancer treatment. Recommended for consumer health and public libraries."

—*Library Journal*, Aug 1 '07

"*Cancer Survivorship Sourcebook* will be useful to anyone who has a friend or loved one with a cancer diagnosis."

—*American Reference Books Annual*, 2008

SEE ALSO Cancer Sourcebook, 5th Edition

# Cardiovascular Diseases and Disorders Sourcebook, 3rd Edition

*Basic Consumer Health Information about Heart and Vascular Diseases and Disorders, Such as Angina, Heart Attacks, Arrhythmias, Cardiomyopathy, Valve Disease, Atherosclerosis, and Aneurysms, with Information about Managing Cardiovascular Risk Factors and Maintaining Heart Health, Medications and Procedures Used to Treat Cardiovascular Disorders, and Concerns of Special Significance to Women*

*Along with Reports on Current Research Initiatives, a Glossary of Related Medical Terms, and a Directory of Sources for Further Help and Information*

Edited by Sandra J. Judd. 687 pages. 2005. 978-0-7808-0739-6.

"This updated sourcebook is still the best first stop for comprehensive introductory information on cardiovascular diseases."

—*American Reference Books Annual*, 2006

"Recommended for public libraries and libraries supporting health care professionals."

—*E-Streams*, Sep '05

# Caregiving Sourcebook

*Basic Consumer Health Information for Caregivers, Including a Profile of Caregivers, Caregiving Responsibilities and Concerns, Tips for Specific Conditions, Care Environments, and the Effects of Caregiving*

*Along with Facts about Legal Issues, Financial Information, and Future Planning, a Glossary, and a Listing of Additional Resources*

Edited by Joyce Brennfleck Shannon. 583 pages. 2001. 978-0-7808-0331-2.

**"Essential for most collections."**
—*Library Journal, Apr 1 '02*

**"An ideal addition to the reference collection of any public library. Health sciences information professionals may also want to acquire the *Caregiving Sourcebook* for their hospital or academic library for use as a ready reference tool by health care workers interested in aging and caregiving."**
—*E-Streams, Jan '02*

# Child Abuse Sourcebook, 2nd Edition

*Basic Consumer Health Information about the Physical, Sexual, and Emotional Abuse of Children, Neglect, Münchhausen Syndrome by Proxy (MSBP), and Shaken Baby Syndrome, and Featuring Facts about Withholding Medical Care, Corporal Punishment, Child Maltreatment in Youth Sports, and Parental Substance Abuse*

*Along with Information about Child Protective Services, Foster Care, Adoption, Parenting Challenges, Abuse Prevention Programs, and Intervention, Treatment, and Recovery Guidelines, a Glossary of Related Terms, and Resources for Additional Help and Information*

Edited by Joyce Brennfleck Shannon. 600 pages. 2009. 978-0-7808-1037-2.

*SEE ALSO Domestic Violence Sourcebook, 3rd Edition*

# Childhood Diseases and Disorders Sourcebook, 2nd Edition

*Basic Consumer Health Information about the Physical, Mental, and Developmental Health of Pre-Adolescent Children, Including Facts about Infectious Diseases, Asthma, Allergies, Diabetes, and Other Acute and Chronic Conditions Affecting the Gastrointestinal Tract, Ears, Nose, Throat, Liver, Kidneys, Heart, Blood, Brain, Muscles, Bones, and Skin*

*Along with Reports on Recommended Childhood Vaccinations, Wellness Guidelines, a Glossary of Related Medical Terms, and a List of Resources for Parents*

Edited by Sandra J. Judd. 694 pages. 2009. 978-0-7808-1031-0.

*SEE ALSO Healthy Children Sourcebook*

# Colds, Flu and Other Common Ailments Sourcebook

*Basic Consumer Health Information about Common Ailments and Injuries, Including Colds, Coughs, the Flu, Sinus Problems, Headaches, Fever, Nausea and Vomiting, Menstrual Cramps, Diarrhea, Constipation, Hemorrhoids, Back Pain, Dandruff, Dry and Itchy Skin, Cuts, Scrapes, Sprains, Bruises, and More*

*Along with Information about Prevention, Self-Care, Choosing a Doctor, Over-the-Counter Medications, Folk Remedies, and Alternative Therapies, and Including a Glossary of Important Terms and a Directory of Resources for Further Help and Information*

Edited by Chad T. Kimball. 622 pages. 2001. 978-0-7808-0435-7.

**"A good starting point for research on common illnesses. It will be a useful addition to public and consumer health library collections."**
—*American Reference Books Annual, 2002*

**"Will prove valuable to any library seeking to maintain a current, comprehensive reference collection of health resources. . . Excellent reference."**
—*The Bookwatch, Aug '01*

# Communication Disorders Sourcebook

*Basic Information about Deafness and Hearing Loss, Speech and Language Disorders, Voice Disorders, Balance and Vestibular Disorders, and Disorders of Smell, Taste, and Touch*

Edited by Linda M. Ross. 533 pages. 1996. 978-0-7808-0077-9.

"This is skillfully edited and is a welcome resource for the layperson. It should be found in every public and medical library."
—*Booklist Health Sciences Supplement, Oct '97*

# Complementary and Alternative Medicine Sourcebook, 3rd Edition

*Basic Consumer Health Information about Complementary and Alternative Medical Therapies, Including Acupuncture, Ayurveda, Traditional Chinese Medicine, Herbal Medicine, Homeopathy, Naturopathy, Biofeedback, Hypnotherapy, Yoga, Art Therapy, Aromatherapy, Clinical Nutrition, Vitamin and Mineral Supplements, Chiropractic, Massage, Reflexology, Crystal Therapy, Therapeutic Touch, and More*

*Along with Facts about Alternative and Complementary Treatments for Specific Conditions Such as Cancer, Diabetes, Osteoarthritis, Chronic Pain, Menopause, Gastrointestinal Disorders, Headaches, and Mental Illness, a Glossary, and a Resource List for Additional Help and Information*

Edited by Sandra J. Judd. 630 pages. 2006. 978-0-7808-0864-5.

"A 'must' reference for any serious healthcare collection. Public library holdings, too, will welcome it as a popular reference."
—*California Bookwatch, Oct '06*

"Both basic and informative at the same time. . . a useful resource for health care professionals as well as consumers interested in learning more information about CAM therapies."
—*AORN Journal, Jan '08*

"A quality, indexed, referenced guideline for many alternative practices that are quite popular around the world...It is neatly organized to find facts quickly, is peer-reviewed, and stays current with the most recent advances."
—*Journal of Dental Hygiene, Jul '07*

# Congenital Disorders Sourcebook, 2nd Edition

*Basic Consumer Health Information about Non-hereditary Birth Defects and Disorders Related to Prematurity, Gestational Injuries, Congenital Infections, and Birth Complications, Including Heart Defects, Hydrocephalus, Spina Bifida, Cleft Lip and Palate, Cerebral Palsy, and More*

*Along with Facts about the Prevention of Birth Defects, Fetal Surgery and Other Treatment Options, Research Initiatives, a Glossary of Related Terms, and Resources for Additional Information and Support*

Edited by Sandra J. Judd. 619 pages. 2007. 978-0-7808-0945-1.

"Congenital Disorders Sourcebook provides an excellent, non-technical overview of many aspects of pregnancy with the focus on congenital disorders."
—*American Reference Books Annual, 2008*

"An excellent readable reference aimed at the lay public for difficult to understand medical problems. An excellent starting point for the interested parent or family member who may then be motivated to seek more information."
—*Doody's Review Service, 2007*

**SEE ALSO** *Pregnancy and Birth Sourcebook, 2nd Edition*

# Contagious Diseases Sourcebook, 2nd Edition

*Basic Consumer Health Information about Diseases Spread from Person to Person through Direct Physical Contact, Airborne Transmissions, Sexual Contact, or Contact with Blood or Other Body Fluids, Including Pneumococcal, Staphylococcal, and Streptococcal Diseases, Colds, Influenza, Lice, Measles, Mumps, Tuberculosis, and Others*

*Along with Facts about Self-Care and Over-the-Counter Medications, Antibiotics and Drug Resistance, Disease Prevention, Vaccines, and Bioterrorism, a Glossary, and a Directory of Resources for More Information*

Edited by Joyce Brennfleck Shannon. 600 pages. 2009. 978-0-7808-1075-4.

**SEE ALSO** *AIDS Sourcebook, 4th Edition, Hepatitis Sourcebook*

# Cosmetic and Reconstructive Surgery Sourcebook, 2nd Edition

*Basic Consumer Information about Plastic Surgery and Non-Surgical Appearance-Enhancing Procedures, Including Facts about Botulinum Toxin, Collagen Replacement, Dermabrasion,*

Chemical Peels, Eyelid Surgery, Nose Reshaping, Lip Augmentation, Liposuction, Breast Enlargement and Reduction, Tummy Tucking, and Other Skin, Hair, Facial, and Body Shaping Procedures

Along with Information about Reconstructive Procedures for Congenital Disorders, Disfiguring Diseases, Burns, and Traumatic Injuries, a Glossary of Related Terms, and a Directory of Additional Resources

Edited by Karen Bellenir. 483 pages. 2007. 978-0-7808-0951-2.

"A practical guide for health care consumers and health care workers. . . . This easy-to-read reference guide would be useful for novice and veteran health care consumers, surgical technology students, nursing students, and perioperative nurses new to plastic and reconstructive surgery. It also may be helpful for medical-surgical nurses as a guide for patient teaching in their practices."

—*AORN Journal*, Aug '08

**SEE ALSO** *Surgery Sourcebook, 2nd Edition*

# Death and Dying Sourcebook, 2nd Edition

Basic Consumer Health Information about End-of-Life Care and Related Perspectives and Ethical Issues, Including End-of-Life Symptoms and Treatments, Pain Management, Quality-of-Life Concerns, the Use of Life Support, Patients' Rights and Privacy Issues, Advance Directives, Physician-Assisted Suicide, Caregiving, Organ and Tissue Donation, Autopsies, Funeral Arrangements, and Grief

Along with Statistical Data, Information about the Leading Causes of Death, a Glossary, and Directories of Support Groups and Other Resources

Edited by Joyce Brennfleck Shannon. 626 pages. 2006. 978-0-7808-0871-3.

# Dental Care and Oral Health Sourcebook, 3rd Edition

Basic Consumer Health Information about Dental Care and Oral Health Throughout the Lifespan, Including Facts about Cavities, Bad Breath, Cold and Canker Sores, Dry Mouth,

Toothaches, Gum Disease, Malocclusion, Temporomandibular Joint and Muscle Disorders, Oral Cancers, and Dental Emergencies

Along with Information about Mouth Hygiene, Crowns, Bridges, Implants, and Fillings, Surgical, Orthodontic, and Cosmetic Dental Procedures, Pain Management, Health Conditions that Impact Oral Care, a Glossary of Related Terms, and a Directory of Additional Resources

Edited by Amy L. Sutton. 619 pages. 2008. 978-0-7808-1032-7.

# Depression Sourcebook, 2nd Edition

Basic Consumer Health Information about Unipolar Depression, Bipolar Disorder, Dysthymia, Seasonal Affective Disorder, Postpartum Depression, and Other Depressive Disorders, Including Facts about Populations at Special Risk, Coexisting Medical Conditions, Symptoms, Treatment Options, and Suicide Prevention

Along with Statistical Data, a Glossary of Related Terms, and a Directory of Resources for Additional Help and Information

Edited by Sandra J. Judd. 646 pages. 2008. 978-0-7808-1003-7.

**"Recommended for public libraries."**
—*ARBAonline*, Nov '08

**SEE ALSO** *Mental Health Disorders Sourcebook, 4th Edition*

# Dermatological Disorders Sourcebook, 2nd Edition

Basic Consumer Health Information about Conditions and Disorders Affecting the Skin, Hair, and Nails, Such as Acne, Rosacea, Rashes, Dermatitis, Pigmentation Disorders, Birthmarks, Skin Cancer, Skin Injuries, Psoriasis, Scleroderma, and Hair Loss, Including Facts about Medications and Treatments for Dermatological Disorders and Tips for Maintaining Healthy Skin, Hair, and Nails

Along with Information about How Aging Affects the Skin, a Glossary of Related Terms, and a Directory of Resources for Additional Help and Information

Edited by Amy L. Sutton. 617 pages. 2006. 978-0-7808-0795-2.

"Helpfully brings together. . . sources in one convenient place, saving the user hours of research time."
—American Reference Books Annual, 2006

SEE ALSO Burns Sourcebook

# Diabetes Sourcebook, 4th Edition

Basic Consumer Health Information about Type 1 and Type 2 Diabetes Mellitus, Gestational Diabetes, Monogenic Forms of Diabetes, and Insulin Resistance, with Guidelines for Lifestyle Modifications and the Medical Management of Diabetes, Including Facts about Insulin, Insulin Delivery Devices, Oral Diabetes Medications, Self-Monitoring of Blood Glucose, Meal Planning, Physical Activity Recommendations, Foot Care, and Treatment Options for People with Kidney Failure

Along with a Section about Diabetes Complications and Co-Occurring Conditions, a Glossary of Related Terms, and Directories of Resources for Additional Help and Information

Edited by Karen Bellenir. 627 pages. 2008. 978-0-7808-1005-1.

"Completely and comprehensively covering almost everything a student or physician would need to know.... well worth the investment."
—Internet Bookwatch, Dec '08

SEE ALSO Endocrine and Metabolic Disorders Sourcebook, 2nd Edition

# Diet and Nutrition Sourcebook, 3rd Edition

Basic Consumer Health Information about Dietary Guidelines and the Food Guidance System, Recommended Daily Nutrient Intakes, Serving Proportions, Weight Control, Vitamins and Supplements, Nutrition Issues for Different Life Stages and Lifestyles, and the Needs of People with Specific Medical Concerns, Including Cancer, Celiac Disease, Diabetes, Eating Disorders, Food Allergies, and Cardiovascular Disease

Along with Facts about Federal Nutrition Support Programs, a Glossary of Nutrition and Dietary Terms, and Directories of Additional Resources for More Information about Nutrition

Edited by Joyce Brennfleck Shannon. 605 pages. 2006. 978-0-7808-0800-3.

"A valuable resource tool for any individual."
—Journal of Dental Hygiene, Apr '07

"From different recommended eating habits to reduce disease and common ailments to nutrition advice for those with specific conditions, Diet and Nutrition Sourcebook is especially important because so much is changing in this area, and so rapidly."
—California Bookwatch, Jun '06

SEE ALSO Digestive Diseases and Disorders Sourcebook, Eating Disorders Sourcebook, 2nd Edition, Gastrointestinal Diseases and Disorders Sourcebook, 2nd Edition, Vegetarian Sourcebook

# Digestive Diseases and Disorders Sourcebook

Basic Consumer Health Information about Diseases and Disorders that Impact the Upper and Lower Digestive System, Including Celiac Disease, Constipation, Crohn's Disease, Cyclic Vomiting Syndrome, Diarrhea, Diverticulosis and Diverticulitis, Gallstones, Heartburn, Hemorrhoids, Hernias, Indigestion (Dyspepsia), Irritable Bowel Syndrome, Lactose Intolerance, Ulcers, and More

Along with Information about Medications and Other Treatments, Tips for Maintaining a Healthy Digestive Tract, a Glossary, and Directory of Digestive Diseases Organizations

Edited by Karen Bellenir. 323 pages. 2000. 978-0-7808-0327-5.

"An excellent addition to all public or patient-research libraries."
—American Reference Books Annual, 2001

"Recommended reference source."
—Booklist, May '00

SEE ALSO Diet and Nutrition Sourcebook, 3rd Edition, Gastrointestinal Diseases and Disorders Sourcebook, 2nd Edition

# Disabilities Sourcebook

Basic Consumer Health Information about Physical and Psychiatric Disabilities, Including Descriptions of Major Causes of Disability, Assistive and Adaptive Aids, Workplace Issues, and Accessibility Concerns

Along with Information about the Americans with Disabilities Act, a Glossary, and Resources for Additional Help and Information

Edited by Dawn D. Matthews. 602 pages. 2000. 978-0-7808-0389-3.

"A must for libraries with a consumer health section."
—*American Reference Books Annual, 2002*

"A much needed addition to the Omnigraphics **Health Reference Series**. A current reference work to provide people with disabilities, their families, caregivers or those who work with them, a broad range of information in one volume, has not been available until now. . . . It is recommended for all public and academic library reference collections."
—*E-Streams, May '01*

"An excellent source book in easy-to-read format covering many current topics; highly recommended for all libraries."
—*CHOICE, Jan '01*

# Disease Management Sourcebook

*Basic Consumer Health Information about Coping with Chronic and Serious Illnesses, Navigating the Health Care System, Communicating with Health Care Providers, Assessing Health Care Quality, and Making Informed Health Care Decisions, Including Facts about Second Opinions, Hospitalization, Surgery, and Medications*

*Along with a Section about Children with Chronic Conditions, Information about Legal, Financial, and Insurance Issues, a Glossary of Related Terms, and Directories of Additional Resources*

Edited by Joyce Brennfleck Shannon. 621 pages. 2008. 978-0-7808-1002-0.

"Consumers need to know how to manage their health care the same way they manage anything else in their lives. The text is very readable and is written for the layperson and consumer. The cost is not prohibitive. This book should be in all collections of health care libraries and public libraries."
—*ARBAonline, Jul '08*

"The information is very current, and the selection of font and layout make the book easy to read. A hardback that will stand up to much usage, this is an excellent resource for

consumers. . . . Recommended. General readers."
—*CHOICE, Nov '08*

"Intended for lay readers, this resource clarifies the many confusing and overwhelming details associated with chronic disease care. Meticulous and clearly explained, the book even includes diagrams intended to ease comprehension of over-the-counter medication labels. An essential guide to navigating the health-care rapids."
—*Library Journal, Aug '08*

# Domestic Violence Sourcebook, 3rd Edition

*Basic Consumer Health Information about Warning Signs, Risk Factors, and Health Consequences of Intimate Partner Violence, Sexual Violence and Rape, Stalking, Human Trafficking, Child Maltreatment, Teen Dating Violence, and Elder Abuse*

*Along with Facts about Victims and Perpetrators, Strategies for Violence Prevention, and Emergency Interventions, Safety Plans, and Financial and Legal Tips for Victims, a Glossary of Related Terms, and Directories of Resources for Additional Information and Support*

Edited by Joyce Brennfleck Shannon. 600 pages. 2009. 978-0-7808-1038-9.

*SEE ALSO Child Abuse Sourcebook, 2nd Edition*

# Drug Abuse Sourcebook, 2nd Edition

*Basic Consumer Health Information about Illicit Substances of Abuse and the Misuse of Prescription and Over-the-Counter Medications, Including Depressants, Hallucinogens, Inhalants, Marijuana, Stimulants, and Anabolic Steroids*

*Along with Facts about Related Health Risks, Treatment Programs, Prevention Programs, a Glossary of Abuse and Addiction Terms, a Glossary of Drug-Related Street Terms, and a Directory of Resources for More Information*

Edited by Catherine Ginther. 581 pages. 2004. 978-0-7808-0740-2.

"Commendable for organizing useful, normally scattered government and association-produced data into a logical sequence."
—*American Reference Books Annual, 2006*

SEE ALSO Alcoholism Sourcebook, 2nd Edition

# Ear, Nose, and Throat Disorders Sourcebook, 2nd Edition

Basic Consumer Health Information about Disorders of the Ears, Hearing Loss, Vestibular Disorders, Nasal and Sinus Problems, Throat and Vocal Cord Disorders, and Otolaryngologic Cancers, Including Facts about Ear Infections and Injuries, Genetic and Congenital Deafness, Sensorineural Hearing Disorders, Tinnitus, Vertigo, Ménière Disease, Rhinitis, Sinusitis, Snoring, Sore Throats, Hoarseness, and More

Along with Reports on Current Research Initiatives, a Glossary of Related Medical Terms, and a Directory of Sources for Further Help and Information

Edited by Sandra J. Judd. 631 pages. 2007. 978-0-7808-0872-0.

"A resource book for the general public that provides comprehensive coverage of basic up-to-date medical information about the causes, symptoms, diagnosis, and treatment of diseases and disorders that affect the ears, nose, sinuses, throat, and voice. . . . The majority of information is presented in question and answer format, much like questions a patient might ask of a health care provider. An extensive index facilitates the reader's ability to easily access information on any specific topic."
—Journal of Dental Hygiene, Oct '07

"A handy compilation of information on common and some not so common ailments of the ears, nose, and throat."
—Doody's Review Service, 2007

# Eating Disorders Sourcebook, 2nd Edition

Basic Consumer Health Information about Anorexia Nervosa, Bulimia, Binge Eating, Compulsive Exercise, Female Athlete Triad, and Other Eating Disorders, Including Facts about Body Image and Other Cultural and Age-Related Risk Factors, Prevention Efforts, Adverse Health Effects, Treatment Options, and the Recovery Process

Along with Guidelines for Healthy Weight Control, a Glossary, and Directories of Additional Resources

Edited by Joyce Brennfleck Shannon. 557 pages. 2007. 978-0-7808-0948-2.

"Recommended for the reference collection of large public libraries."
—American Reference Books Annual, 2008

"A basic health reference any health or general library needs."
—Internet Bookwatch, Jun '07

SEE ALSO Diet and Nutrition Sourcebook, 3rd Edition, Mental Health Disorders Sourcebook, 4th Edition

# Emergency Medical Services Sourcebook

Basic Consumer Health Information about Preventing, Preparing for, and Managing Emergency Situations, When and Who to Call for Help, What to Expect in the Emergency Room, the Emergency Medical Team, Patient Issues, and Current Topics in Emergency Medicine

Along with Statistical Data, a Glossary, and Sources of Additional Help and Information

Edited by Jenni Lynn Colson. 472 pages. 2002. 978-0-7808-0420-3.

"Handy and convenient for home, public, school, and college libraries. Recommended."
—CHOICE, Apr '03

"This reference can provide the consumer with answers to most questions about emergency care in the United States, or it will direct them to a resource where the answer can be found."
—American Reference Books Annual, 2003

SEE ALSO Injury and Trauma Sourcebook

# Endocrine and Metabolic Disorders Sourcebook, 2nd Edition

Basic Consumer Health Information about Hormonal and Metabolic Disorders that Affect the Body's Growth, Development, and Functioning, Including Disorders of the Pancreas, Ovaries and Testes, and Pituitary, Thyroid, Parathyroid, and Adrenal Glands, with Facts about *Growth Disorders, Addison Disease, Cushing Syndrome, Conn Syndrome, Diabetic Disorders, Multiple Endocrine Neoplasia, Inborn Errors of Metabolism, and More*

*Along with Information about Endocrine Functioning, Diagnostic and Screening Tests, a Glossary of Related Terms, and Directories of Additional Resources*

Edited by Joyce Brennfleck Shannon. 597 pages. 2007. 978-0-7808-0952-9.

**SEE ALSO** *Diabetes Sourcebook, 4th Edition*

# Environmental Health Sourcebook, 2nd Edition

*Basic Consumer Health Information about the Environment and Its Effect on Human Health, Including the Effects of Air Pollution, Water Pollution, Hazardous Chemicals, Food Hazards, Radiation Hazards, Biological Agents, Household Hazards, Such as Radon, Asbestos, Carbon Monoxide, and Mold, and Information about Associated Diseases and Disorders, Including Cancer, Allergies, Respiratory Problems, and Skin Disorders*

*Along with Information about Environmental Concerns for Specific Populations, a Glossary of Related Terms, and Resources for Further Help and Information*

Edited by Dawn D. Matthews. 650 pages. 2003. 978-0-7808-0632-0.

"Recommended for teenage and adult students and readers, and for public and academic libraries, as well as any library focusing on consumer health."

*—E-Streams, May '04*

"This recently updated edition continues the level of quality and the reputation of the numerous other volumes in Omnigraphics' Health Reference Series."

*—American Reference Books Annual, 2004*

# Ethnic Diseases Sourcebook

*Basic Consumer Health Information for Ethnic and Racial Minority Groups in the United States, Including General Health Indicators and Behaviors, Ethnic Diseases, Genetic Testing, the Impact of Chronic Diseases, Women's Health, Mental Health Issues, and Preventive Health Care Services*

*Along with a Glossary and a Listing of Additional Resources*

Edited by Joyce Brennfleck Shannon. 648 pages. 2001. 978-0-7808-0336-7.

"Not many books have been written on this topic to date, and the *Ethnic Diseases Sourcebook* is a strong addition to the list. It will be an important introductory resource for health consumers, students, health care personnel, and social scientists. It is recommended for public, academic, and large hospital libraries."

*—American Reference Books Annual, 2002*

"Will prove valuable to any library seeking to maintain a current, comprehensive reference collection of health resources. . . . An excellent source of health information about genetic disorders which affect particular ethnic and racial minorities in the U.S."

*—The Bookwatch, Aug '01*

# Eye Care Sourcebook, 3rd Edition

*Basic Consumer Health Information about Eye Care and Eye Disorders, Including Facts about the Diagnosis, Prevention, and Treatment of Refractive Disorders, Cataracts, Glaucoma, Macular Degeneration, and Problems Affecting the Cornea, Retina, and Lacrimal Glands*

*Along with Advice about Preventing Eye Injuries and Tips for Living with Low Vision or Blindness, a Glossary of Related Terms, and Directories of Resources for More Help and Information*

Edited by Amy L. Sutton. 646 pages. 2008. 978-0-7808-1000-6.

# Family Planning Sourcebook

*Basic Consumer Health Information about Planning for Pregnancy and Contraception, Including Traditional Methods, Barrier Methods, Hormonal Methods, Permanent Methods, Future Methods, Emergency Contraception, and Birth Control Choices for Women at Each Stage of Life*

*Along with Statistics, a Glossary, and Sources of Additional Information*

Edited by Amy Marcaccio Keyzer. 503 pages. 2001. 978-0-7808-0379-4.

"Recommended for public, health, and undergraduate libraries as part of the circulating collection."

*—E-Streams, Mar '02*

"Will prove valuable to any library seeking to maintain a current, comprehensive reference collection of health resources. . . . Excellent reference."

—*The Bookwatch, Aug '01*

**SEE ALSO** *Pregnancy and Birth Sourcebook, 2nd Edition*

---

# Fitness and Exercise Sourcebook, 3rd Edition

*Basic Consumer Health Information about the Physical and Mental Benefits of Fitness, Including Cardiorespiratory Endurance, Muscular Strength, Muscular Endurance, and Flexibility, with Facts about Sports Nutrition and Exercise-Related Injuries and Tips about Physical Activity and Exercises for People of All Ages and for People with Health Concerns*

*Along with Advice on Selecting and Using Exercise Equipment, Maintaining Exercise Motivation, a Glossary of Related Terms, and a Directory of Resources for More Help and Information*

Edited by Amy L. Sutton. 635 pages. 2007. 978-0-7808-0946-8.

"Updates the consumer information on the physical and mental benefits of physical activity throughout the lifespan offered in earlier editions. . . . Recommended. All readers; all levels."

—*CHOICE, Oct '07*

"An exceptionally well-rounded coverage perfect for any concerned about developing and understanding a fitness program."

—*California Bookwatch, Jun '07*

**SEE ALSO** *Sports Injuries Sourcebook, 3rd Edition*

---

# Food Safety Sourcebook

*Basic Consumer Health Information about the Safe Handling of Meat, Poultry, Seafood, Eggs, Fruit Juices, and Other Food Items, and Facts about Pesticides, Drinking Water, Food Safety Overseas, and the Onset, Duration, and Symptoms of Foodborne Illnesses, Including Types of Pathogenic Bacteria, Parasitic Protozoa, Worms, Viruses, and Natural Toxins*

*Along with the Role of the Consumer, the Food Handler, and the Government in Food Safety; a Glossary, and Resources for Additional Help and Information*

Edited by Dawn D. Matthews. 327 pages. 1999. 978-0-7808-0326-8.

"Recommended reference source."

—*Booklist, May '00*

"This book takes the complex issues of food safety and foodborne pathogens and presents them in an easily understood manner. [It does] an excellent job of covering a large and often confusing topic."

— *American Reference Books Annual, 2000*

---

# Forensic Medicine Sourcebook

*Basic Consumer Information for the Layperson about Forensic Medicine, Including Crime Scene Investigation, Evidence Collection and Analysis, Expert Testimony, Computer-Aided Criminal Identification, Digital Imaging in the Courtroom, DNA Profiling, Accident Reconstruction, Autopsies, Ballistics, Drugs and Explosives Detection, Latent Fingerprints, Product Tampering, and Questioned Document Examination*

*Along with Statistical Data, a Glossary of Forensics Terminology, and Listings of Sources for Further Help and Information*

Edited by Annemarie S. Muth. 574 pages. 1999. 978-0-7808-0232-2.

"Given the expected widespread interest in its content and its easy to read style, this book is recommended for most public and all college and university libraries."

—*E-Streams, Feb '01*

"A wealth of information, useful statistics, references are up-to-date and extremely complete. This wonderful collection of data will help students who are interested in a career in any type of forensic field. It is a great resource for attorneys who need information about types of expert witnesses needed in a particular case. It also offers useful information for fiction and nonfiction writers whose work involves a crime. A fascinating compilation. All levels."

—*CHOICE, Jan '00*

"There are several items that make this book attractive to consumers who are seeking certain forensic data. . . . This is a useful current

source for those seeking general forensic medical answers."
—*American Reference Books Annual, 2000*

# Gastrointestinal Diseases and Disorders Sourcebook, 2nd Edition

*Basic Consumer Health Information about the Upper and Lower Gastrointestinal (GI) Tract, Including the Esophagus, Stomach, Intestines, Rectum, Liver, and Pancreas, with Facts about Gastroesophageal Reflux Disease, Gastritis, Hernias, Ulcers, Celiac Disease, Diverticulitis, Irritable Bowel Syndrome, Hemorrhoids, Gastrointestinal Cancers, and Other Diseases and Disorders Related to the Digestive Process*

*Along with Information about Commonly Used Diagnostic and Surgical Procedures, Statistics, Reports on Current Research Initiatives and Clinical Trials, a Glossary, and Resources for Additional Help and Information*

Edited by Sandra J. Judd. 654 pages. 2006. 978-0-7808-0798-3.

"The text is designed for the general reader seeking information on prevention, disease warning signs, diagnostic and therapeutic questions. . . . It is an excellent resource for the general reader to conveniently locate credible, coordinated and indexed information. . . . The sourcebook will prove very helpful for patients, caregivers and should be available in every physician waiting room."
—*Doody's Review Service, 2006*

**SEE ALSO** *Diet and Nutrition Sourcebook, 3rd Edition, Digestive Diseases and Disorders Sourcebook*

# Genetic Disorders Sourcebook, 4th Edition

*Basic Consumer Health Information about Hereditary Diseases and Disorders, Including Facts about the Human Genome, Genetic Inheritance Patterns, Disorders Associated with Specific Genes, Such as Sickle Cell Disease, Hemophilia, and Cystic Fibrosis, Chromosome Disorders, Such as Down Syndrome, Fragile X Syndrome, and Turner Syndrome, and Complex Diseases and Disorders Resulting from the Interaction of Environmental and Genetic Factors, Such as Allergies, Cancer, and Obesity*

*Along with Facts about Genetic Testing, Suggestions for Parents of Children with Special Needs, Reports on Current Research Initiatives, a Glossary of Genetic Terminology, and Resources for Additional Help and Information*

Edited by Sandra J. Judd. 600 pages. 2009. 978-0-7808-1076-1.

# Head Trauma Sourcebook

*Basic Information for the Layperson about Open-Head and Closed-Head Injuries, Treatment Advances, Recovery, and Rehabilitation*

*Along with Reports on Current Research Initiatives*

Edited by Karen Bellenir. 414 pages. 1997. 978-0-7808-0208-7.

# Headache Sourcebook

*Basic Consumer Health Information about Migraine, Tension, Cluster, Rebound and Other Types of Headaches, with Facts about the Cause and Prevention of Headaches, the Effects of Stress and the Environment, Headaches during Pregnancy and Menopause, and Childhood Headaches*

*Along with a Glossary and Other Resources for Additional Help and Information*

Edited by Dawn D. Matthews. 342 pages. 2002. 978-0-7808-0337-4.

"Highly recommended for academic and medical reference collections."
—*Library Bookwatch, Sep '02*

**SEE ALSO** *Pain Sourcebook, 3rd Edition*

# Healthy Aging Sourcebook

*Basic Consumer Health Information about Maintaining Health through the Aging Process, Including Advice on Nutrition, Exercise, and Sleep, Help in Making Decisions about Midlife Issues and Retirement, and Guidance Concerning Practical and Informed Choices in Health Consumerism*

*Along with Data Concerning the Theories of Aging, Different Experiences in Aging by Minority Groups, and Facts about Aging Now and Aging in the Future; and Featuring a Glossary, a Guide to Consumer Help, Additional Suggested Reading, and Practical Resource Directory*

Edited by Jenifer Swanson. 537 pages. 1999. 978-0-7808-0390-9.

"Recommended reference source."
— *Booklist, Feb '00*

*SEE ALSO Physical and Mental Issues in Aging Sourcebook*

## Healthy Children Sourcebook

*Basic Consumer Health Information about the Physical and Mental Development of Children between the Ages of 3 and 12, Including Routine Health Care, Preventative Health Services, Safety and First Aid, Healthy Sleep, Dental Care, Nutrition, and Fitness, and Featuring Parenting Tips on Such Topics as Bedwetting, Choosing Day Care, Monitoring TV and Other Media, and Establishing a Foundation for Substance Abuse Prevention*

*Along with a Glossary of Commonly Used Pediatric Terms and Resources for Additional Help and Information.*

Edited by Chad T. Kimball. 624 pages. 2003. 978-0-7808-0247-6.

"Should be required reading for parents and teachers."
— *E-Streams, Jun '04*

"It is hard to imagine that any other single resource exists that would provide such a comprehensive guide of timely information on health promotion and disease prevention for children aged 3 to 12."
— *American Reference Books Annual, 2004*

"This easy-to-read volume is a tremendous resource."
— *AORN Journal, May '05*

*SEE ALSO Childhood Diseases and Disorders Sourcebook, 2nd Edition*

## Healthy Heart Sourcebook for Women

*Basic Consumer Health Information about Cardiac Issues Specific to Women, Including Facts about Major Risk Factors and Prevention, Treatment and Control Strategies, and Important Dietary Issues*

*Along with a Special Section Regarding the Pros and Cons of Hormone Replacement Therapy and Its Impact on Heart Health, and Additional Help, Including Recipes, a Glossary, and a Directory of Resources*

Edited by Dawn D. Matthews. 321 pages. 2000. 978-0-7808-0329-9.

"A good reference source and recommended for all public, academic, medical, and hospital libraries."
— *Medical Reference Services Quarterly, Summer '01*

"Contains very important information about coronary artery disease that all women should know. The information is current and presented in an easy-to-read format. The book will make a good addition to any library."
— *American Medical Writers Association Journal, Summer '00*

*SEE ALSO Cardiovascular Diseases and Disorders Sourcebook, 3rd Edition, Women's Health Concerns Sourcebook, 3rd Edition*

## Hepatitis Sourcebook

*Basic Consumer Health Information about Hepatitis A, Hepatitis B, Hepatitis C, and Other Forms of Hepatitis, Including Autoimmune Hepatitis, Alcoholic Hepatitis, Nonalcoholic Steatohepatitis, and Toxic Hepatitis, with Facts about Risk Factors, Screening Methods, Diagnostic Tests, and Treatment Options*

*Along with Information on Liver Health, Tips for People Living with Chronic Hepatitis, Reports on Current Research Initiatives, a Glossary of Terms Related to Hepatitis, and a Directory of Sources for Further Help and Information*

Edited by Sandra J. Judd. 570 pages. 2006. 978-0-7808-0749-5.

"The breadth of information found in this one book would not be readily found in another source. Highly recommended."
— *American Reference Books Annual, 2006*

*SEE ALSO Contagious Diseases Sourcebook*

## Household Safety Sourcebook

*Basic Consumer Health Information about Household Safety, Including Information about Poisons, Chemicals, Fire, and Water Hazards in the Home*

*Along with Advice about the Safe Use of Home Maintenance Equipment, Choosing Toys and Nursery Furniture, Holiday and Recreation Safety, a Glossary, and Resources for Further Help and Information*

Edited by Dawn D. Matthews. 587 pages. 2002. 978-0-7808-0338-1.

"As a sourcebook on household safety this book meets its mark. It is encyclopedic in scope and covers a wide range of safety issues that are commonly seen in the home."
—*E-Streams, Jul '02*

## Hypertension Sourcebook

*Basic Consumer Health Information about the Causes, Diagnosis, and Treatment of High Blood Pressure, with Facts about Consequences, Complications, and Co-Occurring Disorders, Such as Coronary Heart Disease, Diabetes, Stroke, Kidney Disease, and Hypertensive Retinopathy, and Issues in Blood Pressure Control, Including Dietary Choices, Stress Management, and Medications*

*Along with Reports on Current Research Initiatives and Clinical Trials, a Glossary, and Resources for Additional Help and Information*

Edited by Dawn D. Matthews and Karen Bellenir. 588 pages. 2004. 978-0-7808-0674-0.

"Academic, public, and medical libraries will want to add the *Hypertension Sourcebook* to their collections."
—*E-Streams, Aug '05*

"The strength of this source is the wide range of information given about hypertension."
—*American Reference Books Annual, 2005*

**SEE ALSO** *Stroke Sourcebook, 2nd Edition*

## Immune System Disorders Sourcebook, 2nd Edition

*Basic Consumer Health Information about Disorders of the Immune System, Including Immune System Function and Response, Diagnosis of Immune Disorders, Information about Inherited Immune Disease, Acquired Immune Disease, and Autoimmune Diseases, Including Primary Immune Deficiency, Acquired Immunodeficiency Syndrome (AIDS), Lupus, Multiple Sclerosis, Type 1 Diabetes, Rheumatoid Arthritis, and Graves' Disease*

*Along with Treatments, Tips for Coping with Immune Disorders, a Glossary, and a Directory of Additional Resources*

Edited by Joyce Brennfleck Shannon. 643 pages. 2005. 978-0-7808-0748-8.

"Highly recommended for academic and public libraries."
—*American Reference Books Annual, 2006*

"The updated second edition is a 'must' for any consumer health library seeking a solid resource covering the treatments, symptoms, and options for immune disorder sufferers. . . . An excellent guide."
—*MBR Bookwatch, Jan '06*

**SEE ALSO** *AIDS Sourcebook, 4th Edition, Arthritis Sourcebook, 2nd Edition*

## Infant and Toddler Health Sourcebook

*Basic Consumer Health Information about the Physical and Mental Development of Newborns, Infants, and Toddlers, Including Neonatal Concerns, Nutrition Recommendations, Immunization Schedules, Common Pediatric Disorders, Assessments and Milestones, Safety Tips, and Advice for Parents and Other Caregivers*

*Along with a Glossary of Terms and Resource Listings for Additional Help*

Edited by Jenifer Swanson. 570 pages. 2000. 978-0-7808-0246-9.

"As a reference for the general public, this would be useful in any library."
—*E-Streams, May '01*

"Recommended reference source."
—*Booklist, Feb '01*

## Infectious Diseases Sourcebook

*Basic Consumer Health Information about Non-Contagious Bacterial, Viral, Prion, Fungal, and Parasitic Diseases Spread by Food and Water, Insects and Animals, or Environmental Contact, Including Botulism, E. Coli, Encephalitis, Legionnaires' Disease, Lyme Disease, Malaria, Plague, Rabies, Salmonella, Tetanus, and Others, and Facts about Newly Emerging Diseases, Such as Hantavirus, Mad Cow Disease, Monkeypox, and West Nile Virus*

*Along with Information about Preventing Disease Transmission, the Threat of Bioterrorism, and Current Research Initiatives, with a Glossary and Directory of Resources for More Information*

Edited by Karen Bellenir. 610 pages. 2004. 978-0-7808-0675-7.

"This reference continues the excellent tradition of the *Health Reference Series* in consolidating a wealth of information on a selected topic into a format that is easy to use and accessible to the general public."
—*American Reference Books Annual, 2005*

"Recommended for public and academic libraries."
—*E-Streams, Jan '05*

## Injury and Trauma Sourcebook

*Basic Consumer Health Information about the Impact of Injury, the Diagnosis and Treatment of Common and Traumatic Injuries, Emergency Care, and Specific Injuries Related to Home, Community, Workplace, Transportation, and Recreation*

*Along with Guidelines for Injury Prevention, a Glossary, and a Directory of Additional Resources*

Edited by Joyce Brennfleck Shannon. 675 pages. 2002. 978-0-7808-0421-0.

"Practitioners should be aware of guides such as this in order to facilitate their use by patients and their families."
—*Doody's Health Sciences Book Review Journal, Sep-Oct '02*

"Recommended reference source."
—*Booklist, Sep '02*

"Highly recommended for academic and medical reference collections."
—*Library Bookwatch, Sep '02*

**SEE ALSO** *Emergency Medical Services Sourcebook, Sports Injuries Sourcebook, 3rd Edition*

## Learning Disabilities Sourcebook, 3rd Edition

*Basic Consumer Health Information about Dyslexia, Auditory and Visual Processing Disorders, Communication Disorders, Dyscalculia, Dysgraphia, and Other Conditions That Impede Learning, Including Attention Deficit/Hyperactivity Disorder, Autism Spectrum Disorders, Hearing and Visual Impairments, Chromosome-Based Disorders, and Brain Injury*

*Along with Facts about Brain Function, Assessment, Therapy and Remediation, Accommodations, Assistive Technology, Legal Protections, and Tips about Family Life, School Transitions, and Employment Strategies, a Glossary of Related Terms, and Directories of Additional Resources*

Edited by Joyce Brennfleck Shannon. 613 pages. 2009. 978-0-7808-1039-6.

**SEE ALSO** *Attention Deficit Disorder Sourcebook, Autism and Pervasive Developmental Disorders Sourcebook*

## Leukemia Sourcebook

*Basic Consumer Health Information about Adult and Childhood Leukemias, Including Acute Lymphocytic Leukemia (ALL), Chronic Lymphocytic Leukemia (CLL), Acute Myelogenous Leukemia (AML), Chronic Myelogenous Leukemia (CML), and Hairy Cell Leukemia, and Treatments Such as Chemotherapy, Radiation Therapy, Peripheral Blood Stem Cell and Marrow Transplantation, and Immunotherapy*

*Along with Tips for Life During and After Treatment, a Glossary, and Directories of Additional Resources*

Edited by Joyce Brennfleck Shannon. 564 pages. 2003. 978-0-7808-0627-6.

"Unlike other medical books for the layperson, . . . the language does not talk down to the reader. . . . This volume is highly recommended for all libraries."
—*American Reference Books Annual, 2004*

"A fine title which ranges from diagnosis to alternative treatments, staging, and tips for life during and after diagnosis."
—*The Bookwatch, Dec '03*

**SEE ALSO** *Cancer Sourcebook, 5th Edition*

## Liver Disorders Sourcebook

*Basic Consumer Health Information about the Liver and How It Works; Liver Diseases, Including Cancer, Cirrhosis, Hepatitis, and Toxic and Drug Related Diseases; Tips for Maintaining a Healthy Liver; Laboratory Tests, Radiology Tests, and Facts about Liver Transplantation*

*Along with a Section on Support Groups, a Glossary, and Resource Listings*

Edited by Joyce Brennfleck Shannon. 580 pages. 2000. 978-0-7808-0383-1.

"This title is recommended for health sciences and public libraries with consumer health collections."
—*E-Streams, Oct '00*

"Recommended reference source."
—*Booklist, Jun '00*

*SEE ALSO Gastrointestinal Diseases and Disorders Sourcebook, 2nd Edition, Hepatitis Sourcebook*

# Lung Disorders Sourcebook

*Basic Consumer Health Information about Emphysema, Pneumonia, Tuberculosis, Asthma, Cystic Fibrosis, and Other Lung Disorders, Including Facts about Diagnostic Procedures, Treatment Strategies, Disease Prevention Efforts, and Such Risk Factors as Smoking, Air Pollution, and Exposure to Asbestos, Radon, and Other Agents*

*Along with a Glossary and Resources for Additional Help and Information*

Edited by Dawn D. Matthews. 657 pages. 2002. 978-0-7808-0339-8.

"Highly recommended for academic and medical reference collections."
—*Library Bookwatch, Sep '02*

*SEE ALSO Respiratory Disorders Sourcebook, 2nd Edition*

# Medical Tests Sourcebook, 3rd Edition

*Basic Consumer Health Information about X-Rays, Blood Tests, Stool and Urine Tests, Biopsies, Mammography, Endoscopic Procedures, Ultrasound Exams, Computed Tomography, Magnetic Resonance Imaging (MRI), Nuclear Medicine, Genetic Testing, Home-Use Tests, and More*

*Along with Facts about Preventive Care and Screening Test Guidelines, Screening and Assessment Tests Associated with Such Specific Concerns as Cancer, Heart Disease, Allergies, Diabetes, Thyroid Disfunction, and Infertility, a Glossary of Related Terms, and a Directory of Resources for Additional Help and Information*

Edited by Karen Bellenir. 627 pages. 2008. 978-0-7808-1040-2

"This volume has a wide scope that makes it useful . . . Can be a valuable reference guide."
—*ARBAonline, Nov '08*

# Men's Health Concerns Sourcebook, 3rd Edition

*Basic Consumer Health Information about Wellness in Men and Gender-Related Differences in Health, With Facts about Heart Disease, Cancer, Traumatic Injury, and Other Leading Causes of Death in Men, Reproductive Concerns, Sexual Dysfunction, Disorders of the Prostate, Penis, and Testes, Sex-Linked Genetic Disorders, and Other Medical and Mental Concerns of Men*

*Along with Statistical Data, a Glossary of Related Terms, and a Directory of Resources for Additional Information*

Edited by Sandra J. Judd. 600 pages. 2009. 978-0-7808-1033-4.

*SEE ALSO Prostate and Urological Disorders Sourcebook*

# Mental Health Disorders Sourcebook, 4th Edition

*Basic Consumer Health Information about the Causes and Symptoms of Mental Health Problems, Including Depression, Bipolar Disorder, Anxiety Disorders, Posttraumatic Stress Disorder, Obsessive-Compulsive Disorder, Eating Disorders, Addictions, and Personality and Psychotic Disorders*

*Along with Information about Medications and Treatments, Mental Health Concerns in Children, Adolescents, and Adults, Tips on Living with Mental Health Disorders, a Glossary of Related Terms, and a Directory of Resources for Additional Help and Information*

Edited by Amy L. Sutton. 600 pages. 2009. 978-0-7808-1041-9.

*SEE ALSO Depression Sourcebook, 2nd Edition, Stress-Related Disorders Sourcebook, 2nd Edition*

# Mental Retardation Sourcebook

*Basic Consumer Health Information about Mental Retardation and Its Causes, Including*

Down Syndrome, Fetal Alcohol Syndrome, Fragile X Syndrome, Genetic Conditions, Injury, and Environmental Sources

Along with Preventive Strategies, Parenting Issues, Educational Implications, Health Care Needs, Employment and Economic Matters, Legal Issues, a Glossary, and a Resource Listing for Additional Help and Information

Edited by Joyce Brennfleck Shannon. 627 pages. 2000. 978-0-7808-0377-0.

"Public libraries will find the book useful for reference and as a beginning research point for students, parents, and caregivers."
—American Reference Books Annual, 2001

"The strength of this work is that it compiles many basic fact sheets and addresses for further information in one volume. It is intended and suitable for the general public."
—E-Streams, Nov '00

"An invaluable overview."
—Reviewer's Bookwatch, Jul '00

## Movement Disorders Sourcebook, 2nd Edition

Basic Consumer Health Information about the Symptoms and Causes of Movement Disorders, Including Parkinson Disease, Amyotrophic Lateral Sclerosis, Cerebral Palsy, Muscular Dystrophy, Multiple Sclerosis, Myasthenia, Myoclonus, Spina Bifida, Dystonia, Essential Tremor, Choreatic Disorders, Huntington Disease, Tourette Syndrome, and Other Disorders That Cause Slowed, Absent, or Excessive Movements

Along with Information about Surgical and Nonsurgical Interventions, Physical Therapies, Strategies for Independent Living, a Glossary of Related Terms, and a Directory of Resources for Additional Help and Information

Edited by Amy L. Sutton. 600 pages. 2009. 978-0-7808-1034-1.

SEE ALSO Multiple Sclerosis Sourcebook, Muscular Dystrophy Sourcebook

## Multiple Sclerosis Sourcebook

Basic Consumer Health Information about Multiple Sclerosis (MS) and Its Effects on Mobility, Vision, Bladder Function, Speech, Swallowing, and Cognition, Including Facts about Risk Factors, Causes, Diagnostic Procedures, Pain Management, Drug Treatments, and Physical and Occupational Therapies

Along with Guidelines for Nutrition and Exercise, Tips on Choosing Assistive Equipment, Information about Disability, Work, Financial, and Legal Issues, a Glossary of Related Terms, and a Directory of Additional Resources

Edited by Joyce Brennfleck Shannon. 553 pages. 2007. 978-0-7808-0998-7.

SEE ALSO Movement Disorders Sourcebook, 2nd Edition

## Muscular Dystrophy Sourcebook

Basic Consumer Health Information about Congenital, Childhood-Onset, and Adult-Onset Forms of Muscular Dystrophy, Such as Duchenne, Becker, Emery-Dreifuss, Distal, Limb-Girdle, Facioscapulohumeral (FSHD), Myotonic, and Ophthalmoplegic Muscular Dystrophies, Including Facts about Diagnostic Tests, Medical and Physical Therapies, Management of Co-Occurring Conditions, and Parenting Guidelines

Along with Practical Tips for Home Care, a Glossary, and Directories of Additional Resources

Edited by Joyce Brennfleck Shannon. 552 pages. 2004. 978-0-7808-0676-4.

"This book is highly recommended for public and academic libraries as well as health care offices that support the information needs of patients and their families."
—E-Streams, Apr '05

"Excellent reference."
—The Bookwatch, Jan '05

SEE ALSO Movement Disorders Sourcebook, 2nd Edition

## Obesity Sourcebook

Basic Consumer Health Information about Diseases and Other Problems Associated with Obesity, and Including Facts about Risk Factors, Prevention Issues, and Management Approaches

Along with Statistical and Demographic Data, Information about Special Populations,

Research Updates, a Glossary, and Source Listings for Further Help and Information

Edited by Wilma Caldwell and Chad T. Kimball. 360 pages. 2001. 978-0-7808-0333-6.

"The book synthesizes the reliable medical literature on obesity into one easy-to-read and useful resource for the general public."
—American Reference Books Annual, 2002

"Well suited for the health reference collection of a public library or an academic health science library that serves the general population."
—E-Streams, Sep '01

## Osteoporosis Sourcebook

Basic Consumer Health Information about Primary and Secondary Osteoporosis and Juvenile Osteoporosis and Related Conditions, Including Fibrous Dysplasia, Gaucher Disease, Hyperthyroidism, Hypophosphatasia, Myeloma, Osteopetrosis, Osteogenesis Imperfecta, and Paget's Disease

Along with Information about Risk Factors, Treatments, Traditional and Non-Traditional Pain Management, a Glossary of Related Terms, and a Directory of Resources

Edited by Allan R. Cook. 568 pages. 2001. 978-0-7808-0239-1.

"This resource is recommended as a great reference source for public, health, and academic libraries, and is another triumph for the editors of Omnigraphics."
—American Reference Books Annual, 2002

"Will prove valuable to any library seeking to maintain a current, comprehensive reference collection of health resources. . . . From prevention to treatment and associated conditions, this provides an excellent survey."
—The Bookwatch, Aug '01

SEE ALSO Healthy Aging Sourcebook, Women's Health Concerns Sourcebook, 3rd Edition

## Pain Sourcebook, 3rd Edition

Basic Consumer Health Information about Acute and Chronic Pain, Including Nerve Pain, Bone Pain, Muscle Pain, Cancer Pain, and Disorders Characterized by Pain, Such as Arthritis, Temporomandibular Muscle and Joint (TMJ) Disorder, Carpal Tunnel Syndrome,

Headaches, Heartburn, Sciatica, and Shingles, and Facts about Diagnostic Tests and Treatment Options for Pain, Including Over-the-Counter and Prescription Drugs, Physical Rehabilitation, Injection and Infusion Therapies, Implantable Technologies, and Complementary Medicine

Along with Tips for Living with Pain, a Glossary of Related Terms, and a Directory of Additional Resources

Edited by Joyce Brennfleck Shannon. 644 pages. 2008. 978-0-7808-1006-8.

"Excellent for ready-reference users and can be used for beginning students in health fields . . . appropriate for the consumer health collection in both public and academic libraries."
—ARBAonline, Nov '08

## Pediatric Cancer Sourcebook

Basic Consumer Health Information about Leukemias, Brain Tumors, Sarcomas, Lymphomas, and Other Cancers in Infants, Children, and Adolescents, Including Descriptions of Cancers, Treatments, and Coping Strategies

Along with Suggestions for Parents, Caregivers, and Concerned Relatives, a Glossary of Cancer Terms, and Resource Listings

Edited by Edward J. Prucha. 575 pages. 1999. 978-0-7808-0245-2.

"An excellent source of information. Recommended for public, hospital, and health science libraries with consumer health collections."
—E-Streams, Jun '00

"A valuable addition to all libraries specializing in health services and many public libraries."
—American Reference Books Annual, 2000

SEE ALSO Childhood Diseases and Disorders Sourcebook, 2nd Edition, Healthy Children Sourcebook

## Physical and Mental Issues in Aging Sourcebook

Basic Consumer Health Information on Physical and Mental Disorders Associated with the Aging Process, Including Concerns about Cardiovascular Disease, Pulmonary Disease, Oral Health, Digestive Disorders, Musculoskeletal and Skin Disorders, Metabolic

Changes, Sexual and Reproductive Issues, and Changes in Vision, Hearing, and Other Senses

Along with Data about Longevity and Causes of Death, Information on Acute and Chronic Pain, Descriptions of Mental Concerns, a Glossary of Terms, and Resource Listings for Additional Help

Edited by Jenifer Swanson. 660 pages. 1999. 978-0-7808-0233-9.

"This is a treasure of health information for the layperson."
—*CHOICE Health Sciences Supplement, May '00*

"Recommended for public libraries."
—*American Reference Books Annual, 2000*

*SEE ALSO* Healthy Aging Sourcebook

## Podiatry Sourcebook, 2nd Edition

*Basic Consumer Health Information about Disorders, Diseases, and Deformities that Affect the Foot and Ankle, Including Sprains, Corns, Calluses, Bunions, Plantar Warts, Plantar Fasciitis, Neuromas, Clubfoot, Flat Feet, Achilles Tendonitis, and Much More*

*Along with Information about Selecting a Foot Care Specialist, Foot Fitness, Shoes and Socks, Diagnostic Tests and Corrective Procedures, Financial Assistance for Corrective Devices, a Glossary of Related Terms, and a Directory of Resources for Additional Help and Information*

Edited by Ivy L. Alexander. 516 pages. 2007. 978-0-7808-0944-4.

"An excellent resource. . . . Although there have been various types of 'foot books' published in the past, none are as comprehensive as this one. 5 Stars (out of 5)!"
—*Doody's Review Service, 2007*

"Perfect for both health libraries and general-interest lending collections."
—*Internet Bookwatch, Jul '07*

## Pregnancy and Birth Sourcebook, 3rd Edition

*Basic Consumer Health Information about Pregnancy and Fetal Development, Including Facts about Fertility and Conception, Physical*

and Emotional Changes during Pregnancy, Prenatal Care and Diagnostic Tests, High-Risk Pregnancies and Complications, Labor, Delivery, and the Postpartum Period

*Along with Tips on Maintaining Health and Wellness during Pregnancy and Caring for Newborn Infants, a Glossary of Related Terms, and Directories of Resources for Additional Help and Information*

Edited by Amy L. Sutton. 600 pages. 2009. 978-0-7808-1074-7.

*SEE ALSO* Breastfeeding Sourcebook, Congenital Disorders Sourcebook, 2nd Edition, Family Planning Sourcebook, Women's Health Concerns Sourcebook, 3rd Edition

## Prostate and Urological Disorders Sourcebook

*Basic Consumer Health Information about Urogenital and Sexual Disorders in Men, Including Prostate and Other Andrological Cancers, Prostatitis, Benign Prostatic Hyperplasia, Testicular and Penile Trauma, Cryptorchidism, Peyronie Disease, Erectile Dysfunction, and Male Factor Infertility, and Facts about Commonly Used Tests and Procedures, Such as Prostatectomy, Vasectomy, Vasectomy Reversal, Penile Implants, and Semen Analysis*

*Along with a Glossary of Andrological Terms and a Directory of Resources for Additional Information*

Edited by Karen Bellenir. 604 pages. 2006. 978-0-7808-0797-6.

"Certain to be a popular pick among library reference holdings. . . . No prior knowledge is assumed for any of the conditions or terms herein, making it a most accessible general-interest reference."
—*California Bookwatch, Apr '06*

*SEE ALSO* Men's Health Concerns Sourcebook, 3rd Edition, Urinary Tract and Kidney Diseases and Disorders Sourcebook, 2nd Edition

## Prostate Cancer Sourcebook

*Basic Consumer Health Information about Prostate Cancer, Including Information about the Associated Risk Factors, Detection, Diagnosis, and Treatment of Prostate Cancer*

*Along with Information on Non-Malignant Prostate Conditions, and Featuring a Section*

Listing Support and Treatment Centers and a Glossary of Related Terms

Edited by Dawn D. Matthews. 340 pages. 2001. 978-0-7808-0324-4.

**"Recommended reference source."**
— Booklist, Jan '02

**"A valuable resource for health care consumers seeking information on the subject. . . . All text is written in a clear, easy-to-understand language that avoids technical jargon. Any library that collects consumer health resources would strengthen their collection with the addition of the *Prostate Cancer Sourcebook*."**
— American Reference Books Annual, 2002

**SEE ALSO** *Cancer Sourcebook, 5th Edition, Men's Health Concerns Sourcebook, 3rd Edition*

■

# Rehabilitation Sourcebook

*Basic Consumer Health Information about Rehabilitation for People Recovering from Heart Surgery, Spinal Cord Injury, Stroke, Orthopedic Impairments, Amputation, Pulmonary Impairments, Traumatic Injury, and More, Including Physical Therapy, Occupational Therapy, Speech/Language Therapy, Massage Therapy, Dance Therapy, Art Therapy, and Recreational Therapy*

*Along with Information on Assistive and Adaptive Devices, a Glossary, and Resources for Additional Help and Information*

Edited by Dawn D. Matthews. 519 pages. 2000. 978-0-7808-0236-0.

**"This is an excellent resource for public library reference and health collections."**
— American Reference Books Annual, 2001

**"Recommended reference source."**
— Booklist, May '00

■

# Respiratory Disorders Sourcebook, 2nd Edition

*Basic Consumer Health Information about Infectious, Inflammatory, and Chronic Conditions Affecting the Lungs and Respiratory System, Including Pneumonia, Bronchitis, Influenza, Tuberculosis, Sarcoidosis, Asthma, Cystic Fibrosis, Chronic Obstructive Pulmonary Disease, Lung Abscesses, Pulmonary Embolism, Occupational Lung Diseases, and Other Bacterial, Viral, and Fungal Infections*

*Along with Facts about the Structure and Function of the Lungs and Airways, Methods of Diagnosing Respiratory Disorders, and Treatment and Rehabilitation Options, a Glossary of Related Terms, and a Directory of Resources for Additional Help and Information*

Edited by Sandra L. Judd. 638 pages. 2008. 978-0-7808-1007-5.

**"A great addition for public and school libraries because it provides concise health information . . . readers can start with this reference source and get satisfactory answers before proceeding to other medical reference tools for more in depth information . . . A good guide for health education on lung disorders."**
— ARBAonline, Nov '08

**SEE ALSO** *Lung Disorders Sourcebook*

■

# Sexually Transmitted Diseases Sourcebook, 4th Edition

*Basic Consumer Health Information about Chlamydial Infections, Gonorrhea, Hepatitis, Herpes, HIV/AIDS, Human Papillomavirus, Pubic Lice, Scabies, Syphilis, Trichomoniasis, Vaginal Infections, and Other Sexually Transmitted Diseases, Including Facts about Risk Factors, Symptoms, Diagnosis, Treatment, and the Prevention of Sexually Transmitted Infections*

*Along with Updates on Current Research Initiatives, a Glossary of Related Terms, and Resources for Additional Help and Information*

Edited by Laura Larsen. 600 pages. 2009. 978-0-7808-1073-0.

**SEE ALSO** *AIDS Sourcebook, 4th Edition, Contagious Diseases Sourcebook, 2nd Edition, Men's Health Concerns Sourcebook, 3rd Edition, Women's Health Concerns Sourcebook, 3rd Edition*

■

# Sleep Disorders Sourcebook, 2nd Edition

*Basic Consumer Health Information about Sleep and Sleep Disorders, Including Insomnia, Sleep Apnea, Restless Legs Syndrome, Narcolepsy, Parasomnias, and Other Health Problems That Affect Sleep, Plus Facts about Diagnostic Procedures, Treatment Strategies,*

Sleep Medications, and Tips for Improving Sleep Quality

*Along with a Glossary of Related Terms and Resources for Additional Help and Information*

Edited by Amy L. Sutton. 567 pages. 2005. 978-0-7808-0743-3.

**"This book will be useful for just about everybody, especially the 40 million Americans with sleep disorders."**
—*American Reference Books Annual, 2006*

**"A welcome addition to public libraries and consumer health libraries."**
—*Medical Reference Services Quarterly, Summer '06*

# Smoking Concerns Sourcebook

*Basic Consumer Health Information about Nicotine Addiction and Smoking Cessation, Featuring Facts about the Health Effects of Tobacco Use, Including Lung and Other Cancers, Heart Disease, Stroke, and Respiratory Disorders, Such as Emphysema and Chronic Bronchitis*

*Along with Information about Smoking Prevention Programs, Suggestions for Achieving and Maintaining a Smoke-Free Lifestyle, Statistics about Tobacco Use, Reports on Current Research Initiatives, a Glossary of Related Terms, and Directories of Resources for Additional Help and Information*

Edited by Karen Bellenir. 595 pages. 2004. 978-0-7808-0323-7.

**"Provides everything needed for the student or general reader seeking practical details on the effects of tobacco use."**
—*The Bookwatch, Mar '05*

**"Public libraries and consumer health care libraries will find this work useful."**
—*American Reference Books Annual, 2005*

**SEE ALSO** *Respiratory Disorders Sourcebook, 2nd Edition*

# Sports Injuries Sourcebook, 3rd Edition

*Basic Consumer Health Information about Sprains and Strains, Fractures, Growth Plate Injuries, Overtraining Injuries, and Injuries to* the Head, Face, Shoulders, Elbows, Hands, Spinal Column, Knees, Ankles, and Feet, and with Facts about Heat-Related Illness, Steroids and Sport Supplements, Protective Equipment, Diagnostic Procedures, Treatment Options, and Rehabilitation

*Along with a Glossary of Related Terms and a Directory of Resources for Additional Help and Information*

Edited by Sandra J. Judd. 623 pages. 2007. 978-0-7808-0949-9.

**SEE ALSO** *Fitness and Exercise Sourcebook, 3rd Edition*

# Stress-Related Disorders Sourcebook, 2nd Edition

*Basic Consumer Health Information about Stress and Stress-Related Disorders, Including Types of Stress, Sources of Acute and Chronic Stress, the Impact of Stress on the Body's Systems, and Mental and Emotional Health Problems Associated with Stress, Such as Depression, Anxiety Disorders, Substance Abuse, Posttraumatic Stress Disorder, and Suicide*

*Along with Advice about Getting Help for Stress-Related Disorders, Information about Stress Management Techniques, a Glossary of Stress-Related Terms, and a Directory of Resources for Additional Help and Information*

Edited by Amy L. Sutton. 608 pages. 2007. 978-0-7808-0996-3.

**"Accessible to the lay reader. Highly recommended for medical and psychiatric collections."**
—*Library Journal, Mar '08*

**"Well-written for a general readership, the 2nd Edition of *Stress-Related Disorders Sourcebook* is a useful addition to the health reference literature."**
—*American Reference Books Annual, 2008*

**SEE ALSO** *Mental Health Disorders Sourcebook, 4th Edition*

# Stroke Sourcebook, 2nd Edition

*Basic Consumer Health Information about Stroke, Including Ischemic, Hemorrhagic, and Mini Strokes, as Well as Risk Factors, Prevention Guidelines, Diagnostic Tests, Medications and*

*Surgical Treatments, and Complications of Stroke*

*Along with Rehabilitation Techniques and Innovations, Tips on Staying Healthy and Maintaining Independence after Stroke, a Glossary of Related Terms, and a Directory of Resources for Stroke Survivors and Their Families*

Edited by Amy L. Sutton. 626 pages. 2008. 978-0-7808-1035-8.

**"An encyclopedic handbook on stroke that is written in a language the layperson can understand. . . . This is one of the most helpful, readable books on stroke. This volume is highly recommended and should be in every medical, hospital and public library; in addition, every family practitioner should have a copy in his or her office."**
*—ARBAonline Dec '08*

**SEE ALSO** *Hypertension Sourcebook*

# Surgery Sourcebook, 2nd Edition

*Basic Consumer Health Information about Common Inpatient and Outpatient Surgeries, Including Critical Care and Trauma, Gastrointestinal, Gynecologic and Obstetric, Cardiac and Vascular, Neurologic, Ophthalmologic, Orthopedic, Reconstructive and Cosmetic, and Other Major and Minor Surgeries*

*Along with Information about Anesthesia and Pain Relief Options, Risks and Complications, Postoperative Recovery Concerns, and Innovative Surgical Techniques and Tools, a Glossary of Related Terms, and a Directory of Additional Resources*

Edited by Amy L. Sutton. 645 pages. 2008. 978-0-7808-1004-4.

**"Large public libraries and medical libraries would benefit from this material in their reference collections."**
*—ARBAonline Aug '08*

**SEE ALSO** *Cosmetic and Reconstructive Surgery Sourcebook, 2nd Edition*

# Thyroid Disorders Sourcebook

*Basic Consumer Health Information about Disorders of the Thyroid and Parathyroid Glands, Including Hypothyroidism, Hyperthyroidism,*

*Graves Disease, Hashimoto Thyroiditis, Thyroid Cancer, and Parathyroid Disorders, Featuring Facts about Symptoms, Risk Factors, Tests, and Treatments*

*Along with Information about the Effects of Thyroid Imbalance on Other Body Systems, Environmental Factors That Affect the Thyroid Gland, a Glossary, and a Directory of Additional Resources*

Edited by Joyce Brennfleck Shannon. 573 pages. 2005. 978-0-7808-0745-7.

**"Recommended for consumer health collections."**
*—American Reference Books Annual, 2006*

**"Highly recommended pick for basic consumer health reference holdings at all levels."**
*—The Bookwatch, Aug '05*

**SEE ALSO** *Endocrine and Metabolic Disorders Sourcebook, 2nd Edition*

# Transplantation Sourcebook

*Basic Consumer Health Information about Organ and Tissue Transplantation, Including Physical and Financial Preparations, Procedures and Issues Relating to Specific Solid Organ and Tissue Transplants, Rehabilitation, Pediatric Transplant Information, the Future of Transplantation, and Organ and Tissue Donation*

*Along with a Glossary and Listings of Additional Resources*

Edited by Joyce Brennfleck Shannon. 610 pages. 2002. 978-0-7808-0322-0.

**"Recommended for libraries with an interest in offering consumer health information."**
*—E-Streams, Jul '02*

**"This is a unique and valuable resource for patients facing transplantation and their families."**
*—Doody's Review Service, Jun '02*

# Traveler's Health Sourcebook

*Basic Consumer Health Information for Travelers, Including Physical and Medical Preparations, Transportation Health and Safety, Essential Information about Food and Water, Sun Exposure, Insect and Snake Bites, Camping and Wilderness Medicine, and Travel with Physical or Medical Disabilities*

Along with International Travel Tips, Vaccination Recommendations, Geographical Health Issues, Disease Risks, a Glossary, and a Listing of Additional Resources

Edited by Joyce Brennfleck Shannon. 619 pages. 2000. 978-0-7808-0384-8.

"Recommended reference source."
—*Booklist, Feb '01*

"This book is recommended for any public library, any travel collection, and especially any collection for the physically disabled."
—*American Reference Books Annual, 2001*

**SEE ALSO** *Worldwide Health Sourcebook*

---

# Urinary Tract and Kidney Diseases and Disorders Sourcebook, 2nd Edition

*Basic Consumer Health Information about the Urinary System, Including the Bladder, Urethra, Ureters, and Kidneys, with Facts about Urinary Tract Infections, Incontinence, Congenital Disorders, Kidney Stones, Cancers of the Urinary Tract and Kidneys, Kidney Failure, Dialysis, and Kidney Transplantation*

*Along with Statistical and Demographic Information, Reports on Current Research in Kidney and Urologic Health, a Summary of Commonly Used Diagnostic Tests, a Glossary of Related Terms, and a Directory of Resources for Additional Help and Information*

Edited by Ivy L. Alexander. 621 pages. 2005. 978-0-7808-0750-1.

"A good choice for a consumer health information library or for a medical library needing information to refer to their patients."
—*American Reference Books Annual, 2006*

**SEE ALSO** *Prostate and Urological Disorders Sourcebook*

---

# Vegetarian Sourcebook

*Basic Consumer Health Information about Vegetarian Diets, Lifestyle, and Philosophy, Including Definitions of Vegetarianism and Veganism, Tips about Adopting Vegetarianism, Creating a Vegetarian Pantry, and Meeting Nutritional Needs of Vegetarians, with Facts Regarding Vegetarianism's Effect on Pregnant and Lactating Women, Children, Athletes, and Senior Citizens*

Along with a Glossary of Commonly Used Vegetarian Terms and Resources for Additional Help and Information

Edited by Chad T. Kimball. 337 pages. 2002. 978-0-7808-0439-5.

"Organizes into one concise volume the answers to the most common questions concerning vegetarian diets and lifestyles. This title is recommended for public and secondary school libraries."
—*E-Streams, Apr '03*

"Invaluable reference for public and school library collections alike."
—*Library Bookwatch, Apr '03*

"The articles in this volume are easy to read and come from authoritative sources. The book does not necessarily support the vegetarian diet but instead provides the pros and cons of this important decision. . . . Recommended for public libraries and consumer health libraries."
—*American Reference Books Annual, 2003*

**SEE ALSO** *Diet and Nutrition Sourcebook, 3rd Edition*

---

# Women's Health Concerns Sourcebook, 3rd Edition

*Basic Consumer Health Information about Issues and Trends in Women's Health and Health Conditions of Special Concern to Women, Including Endometriosis, Uterine Fibroids, Menstrual Irregularities, Menopause, Sexual Dysfunction, Infertility, Cancer in Women, and Other Such Chronic Disorders as Lupus, Fibromyalgia, and Thyroid Disease*

*Along with Statistical Data, Tips for Maintaining Wellness, a Glossary, and a Directory of Resources for Further Help and Information*

Edited by Sandra J. Judd. 600 pages. 2009. 978-0-7808-1036-5.

**SEE ALSO** *Breast Cancer Sourcebook, 3rd Edition, Cancer Sourcebook for Women, 3rd Edition, Healthy Heart Sourcebook for Women, Osteoporosis Sourcebook*

---

# Workplace Health and Safety Sourcebook

*Basic Consumer Health Information about Workplace Health and Safety, Including the Effect of Workplace Hazards on the Lungs,*

Skin, Heart, Ears, Eyes, Brain, Reproductive Organs, Musculoskeletal System, and Other Organs and Body Parts

Along with Information about Occupational Cancer, Personal Protective Equipment, Toxic and Hazardous Chemicals, Child Labor, Stress, and Workplace Violence

Edited by Chad T. Kimball. 610 pages. 2000. 978-0-7808-0231-5.

"As a reference for the general public, this would be useful in any library."
—E-Streams, Jun '01

"Provides helpful information for primary care physicians and other caregivers interested in occupational medicine. . . . General readers; professionals."
—CHOICE, May '01

# Worldwide Health Sourcebook

Basic Information about Global Health Issues, Including Malnutrition, Reproductive Health, Disease Dispersion and Prevention, Emerging Diseases, Risky Health Behaviors, and the Leading Causes of Death

Along with Global Health Concerns for Children, Women, and the Elderly, Mental Health Issues, Research and Technology Advancements, and Economic, Environmental, and Political Health Implications, a Glossary, and a Resource Listing for Additional Help and Information

Edited by Joyce Brennfleck Shannon. 597 pages. 2001. 978-0-7808-0330-5.

"Named an Outstanding Academic Title."
—CHOICE, Jan '02

"Yet another handy but also unique compilation in the extensive *Health Reference Series*, this is a useful work because many of the international publications reprinted or excerpted are not readily available. Highly recommended."
—CHOICE, Nov '01

SEE ALSO *Traveler's Health Sourcebook*

# Teen Health Series

## Complete Catalog

List price $69 per volume. School and library price $62 per volume.

## Abuse and Violence Information for Teens

***Health Tips about the Causes and Consequences of Abusive and Violent Behavior***

*Including Facts about the Types of Abuse and Violence, the Warning Signs of Abusive and Violent Behavior, Health Concerns of Victims, and Getting Help and Staying Safe*

Edited by Sandra Augustyn Lawton. 411 pages. 2008. 978-0-7808-1008-2.

**"A useful resource for schools and organizations providing services to teens and may also be a starting point in research projects."**
—*Reference and Research Book News, Aug '08*

**"Violence is a serious problem for teens. . . . This resource gives teens the information they need to face potential threats and get help— either for themselves or for their friends."**
—*ARBAonline, Aug '08*

## Accident and Safety Information for Teens

***Health Tips about Medical Emergencies, Traumatic Injuries, and Disaster Preparedness***

*Including Facts about Motor Vehicle Accidents, Burns, Poisoning, Firearms, Natural Disasters, National Security Threats, and More*

Edited by Karen Bellenir. 420 pages. 2008. 978-0-7808-1046-4.

**SEE ALSO** *Sports Injuries Information for Teens, 2nd Edition*

## Alcohol Information for Teens, 2nd Edition

***Health Tips about Alcohol and Alcoholism***

*Including Facts about Alcohol's Effects on the Body, Brain, and Behavior, the Consequences of Underage Drinking, Alcohol Abuse Prevention and Treatment, and Coping with Alcoholic Parents*

Edited by Lisa Bakewell. 400 pages. 2009. 978-0-7808-1043-3.

**SEE ALSO** *Drug Information for Teens, 2nd Edition*

## Allergy Information for Teens

***Health Tips about Allergic Reactions Such as Anaphylaxis, Respiratory Problems, and Rashes***

*Including Facts about Identifying and Managing Allergies to Food, Pollen, Mold, Animals, Chemicals, Drugs, and Other Substances*

Edited by Karen Bellenir. 410 pages. 2006. 978-0-7808-0799-0.

**"This is a comprehensive, readable text on the subject of allergic diseases in teenagers. 5 Stars (out of 5)!"**
—*Doody's Review Service, Jun '06*

**"This authoritative and useful self-help title is a solid addition to YA collections, whether for personal interest or reports."**
—*School Library Journal, Jul '06*

## Asthma Information for Teens

***Health Tips about Managing Asthma and Related Concerns***

*Including Facts about Asthma Causes, Triggers, Symptoms, Diagnosis, and Treatment*

Edited by Karen Bellenir. 386 pages. 2005. 978-0-7808-0770-9.

**"Highly recommended for medical libraries, public school libraries, and public libraries."**
—*American Reference Books Annual, 2006*

**"Although this volume is nearly 400 pages long, it is so clearly written and well organized that even hesitant readers will be able to find the facts they need, whether for reports or personal information. . . . A succinct but complete resource."**
—*School Library Journal, Sep '05*

## Body Information for Teens

**Health Tips about Maintaining Well-Being for a Lifetime**

*Including Facts about the Development and Functioning of the Body's Systems, Organs, and Structures and the Health Impact of Lifestyle Choices*

Edited by Sandra Augustyn Lawton. 458 pages. 2007. 978-0-7808-0443-2.

## Cancer Information for Teens, 2nd Edition

**Health Tips about Cancer Awareness, Symptoms, Prevention, Diagnosis, and Treatment**

*Including Facts about Common Cancers Affecting Teens, Causes, Detection, Coping Strategies, Clinical Trials, Nutrition and Exercise, Cancer in Friends or Family, and More*

Edited by Karen Bellenir and Lisa Bakewell. 400 pages. 2009. 978-0-7808-1085-3.

## Complementary and Alternative Medicine Information for Teens

**Health Tips about Non-Traditional and Non-Western Medical Practices**

*Including Information about Acupuncture, Chiropractic Medicine, Dietary and Herbal Supplements, Hypnosis, Massage Therapy, Prayer and Spirituality, Reflexology, Yoga, and More*

Edited by Sandra Augustyn Lawton. 407 pages. 2007. 978-0-7808-0966-6.

"This volume covers CAM specifically for teenagers but of general use also. It should be a welcome addition to both public and academic libraries."
—American Reference Books Annual, 2008

"This volume provides a solid foundation for further investigation of the subject, making it useful for both public and high school libraries."
—VOYA: Voice of Youth Advocates, Jun '07

## Diabetes Information for Teens

**Health Tips about Managing Diabetes and Preventing Related Complications**

*Including Information about Insulin, Glucose Control, Healthy Eating, Physical Activity, and Learning to Live with Diabetes*

Edited by Sandra Augustyn Lawton. 410 pages. 2006. 978-0-7808-0811-9.

"A comprehensive instructional guide for teens. . . . some of the material may also be directed towards parents or teachers. 5 stars (out of 5)!"
—Doody's Review Service, 2006

"Students dealing with their own diabetes or that of a friend or family member or those writing reports on the topic will find this a valuable resource."
—School Library Journal, Aug '06

"This text is directed to the teen population and would be an excellent library resource for a health class or for the teacher as a reference for class preparation. It can, however, serve a much wider audience. The clinical educator on diabetes may find it valuable to educate the newly diagnosed client regardless of age. It also would be an excellent reference and education tool for a preventive medicine seminar on diabetes."
—Physical Therapy, Mar '07

## Diet Information for Teens, 2nd Edition

**Health Tips about Diet and Nutrition**

*Including Facts about Dietary Guidelines, Food Groups, Nutrients, Healthy Meals, Snacks, Weight Control, Medical Concerns Related to Diet, and More*

Edited by Karen Bellenir. 432 pages. 2006. 978-0-7808-0820-1.

"A very quick and pleasant read in spite of the fact that it is very detailed in the information it gives. . . . A book for anyone concerned about diet and nutrition."
—American Reference Books Annual, 2007

**SEE ALSO** *Eating Disorders Information for Teens, 2nd Edition*

## Drug Information for Teens, 2nd Edition

**Health Tips about the Physical and Mental Effects of Substance Abuse**

*Including Information about Marijuana, Inhalants, Club Drugs, Stimulants, Hallucinogens,*

628

Opiates, Prescription and Over-the-Counter Drugs, Herbal Products, Tobacco, Alcohol, and More

Edited by Sandra Augustyn Lawton. 468 pages. 2006. 978-0-7808-0862-1.

"As with earlier installments in Omnigraphics' **Teen Health Series, Drug Information for Teens** is designed specifically to meet the needs and interests of middle and high school students. . . . Strongly recommended for both academic and public libraries."
—*American Reference Books Annual,*
*2007*

"Solid thoughtful advice is given about how to handle peer pressure, drug-related health concerns, and treatment strategies."
—*School Library Journal, Dec '06*

*SEE ALSO* Alcohol Information for Teens, 2nd Edition, Tobacco Information for Teens

# Eating Disorders Information for Teens, 2nd Edition
*Health Tips about Anorexia, Bulimia, Binge Eating, And Other Eating Disorders*
*Including Information about Risk Factors, Diagnosis and Treatment, Prevention, Related Health Concerns, and Other Issues*

Edited by Sandra Augustyn Lawton. 377 pages. 2009. 978-0-7808-1044-0.

*SEE ALSO* Diet Information for Teens, 2nd Edition

# Fitness Information for Teens, 2nd Edition
*Health Tips about Exercise, Physical Well-Being, and Health Maintenance*
*Including Facts about Conditioning, Stretching, Strength Training, Body Shape and Body Image, Sports Nutrition, and Specific Activities for Athletes and Non-Athletes*

Edited by Lisa Bakewell. 432 pages. 2009. 978-0-7808-1045-7.

*SEE ALSO* Diet Information for Teens, 2nd Edition, Sports Injuries Information for Teens, 2nd Edition

# Learning Disabilities Information for Teens
*Health Tips about Academic Skills Disorders and Other Disabilities That Affect Learning*
*Including Information about Common Signs of Learning Disabilities, School Issues, Learning to Live with a Learning Disability, and Other Related Issues*

Edited by Sandra Augustyn Lawton. 400 pages. 2006. 978-0-7808-0796-9.

"This book provides a wealth of information for any reader interested in the signs, causes, and consequences of learning disabilities, as well as related legal rights and educational interventions. . . . Public and academic libraries should want this title for both students and general readers."
—*American Reference Books Annual, 2006*

# Mental Health Information for Teens, 2nd Edition
*Health Tips about Mental Wellness and Mental Illness*
*Including Facts about Mental and Emotional Health, Depression and Other Mood Disorders, Anxiety Disorders, Conduct Disorder, Self-Injury, Psychosis, Schizophrenia, and More*

Edited by Karen Bellenir. 424 pages. 2006. 978-0-7808-0863-8.

"This excellent overview of the psychological disorders that affect teens provides clear definitions and descriptions, and discusses resources, therapies, coping mechanisms, and medications."
—*School Library Journal Curriculum Connections, Fall '07*

"A well done reference for a specific, often under-represented group."
—*Doody's Review Service, 2006*

*SEE ALSO* Stress Information for Teens

# Pregnancy Information for Teens
*Health Tips about Teen Pregnancy and Teen Parenting*
*Including Facts about Prenatal Care, Pregnancy Complications, Labor and Delivery,*

Postpartum Care, Pregnancy-Related Lifestyle Concerns, and More

Edited by Sandra Augustyn Lawton. 434 pages. 2007. 978-0-7808-0984-0.

*SEE ALSO* Sexual Health Information for Teens, 2nd Edition

# Sexual Health Information for Teens, 2nd Edition
*Health Tips about Sexual Development, Reproduction, Contraception, and Sexually Transmitted Infections*
*Including Facts about Puberty, Sexuality, Birth Control, Chlamydia, Gonorrhea, Herpes, Human Papillomavirus, Syphilis, and More*

Edited by Sandra Augustyn Lawton. 430 pages. 2008. 978-0-7808-1010-5.

"This offering represents the most up-to-date information available on an array of topics including abstinence-only sexual education and pregnancy-prevention methods. . . . The range of coverage—from puberty and anatomy to sexually transmitted diseases—is thorough and extensive. Each chapter includes a bibliographic citation, and the three back sections containing additional resources, further reading, and the index are all first-rate. . . . This volume will be well used by students in need of the facts, whether for educational or personal reasons."
—*School Library Journal, Nov '08*

*SEE ALSO* Pregnancy Information for Teens

# Skin Health Information for Teens, 2nd Edition
*Health Tips about Dermatological Concerns and Skin Cancer Risks*
*Including Facts about Acne, Warts, Allergies, and Other Conditions and Lifestyle Choices, Such as Tanning, Tattooing, and Piercing, That Affect the Skin, Nails, Scalp, and Hair*

Edited by Edited by Kim Wohlenhaus. 400 pages. 2009. 978-0-7808-1042-6.

# Sleep Information for Teens
*Health Tips about Adolescent Sleep Requirements, Sleep Disorders, and the Effects of Sleep Deprivation*

Including Facts about Why People Need Sleep, Sleep Patterns, Circadian Rhythms, Dreaming, Insomnia, Sleep Apnea, Narcolepsy, and More

Edited by Karen Bellenir. 355 pages. 2008. 978-0-7808-1009-9.

*SEE ALSO* Body Information for Teens

# Sports Injuries Information for Teens, 2nd Edition
*Health Tips about Acute, Traumatic, and Chronic Injuries in Adolescent Athletes*
*Including Facts about Sprains, Fractures, and Overuse Injuries, Treatment, Rehabilitation, Sport-Specific Safety Guidelines, Fitness Suggestions, and More*

Edited by Karen Bellenir. 429 pages. 2008. 978-0-7808-1011-2.

"An engaging selection of informative articles about the prevention and treatment of sports injuries. . . The value of this book is that the articles have been vetted and are often augmented with inserts of useful facts, definitions of technical terms, and quick tips. Sensitive topics like injuries to genitalia are discussed openly and responsibly. This revised edition contains updated articles and defines sport more broadly than the first edition."
—*School Library Journal, Nov '08*

"This work will be useful in the young adult collections of public libraries as well as high school libraries. . . . A useful resource for student research."
—*ARBAonline, Aug '08*

*SEE ALSO* Accident and Safety Information for Teens

# Stress Information for Teens
*Health Tips about the Mental and Physical Consequences of Stress*
*Including Information about the Different Kinds of Stress, Symptoms of Stress, Frequent Causes of Stress, Stress Management Techniques, and More*

Edited by Sandra Augustyn Lawton. 392 pages. 2008. 978-0-7808-1012-9.

"Understanding what stress is, what causes it, how the body and the mind are impacted by it, and what teens can do are the general categories addressed here. . . . The chapters are brief but informative, and the list of community-help organizations is exhaustive. Report writers will find information quickly and easily, as will those who have personal concerns. The print is clear and the format is readable, making this an accessible resource for struggling readers and researchers."

—*School Library Journal, Dec '08*

"The articles selected will specifically appeal to young adults and are designed to answer their most common questions."

—*ARBAonline, Aug '08*

**SEE ALSO** *Mental Health Information for Teens, 2nd Edition*

# Suicide Information for Teens

**Health Tips about Suicide Causes and Prevention**
*Including Facts about Depression, Risk Factors, Getting Help, Survivor Support, and More*

Edited by Joyce Brennfleck Shannon. 368 pages. 2005. 978-0-7808-0737-2.

"Highly Recommended for libraries serving teenagers as well as those who work with them."

—*E-Streams, Apr '06*

**SEE ALSO** *Mental Health Information for Teens, 2nd Edition*

# Tobacco Information for Teens

**Health Tips about the Hazards of Using Cigarettes, Smokeless Tobacco, and Other Nicotine Products**
*Including Facts about Nicotine Addiction, Immediate and Long-Term Health Effects of Tobacco Use, Related Cancers, Smoking Cessation, Tobacco Use Prevention, and Tobacco Use Statistics*

Edited by Karen Bellenir. 440 pages. 2007. 978-0-7808-0976-5.

"A comprehensive resource. Each chapter is written to stand alone, so students can dip in and use the information in each section for reports or to answer personal questions without

having to read the entire book. . . . The book is packed full of statistics, with sources to help students look up more."

—*School Library Journal, Sep '07*

"Pulls together a wide variety of authoritative sources to provide a comprehensive overview of tobacco use for this age group. . . . This reasonably priced reference title should be considered a necessary purchase for all public libraries and school media centers, along with academic libraries supporting teacher education."

—*American Reference Books Annual, 2008*

**SEE ALSO** *Drug Information for Teens, 2nd Edition*

# Health Reference Series

Adolescent Health Sourcebook, 2nd Edition

Adult Health Concerns Sourcebook

AIDS Sourcebook, 4th Edition

Alcoholism Sourcebook, 2nd Edition

Allergies Sourcebook, 3rd Edition

Alzheimer Disease Sourcebook, 4th Edition

Arthritis Sourcebook, 2nd Edition

Asthma Sourcebook, 2nd Edition

Attention Deficit Disorder Sourcebook

Autism & Pervasive Developmental Disorders
    Sourcebook

Back & Neck Sourcebook, 2nd Edition

Blood & Circulatory Disorders Sourcebook, 2nd
    Edition

Brain Disorders Sourcebook, 2nd Edition

Breast Cancer Sourcebook, 3rd Edition

Breastfeeding Sourcebook

Burns Sourcebook

Cancer Sourcebook, 5th Edition

Cancer Sourcebook for Women, 3rd Edition

Cancer Survivorship Sourcebook

Cardiovascular Diseases & Disorders
    Sourcebook, 3rd Edition

Caregiving Sourcebook

Child Abuse Sourcebook

Childhood Diseases & Disorders Sourcebook,
    2nd Edition

Colds, Flu & Other Common Ailments
    Sourcebook

Communication Disorders Sourcebook

Complementary & Alternative Medicine
    Sourcebook, 3rd Edition

Congenital Disorders Sourcebook, 2nd Edition

Contagious Diseases Sourcebook

Cosmetic & Reconstructive Surgery
    Sourcebook, 2nd Edition

Death & Dying Sourcebook, 2nd Edition

Dental Care & Oral Health Sourcebook, 3rd
    Edition

Depression Sourcebook, 2nd Edition

Dermatological Disorders Sourcebook, 2nd Edition

Diabetes Sourcebook, 4th Edition

Diet & Nutrition Sourcebook, 3rd Edition

Digestive Diseases & Disorder Sourcebook

Disabilities Sourcebook

Disease Management Sourcebook

Domestic Violence Sourcebook, 3rd Edition

Drug Abuse Sourcebook, 2nd Edition

Ear, Nose & Throat Disorders Sourcebook, 2nd
    Edition

Eating Disorders Sourcebook, 2nd Edition

Emergency Medical Services Sourcebook

Endocrine & Metabolic Disorders Sourcebook,
    2nd Edition

Environmental Health Sourcebook, 2nd Edition

Ethnic Diseases Sourcebook

Eye Care Sourcebook, 3rd Edition

Family Planning Sourcebook

Fitness & Exercise Sourcebook, 3rd Edition

Food Safety Sourcebook

Forensic Medicine Sourcebook

Gastrointestinal Diseases & Disorders
    Sourcebook, 2nd Edition

Genetic Disorders Sourcebook, 3rd Edition

Head Trauma Sourcebook

Headache Sourcebook

Health Insurance Sourcebook

Healthy Aging Sourcebook

Healthy Children Sourcebook

Healthy Heart Sourcebook for Women

Hepatitis Sourcebook

Household Safety Sourcebook

Hypertension Sourcebook

Immune System Disorders Sourcebook, 2nd
    Edition

Infant & Toddler Health Sourcebook

Infectious Diseases Sourcebook

Injury & Trauma Sourcebook